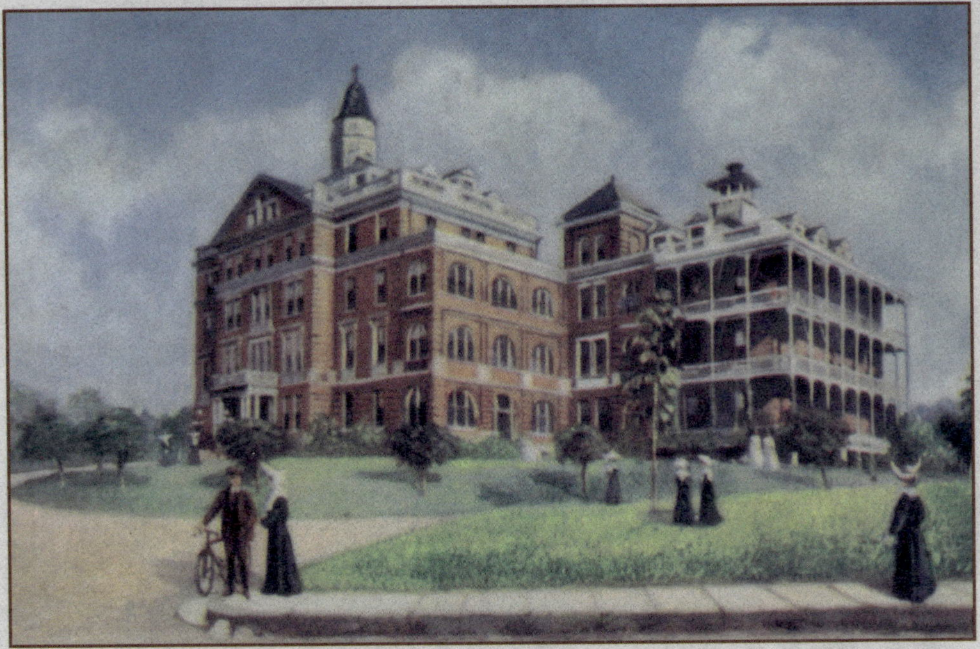

Circa 1908

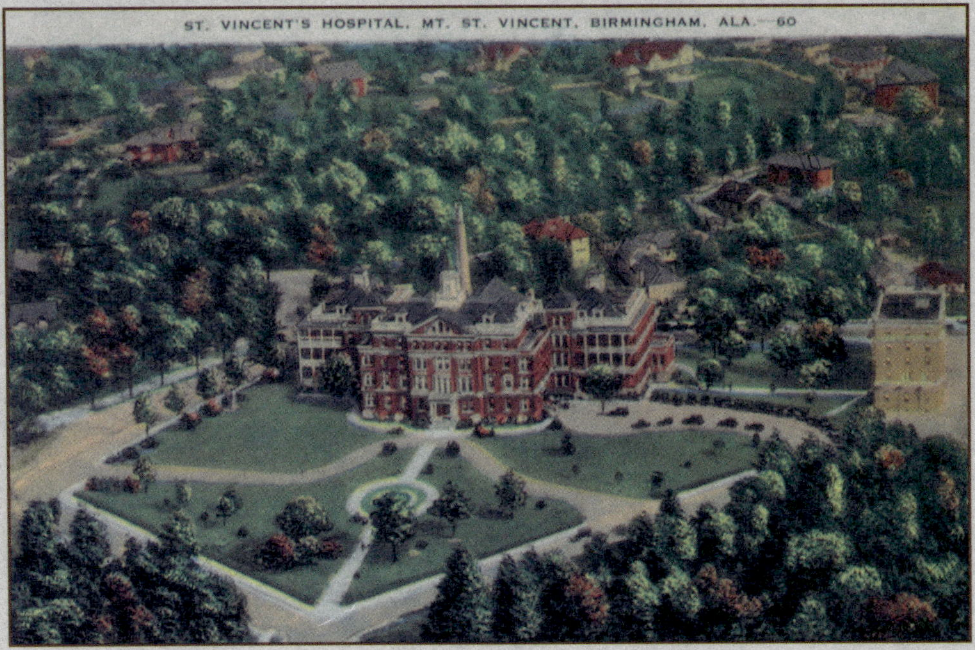

Circa 1940

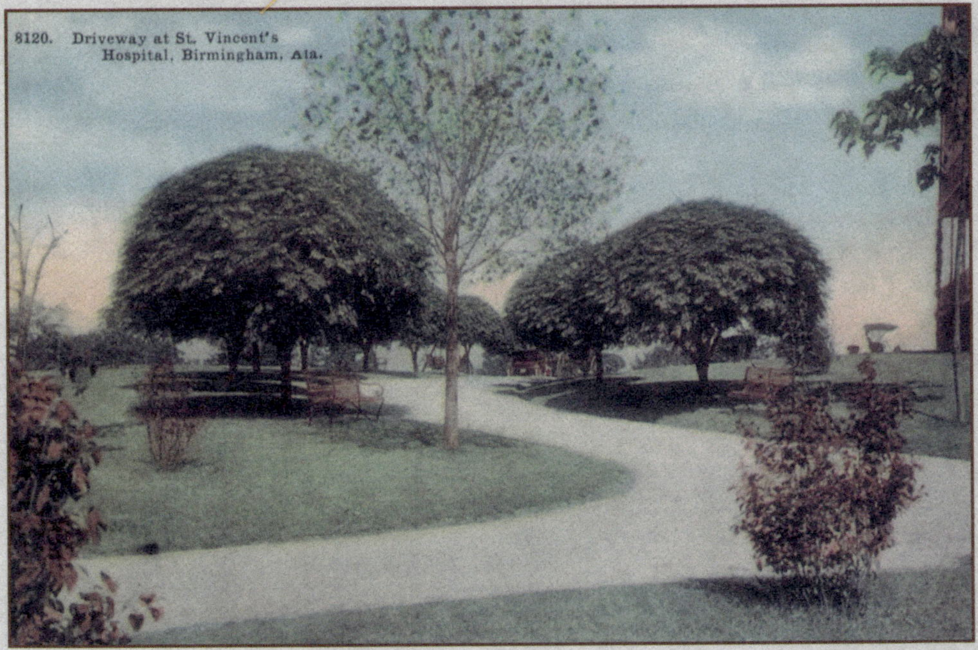

Hospital Driveway, Circa 1910

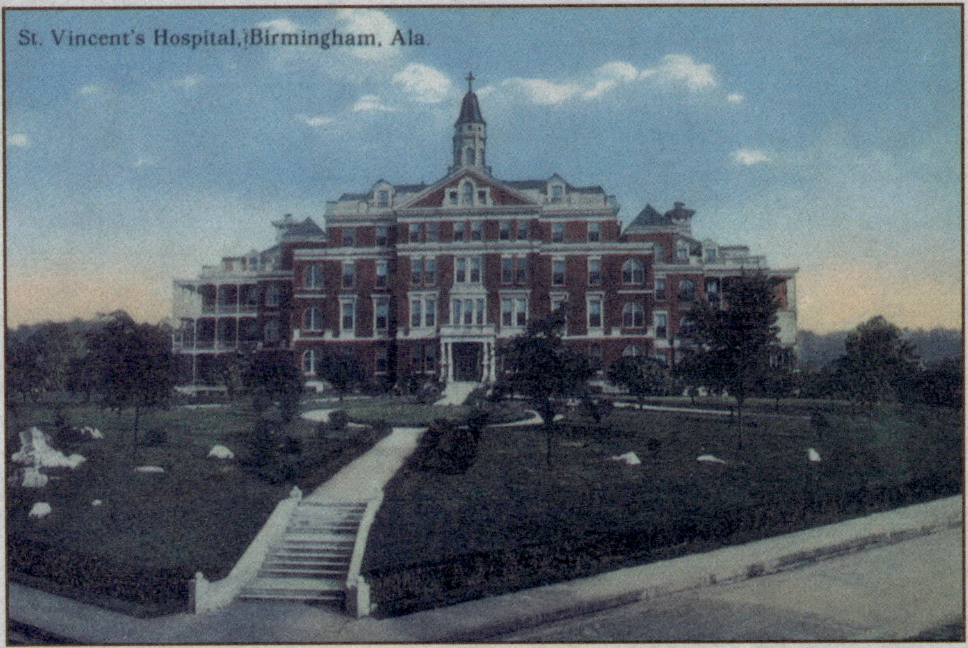

Circa 1919

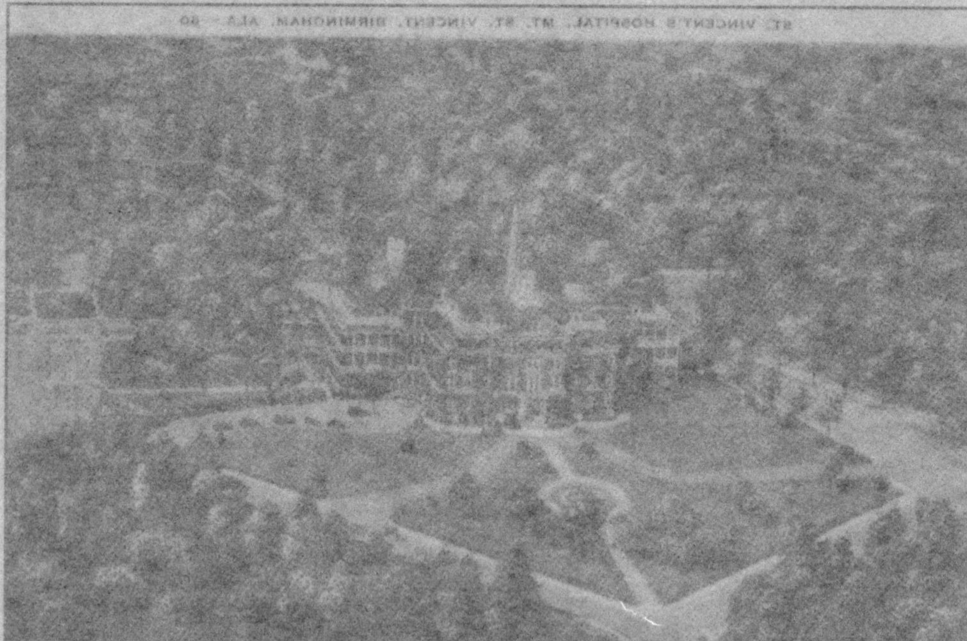

Circa 1940

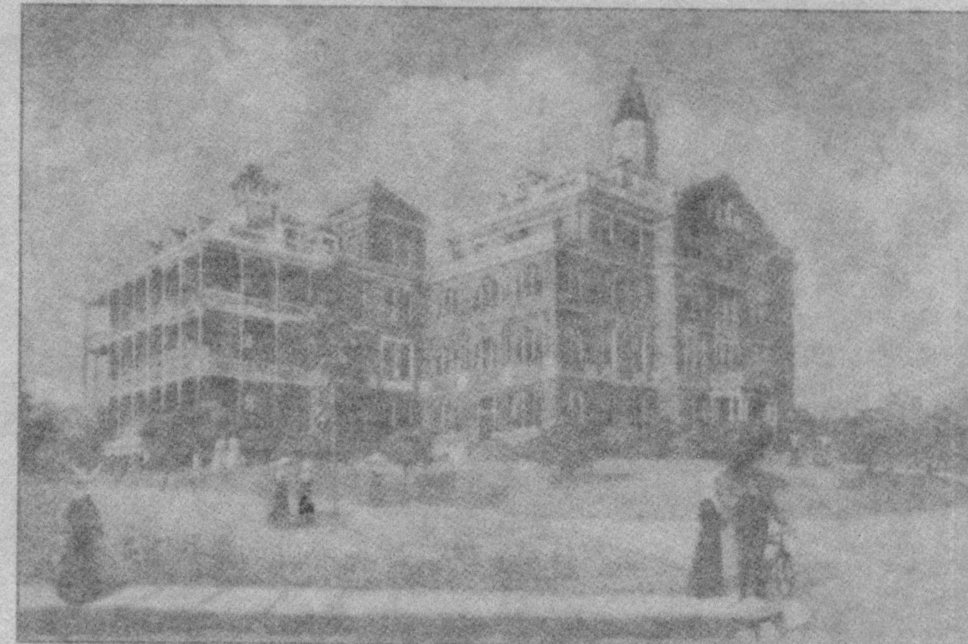

Circa 1908

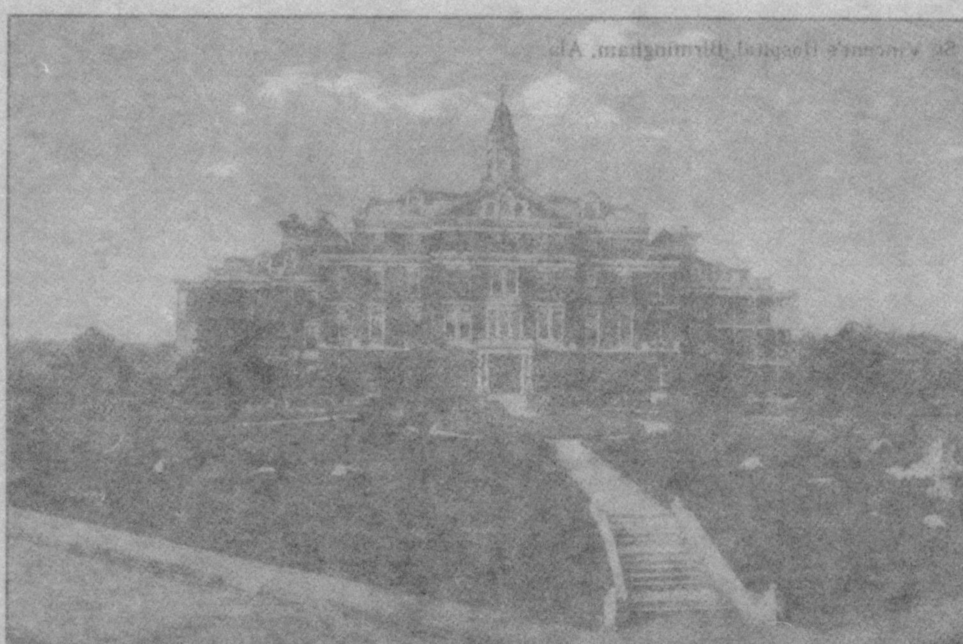

Circa 1919

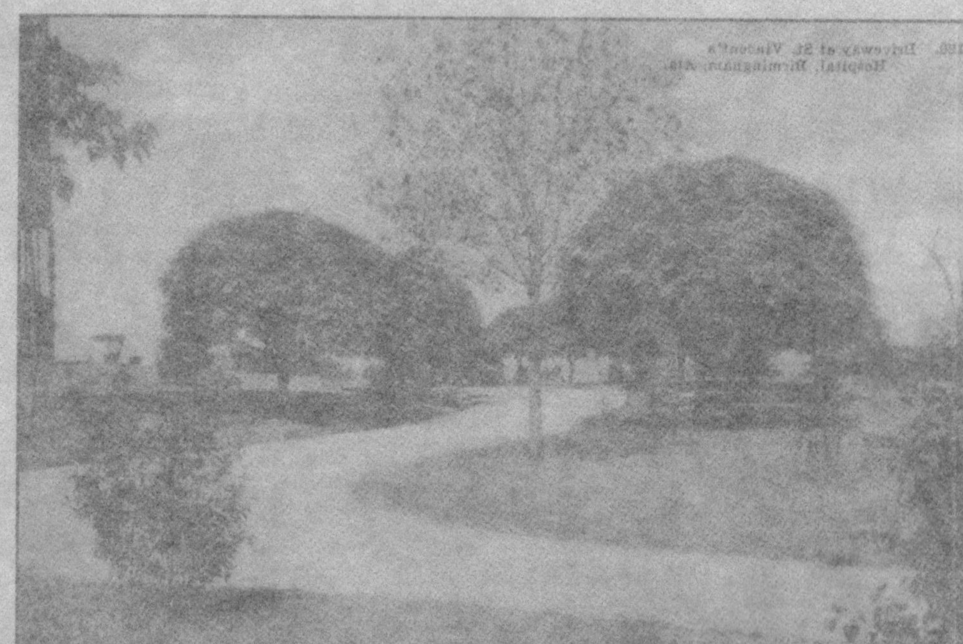

Hospital Driveway, Circa 1910

The St. Vincent's Story

1898 — *A Century of Caring* — 1998

The Daughters of Charity of St. Vincent de Paul
St. Vincent's Hospital, Birmingham, Alabama

This book was commissioned by
St. Vincent's Foundation
in commemoration of 100 years of service
by the Daughters of Charity and
St. Vincent's Hospital
to the people of Birmingham, Alabama.

Author
TOM WOFFORD

Art Director
LORI PITTS RYAN

Project Director
BARBARA TRAYLOR

The cover illustration is from a St. Vincent's souvenir postcard, circa 1908.

 Printed in the United States of America by Birmingham Printing and Publishing.

Library of Congress Catalog Card Number 97-061780
ISBN 0-9660631-0-4

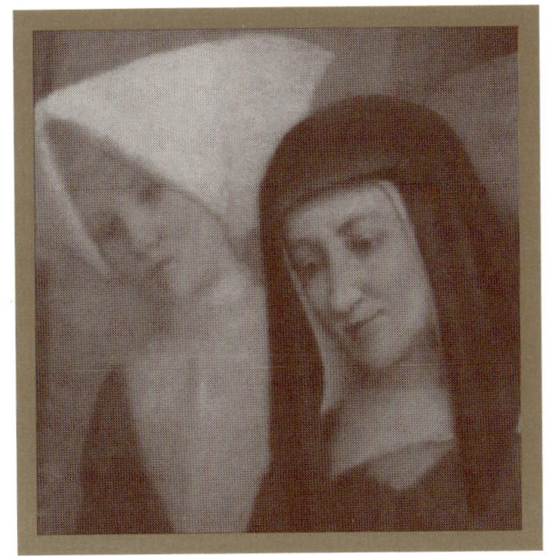

Table of Contents

Archives, St. Vincent's Hospital

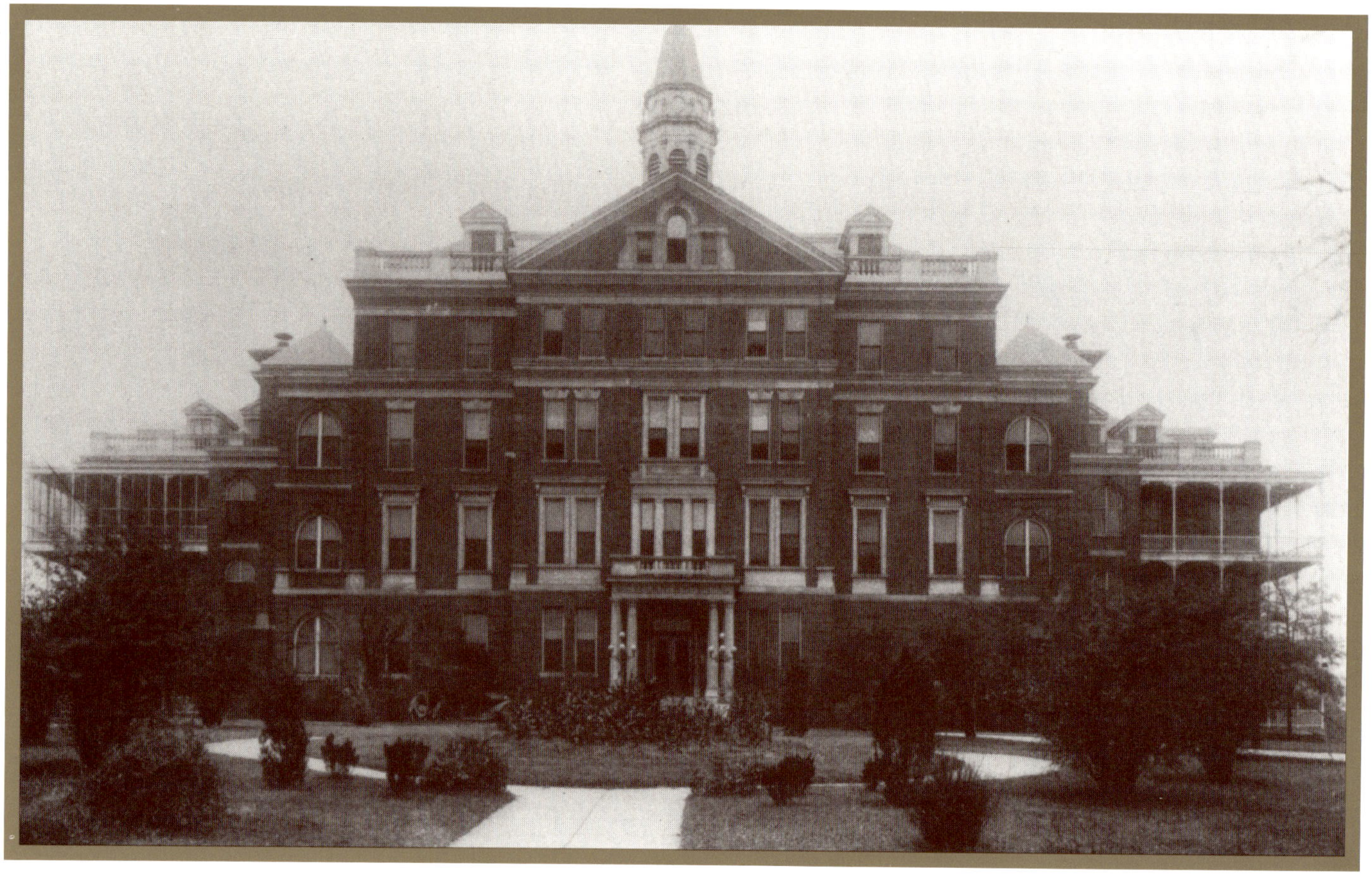

1898	1899	1900	1911	1915	1916	1920	1926	1950	1951	1963
Temporary hospital in the DeBardeleben home	Groundbreaking for the permanent hospital	Original hospital building opens Nursing School established	East Wing	Radiology Department	Sister Chrysostom becomes first registered nurse in Alabama	Pathology Department	Laboure Hall	New East Wing	School of Medical Technology	Hospital Auxiliary

St. Vincent's Hospital Administrators

1898-1899	*Sister Benedicta Roach*
1899-1917	*Sister Chrysostom Moynahan*
1917-1920	*Sister Magdalen Welch*
1920-1927	*Sister Angela O'Brien*
1927-1930	*Sister Alphonsine Casey*
1930-1934	*Sister Alberta Sullivan*
1934-1942	*Sister Lydia Hoffman*
1942	*Sister Clementine Nee*
1942-1945	*Sister Mariana Flynn*
1945-1951	*Sister Mary Alice McCarthy*
1951-1956	*Sister Catherine Wintz*
1956-1961	*Sister Lydia Hoffman*
1961-1966	*Sister Carlos McDonnell*
1966-1972	*Sister Mary Bourke*
1972-1975	*Sister Xavier Ballance*
1975-1985	*Sister Carlos McDonnell*
1985-1987	*Sister Almeda Golson*
1987-1992	*Sister Mary Frances Loftin*
1992-	*Vincent C. Caponi*

1972 — Original hospital replaced by new seven-story structure

1975 — Professional Building I and first parking deck

1981 — West Wing (Barbara Ingalls Shook Pavilion)

1982 — Laboure Hall razed

1984 — St. Vincent's Foundation established

1987 — Professional Building II; Nursing School graduates last class

1989 — Bruno Cancer Center

1992 — Bruno Memorial Heart Care Center; Bruno Rehabilitation Center; Professional Building III; First Lay Administrator

1997 — Women's and Children's Center; Bruno Conference Center

Chapter One

A City in Need

Archives, Birmingham Public Library

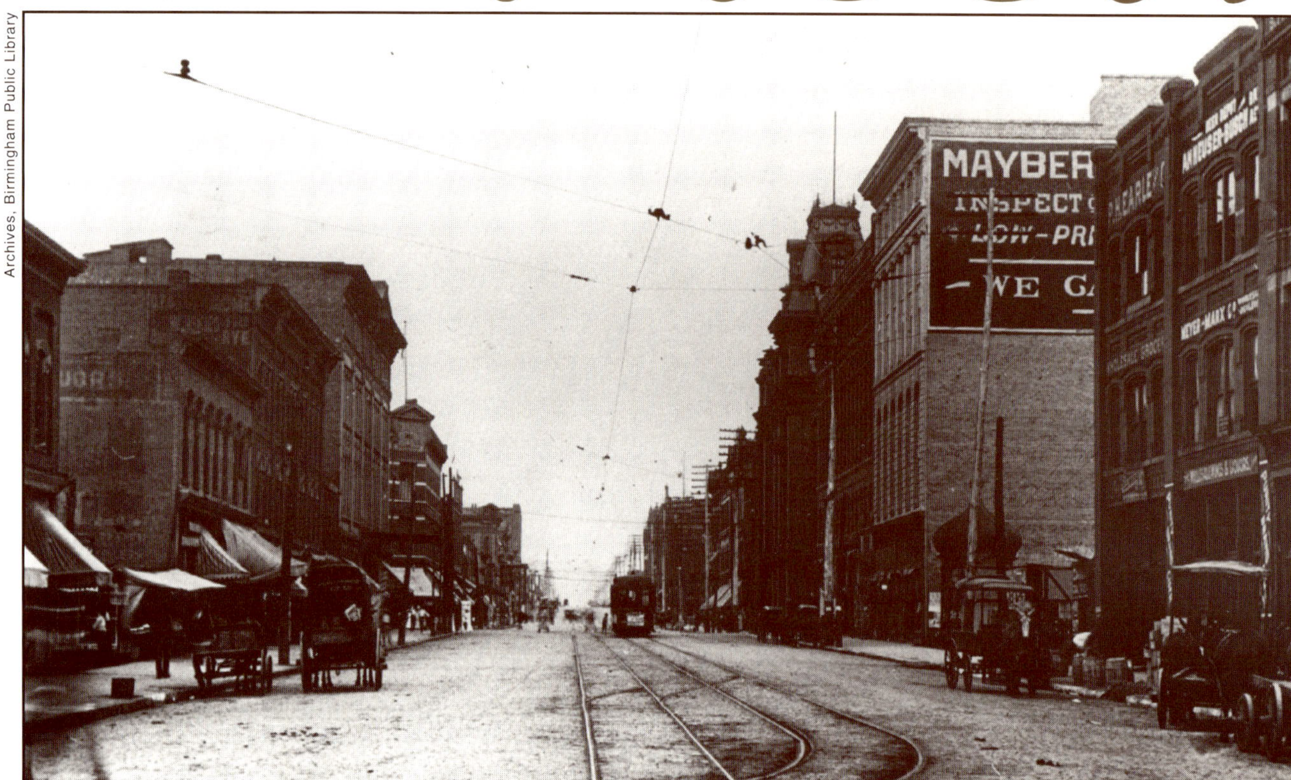

First Avenue North, circa 1895

The Reverend Father Patrick A. O'Reilly of St. Paul's Catholic Church met the train at the old L & N Station that Tuesday evening, a day that had been rainy and windy.

It was November 16, 1898.

Aboard the train, having traveled the long hours from St. Louis, were three passengers whose arrival would realize a dream the energetic young Father O'Reilly had been doggedly pursuing for the community he served and loved. Sisters Benedicta and Magdeline, two members of the Daughters of Charity of St. Vincent de Paul, descended from the train with Father R. A. Lennon, the provincial spiritual director of the Daughters.

They had come to give Birmingham something the bustling young city was desperate for – a hospital.

As the three newcomers left the train station on Morris Avenue with Father O'Reilly for the eight-block trip to the Sisters' temporary quarters, they saw Birmingham in all its rough-hewn glory. The air was smoky. Even at dusk the streets were filled with people, and the rowdiness of the saloons could be heard all the way to 20th Street.

The city, not quite 27 years old, was often compared to a Wild West boomtown. It drew its life's blood from iron and steel and coal, and these industries created a hard-living, grimy atmosphere.

City sewers emptied into Valley and Village Creeks. Much of the city's water supply was unfiltered and polluted. There were frequent mining and furnace accidents, many more serious than the company infirmaries could treat. Tuberculosis and typhoid were common. There had been a smallpox epidemic for the second year in a row.

Birmingham was a city in need. Even though there were more than 100,000 people in the immediate vicinity, the city had no hospital.

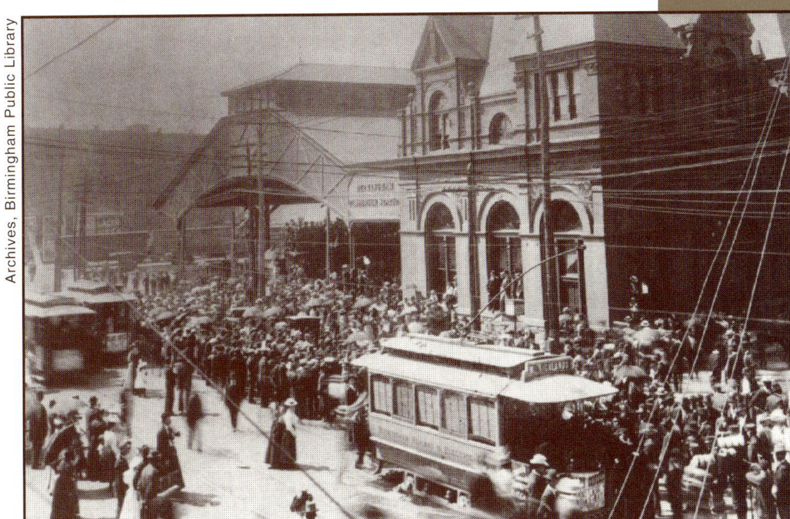

Archives, Birmingham Public Library

Union Station, 1898

The Sisters' first glimpse of Birmingham was the L & N Station, commonly called Union Station.

Built in 1887 to service the Louisville and Nashville Railroad, this gateway to the city bore witness to the massive growth that earned Birmingham the nickname "Magic City." Union Station, which stood at Morris Avenue and 20th Street, predated the grander and more well-known Terminal Station by more than 15 years.

This photograph was taken May 1, 1898, one of Union Station's busiest days at that time, as hundreds of soldiers boarded trains headed for service in the Spanish-American War.

The station was torn down in 1960.

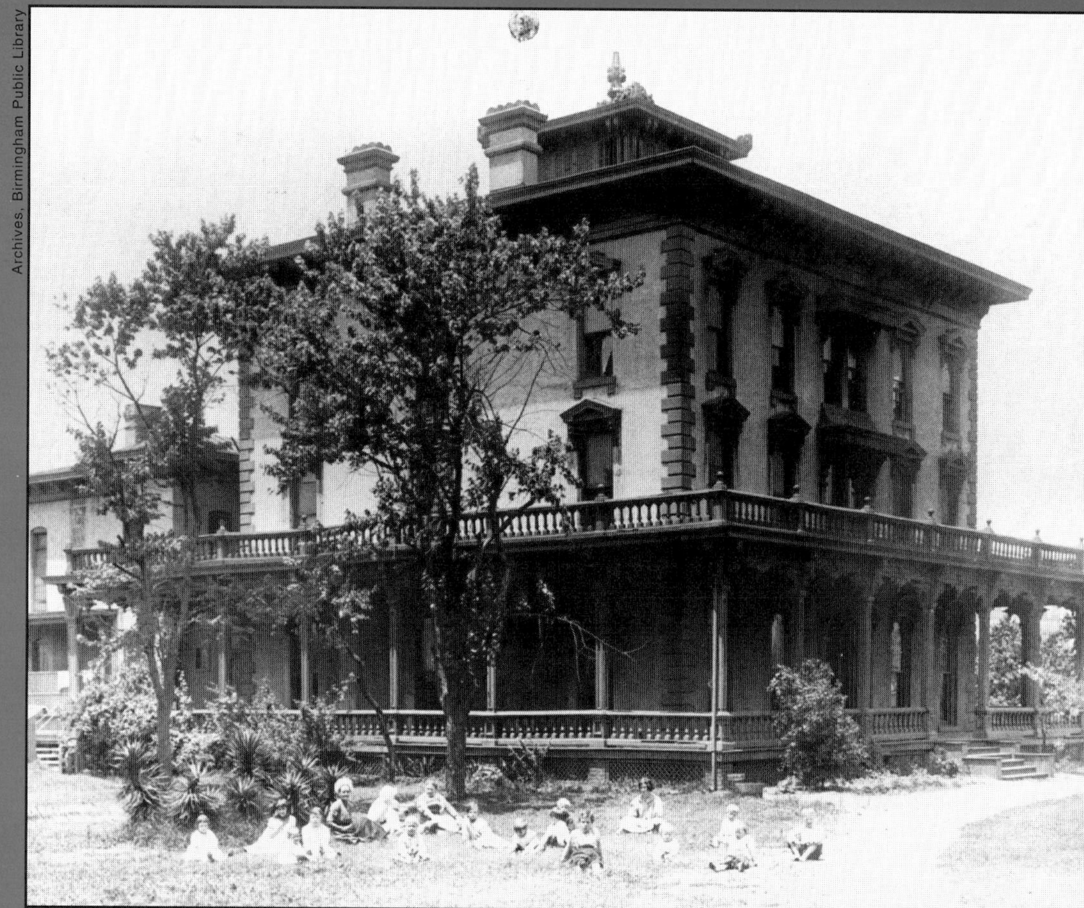

The DeBardeleben Mansion

St. Vincent's opened in this three-story mansion that Henry F. DeBardeleben had built in the 1880s for his family. DeBardeleben, "the king of the Southern iron world," was the son-in-law of famed Alabama industrialist Daniel Pratt and was the wealthiest man in the state at the time, with numerous coal and iron interests in Birmingham and the surrounding area.

DeBardeleben later lost much of his fortune in an unsuccessful attempt to gain control of the Tennessee Coal, Iron and Railroad Company. Sister Benedicta wrote to the Mother House about DeBardeleben the week she arrived: "The building is owned by a gentleman who some years ago lost his fortune by speculation in New York; he lost in Wall Street, New York, over a million of dollars in less than twelve hours." One of the most famous of Birmingham's forefathers, DeBardeleben, however, soon built a new fortune.

This house, which was located between 15th and 16th Streets and Avenues B and C (present-day Second and Third Avenues South), was the first of many grand homes in Birmingham built by Harry F. Wheelock, the city's most noted architect/builder of the day.

The Sisters roomed that first week with the Benedictine Sisters, who were in charge of the Holy Angels Academy, the parish school at St. Paul's. Sister Magdeline would stay in Birmingham only a few days, and then return to St. Louis. Father Lennon's stay would also be relatively brief.

Sister Benedicta Roach, however, had come to stay. She couldn't be sure how long, but at least until the new hospital, St. Vincent's Hospital, was in operation. She was young, energetic and light-hearted, and in her early writings from Birmingham she conveys a practical excitement about the daunting effort before her.

On November 20 she wrote to Mother Mariana, superior of the Daughters of Charity Provincial House in Emmitsburg, Maryland, a cheerful, excited letter about, among other things, the local affordability of furniture, which could be "bought as cheap here as in St. Louis." Her mission, she knew, was to serve the people of this city, and the need was clear.

"The prospects are that much good can be done for the poor and for suffering humanity," she concluded.

"Angels" of the Battlefield

By the time Sister Benedicta arrived in Birmingham, the Daughters of Charity of St. Vincent de Paul had been tending to the needs of the poor for more than 200 years, first in France and then all across the world. St. Vincent founded the order in 1633 with St. Louise de Marillac. The order spread through France and then across Europe.

In 1813 St. Elizabeth Ann Seton founded the Sisters of Charity based upon the rules of the Daughters of Charity. Although this group later unified with the Mother House in Paris, the American group was still often called the Sisters of Charity in the late 19th century.

As early as 1883 a Birmingham alderman had reported the need for a hospital in the fast-growing city.

A cholera epidemic in 1873 had killed 128 people in Birmingham, and it almost killed the town itself as more than half the population fled in only a few months' time.

A phenomenal business explosion during the 1880s led to unprecedented growth in Birmingham, and the need for adequate health care in the crowded city became imperative.

The eventual response, Charity Hospital, began in a floor of the Hughes Building on 20th Street and later moved to a new building in Smithfield, just west of Birmingham and north of Elyton.

The hospital's importance was quickly illustrated; it treated 401 patients in 1892. However, after the hospital burned on December 1, 1894, the trust that funded Charity Hospital was not substantial enough alone to rebuild the hospital. Public funds had been withdrawn following the financial panic of 1893 that caused the First National Bank to close its doors for a time.

Although the Charity Hospital group maintained a small infirmary in a portion of a private physician's practice, Birmingham was effectively without a hospital, and thousands went without medical attention.

St. Vincent de Paul

was born in southern France during the reign of Henry III in 1581. The third of six children born to peasants, Vincent was educated by the Franciscans at Dax and ordained in 1600. He later enjoyed the spiritual guidance of the celebrated Cardinal Pierre de Bérulle, who entrusted him with the parish of Clichy.

Although he knew and associated with a number of people of rank and prominence – Louis XIII asked for him as he lay dying – St. Vincent's concern repeatedly turned to the needs of the poor. He consistently signed his name in the peasant fashion: Vincent Depaul.

France in the days of St. Vincent was a place of war, epidemic and famine. Almost half of all children died in infancy, and the average citizen did not live to see his 13th birthday. Only the middle class and the rich, a small portion of the country's populace, lived beyond middle age.

After founding the Congregation of the Mission in 1625, St. Vincent established the Confraternities of Charity, associations of laywomen who worked among the poor. With their help St. Vincent founded a number of hospitals, and in 1633 he and St. Louise de Marillac founded the Daughters of Charity.

The St. Vincent de Paul Society, founded in Paris in 1833 to carry on his work for the poor, has more than a million members worldwide.

"If we do God's works, He will take care of ours."

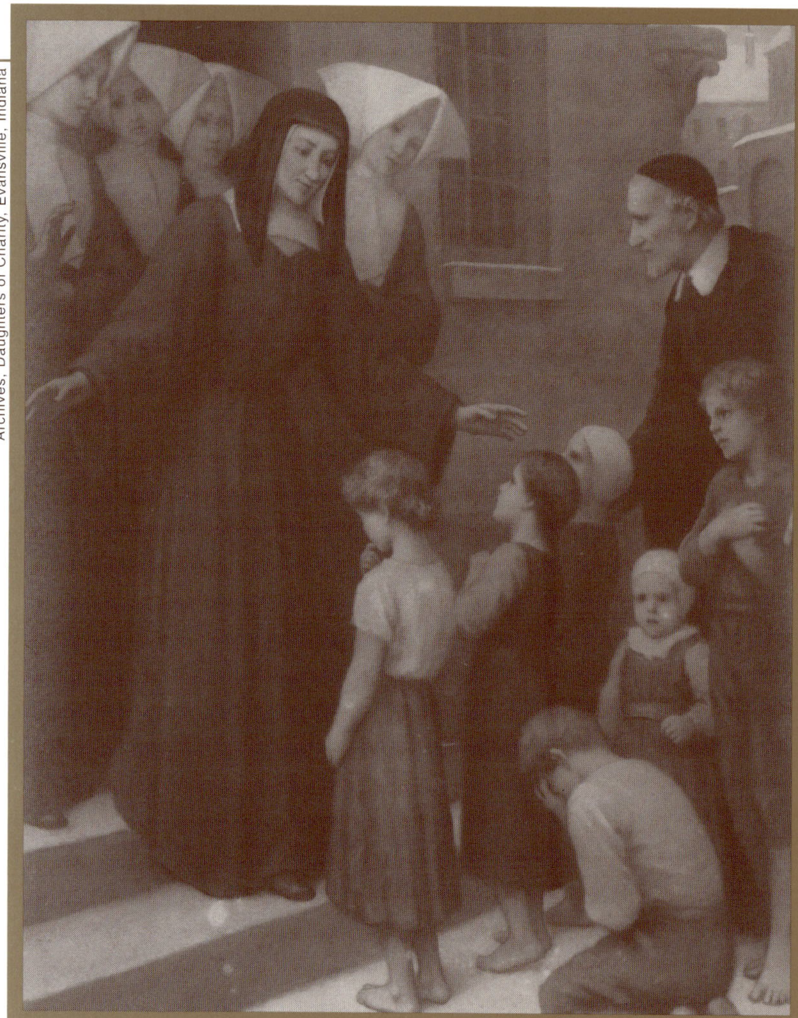

Archives, Daughters of Charity, Evansville, Indiana

St. Vincent de Paul, St. Louise de Marillac and Daughters of Charity, as depicted in a 17th-century French painting

The Daughters of Charity

of St. Vincent de Paul began in Paris in 1633, the first order of women in the Catholic Church that was not cloistered and therefore required to remain within the confines of the church walls.

The first Daughter of Charity was Louise de Marillac, a spiritually hungry widow when she met St. Vincent in the 1620s. Although a member of an illustrious and powerful family, under his guidance this woman of remarkable depth of spirit recruited young women from the French countryside to devote themselves to God and be living signs of Jesus among the poor.

Though at first dedicated to nursing the poor, the Daughters almost immediately undertook the care and teaching of poor children and the management of hospitals.

The Daughters of Charity order was established in the United States by St. Elizabeth Ann Seton in 1809 as the Sisters of Charity, who later became unified with the Mother House in France.

Today there are more than 26,000 Daughters of Charity, the largest Catholic congregation of women, serving the poor in almost every country of the world.

St. Vincent said to the Daughters: "Consider often the excellence of your holy vocation. It is esteemed by all who know it; appreciate it yourselves at its excellent worth. You have received your vocation from God Himself. In performing the work of your holy vocation, you help to save souls, and you imitate the life on earth of our Lord Jesus Christ."

Sister Benedicta's experience as she came to Birmingham was typical of the life of service of the Daughters. In her few years of service, Sister Benedicta had already taught at St. Simeon's School in New Orleans, run an asylum in Pennsylvania and worked with orphans in Dallas. Most recently she had nursed soldiers at Chickamauga, Tennessee, and Lexington, Kentucky, during the Spanish-American War.

The Daughters of Charity's service as wartime nurses had long before earned the order the description "Angels of the Battlefield."

A Welcome "Curiosity"

Two days after Sister Benedicta's arrival, she was joined by another member of the Daughters of Charity whose mission was also to be of a lengthy duration, Sister Patricia Malloy. On November 21 they were joined by Sisters Antonia Hanrahan and Placida Scott. With Sister Benedicta as Sister Servant, these four would comprise the original nursing staff of St. Vincent's.

That same day the four went, in Sister Benedicta's words, "to take up permanent abode in the temporary Hospital," the grand, three-story mansion on South 15th Street that had once been the residence of famed local industrialist Henry F. DeBardeleben. Having recently lost a great deal of money (a temporary setback, it would later turn out), DeBardeleben most recently had been renting the mansion for use as a boarding house.

Sister Benedicta had already "fit up a dormitory" for them and "procured a basket of groceries."

According to Sister Benedicta, the house was "well adapted for its purpose. The [Birmingham] people have taken great interest in the work...The building has been thoroughly cleaned...They have had electric lights put throughout...The house is heated by hot-air furnaces...and is well supplied with water."

Sister Benedicta had grown up in the predominantly Catholic city of New Orleans, and while Birmingham's population was diverse, the city's Catholic population was relatively small. There were only two Catholic churches in Jefferson County.

"We are as much of a curiosity here as we were in Dallas," Sister Benedicta wrote to Mother Mariana.

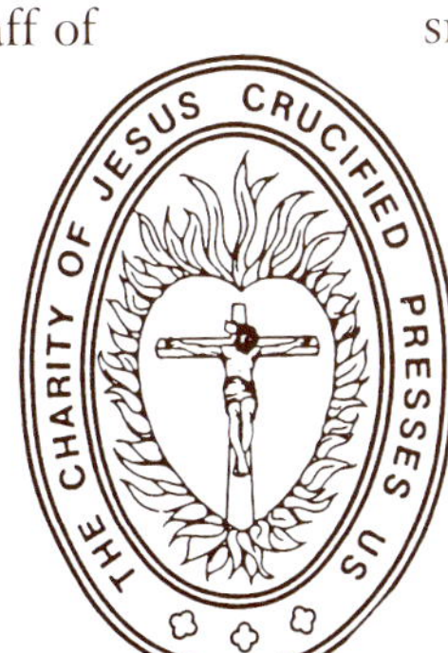

The seal of the Daughters of Charity

Archives. Daughters of Charity, Evansville, Indiana

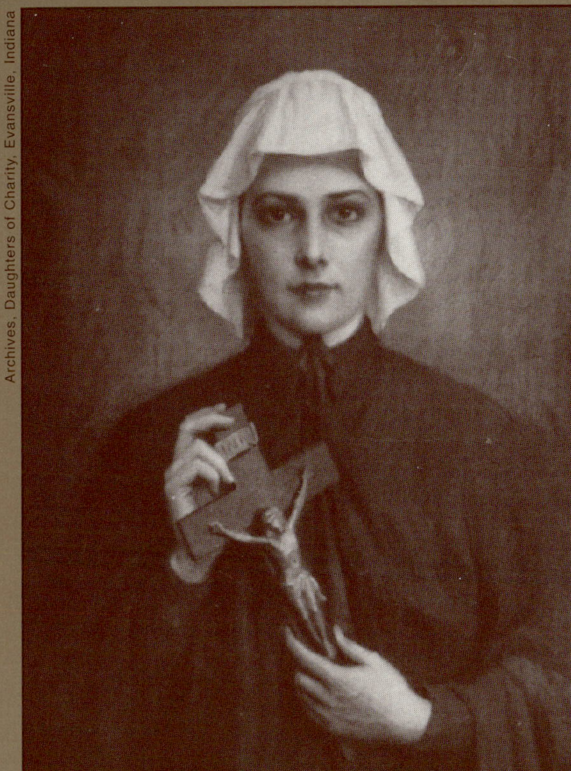

St. Elizabeth Ann Seton

St. Elizabeth Ann Seton was the first native-born American to be recognized as a saint by the Roman Catholic Church.

Reared a Protestant, Mother Seton converted to Catholicism in 1805, two years after the death of her husband, a wealthy New York City shipping merchant.

Mother Seton founded the Sisters of Charity in Emmitsburg, Maryland, the first Catholic religious community in the United States based upon the rules of the Daughters of Charity. The order later unified with the Mother House in Paris.

Known as the mother of the parochial school system in the United States, Mother Seton also founded the nation's first Catholic childcare institution.

She was canonized in 1975.

From the Ashes, a Phoenix

"Magic City" isn't simply a clever promotional slogan dreamed up by civic boosters.

To begin with, Birmingham was unlike other Southern cities in that it had been formed as a business venture: planned and financed by businessmen who saw in some swampy farmland the potential for a great industrial city. Birmingham was an early hope for those in the South who sought to create something great from the ashes of the Civil War.

In 1870 Jefferson County was typical Alabama backwoods, with little more than 12,000 people living in the entire county, 1,000 of them in the county seat, Elyton. Elyton was a stop on the railroad to Chattanooga and a planned stop on a line being built to run north from Montgomery.

Developers had been aware of the rich minerals of the area for more than 20 years, and there had been local iron furnaces at Tannehill, Irondale, Oxmoor and Mount Pinson.

Although the Civil War and the formidable terrain had prevented widespread development of the region, the new railroad would make this mineral wealth accessible on a whole new scale.

In December of 1870 John T. Milner, an engineer involved in planning the course of the new railroad, met with a group of men associated with the new line, the South and North Railroad. These were men with names familiar to any Birmingham resident – Morris, Powell, Caldwell, Nabers and Mudd. This

Birmingham and Jones Valley grew up and grew strong on iron, coal and steel.

Although the natural resources of the area were not immediately used to full advantage, by the Gay '90s Birmingham was an industrial boomtown.

In 1900 the city, not yet 30 years old, produced three-fourths of the pig iron in the United States, and more than 100,000 people lived in Birmingham and its surrounding communities.

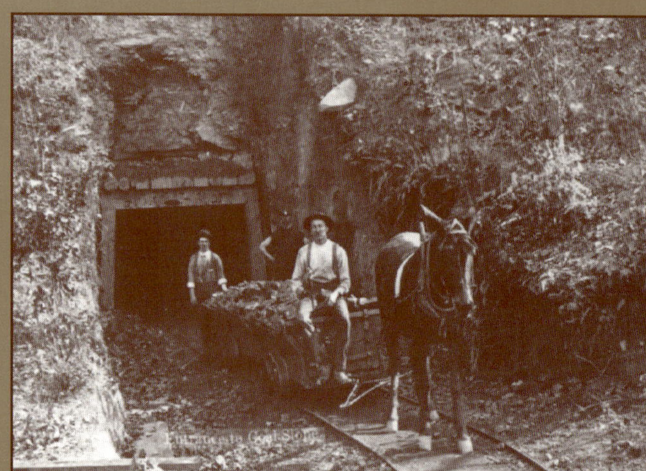

Pratt Mine, circa 1900

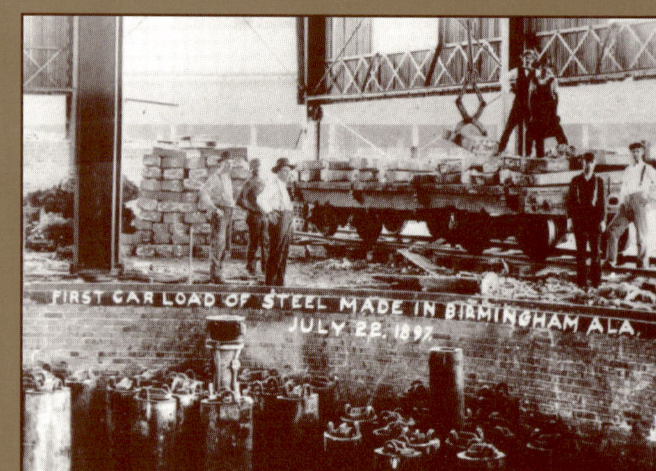

The first carload of Birmingham steel, which shipped July 22, 1897

meeting in Montgomery gave birth to the Elyton Land Company, whose charter was to "build a city in Jefferson County." They drew a new course for the railroad, which bypassed Elyton, and instead crossed Jones Valley through the rabbit-infested cornfields recently optioned by the new company.

The first sale of "lots" began on June 1, 1871 – actually cotton and corn fields, sometimes with rail fences still standing, sometimes in wooded sections that could be reached only on foot. Stakes denoted property lines and planned sidewalks.

A magical rush began. Less than seven months later, Birmingham was incorporated. It had a population of 1,200.

The initial boom continued as the new railroad arrived in 1872, and by the next year the county seat had been moved to the upstart town, where 4,000 people now lived. However, almost as soon as the promise of Birmingham became reality, bad luck struck.

In 1873 the baby boomtown was almost destroyed. A financial panic crippled the nation and cut off investment capital, and a cholera epidemic created a more tragic panic. Half the population fled the town, and 128 people died.

The depression continued, and by 1878 the population had fallen to that of seven years earlier: 1,200.

In 1880, however, the city rose again, aided this time by the smoke and ashes of two new coke furnaces. More furnaces followed during the decade, as did coal and ore mining, a cotton mill and thousands of new people.

During the 1880s the city grew up. Telephones and street lights arrived. Downtown streets were paved. Streetcars pulled by mules were

In the News

What was on the lips of the people of Birmingham when the first Daughters of Charity arrived to open a hospital there? Much of the news reported by the Birmingham Age-Herald *in 1898 was related to the city's need for a hospital:*

- *On August 27 a wagon containing a "pleasure party" was struck by a train, killing five people. Since Birmingham had no hospital, the four injured were taken to the town hall.*
- *The entire state of Alabama was quarantined on August 29 against entry by residents of Galveston, Texas and Franklin, Louisiana, as well as Key West, Florida, because of a yellow fever outbreak in those cities.*
- *On August 31 a railroad car inspector shot a brakeman who was trying to "brain" him with a hammer.*
- *In early October yellow fever was raging throughout the South, particularly in Jackson, Mississippi, where deaths were reported almost daily.*
- *Later in October came an occurrence at the DeBardeleben mansion, which was a rooming house at the time. An argument about the differences between Southern and Northern attitudes toward blacks resulted in one boarder being "carved" by the other, who left him with 15 wounds. Ironically, the Daughters of Charity would treat their first patient in that very house only one month later.*

Other big news stories during the Fall of 1898:

- *The Board of Aldermen voted to draw up a new city charter, because "the old charter was drawn up before the city had reached a very respectable size…and is unsuited to the conduct of a metropolitan city."*
- *A widow sued a local businessman for $10,000, contending he had not followed through on a proposal of marriage.*
- *The "dry goods firm" of Loveman, Joseph and Loeb announced plans to build a four-story building adjoining their present store.*
- *The Carnival Society Committee on Designs decided, but did not announce, the subject to be illustrated by the parade floats in the 1899 Mardi Gras parade. (Note: To compete with Mobile and New Orleans, Birmingham began holding a Mardi Gras celebration in 1896, later with a king who bore the title "Rex Vulcan." Because the typical weather in Birmingham during February is, at the least, inhospitable, Mardi Gras there did not survive the turn of the century.)*

replaced by steam dummies and then by electric streetcars. By 1890 the population within the city limits of Birmingham was more than 26,000, with at least that many more people living nearby.

Despite labor unrest and a national financial panic in 1893, Birmingham burst at its seams all through the Gay '90s. Pig iron, steel and rolling mill facilities went up, as well as a large textile mill. During the decade, the population of the city swelled to almost 40,000, with 60,000 more living in the 16 surrounding communities.

"Bad Birmingham"

Birmingham was now "a man's town," "Bad Birmingham," "murder capital of the world" and "the dustiest city on earth."

There was an outlaw atmosphere. Saloons were plentiful, and prostitution was such a problem that a legal red-light district would soon be established and regulated in an effort to control the spread of related diseases. Shootings, stabbings and injuries from fighting were frequent.

Living conditions were often dreadful. Essentially comprised of a rural population compacted into an urban area, Birmingham continually struggled with outbreaks of various contagious diseases: typhoid, dysentery, pneumonia and tuberculosis. In 1890, adult and infant mortality rates were three times the state average.

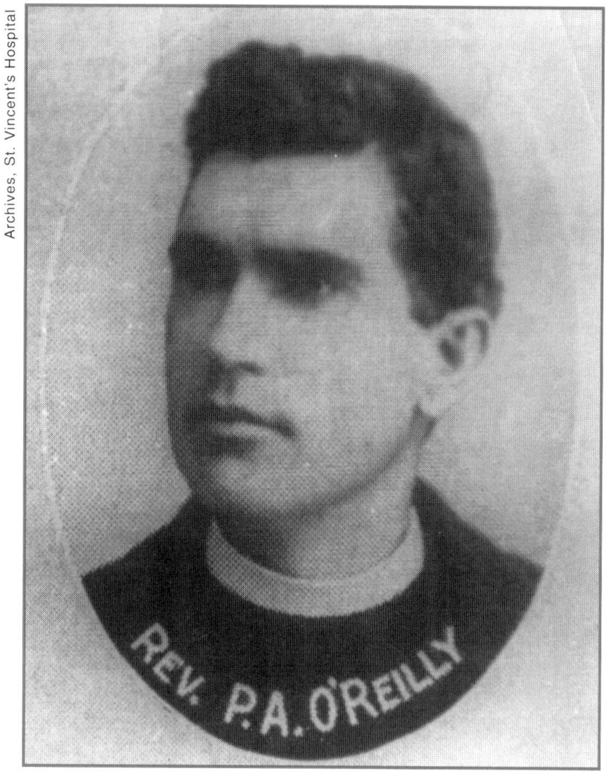

Archives, St. Vincent's Hospital

Father O'Reilly

The Reverend Father Patrick A. O'Reilly was born in County Cavan, Ireland, and came to the United States at the age of 17. After studying at St. Charles College, Father O'Reilly attended the famed La Grande Seminary in Montreal and later the Seminary at St. Bonaventure, Pennsylvania. His only assignment prior to coming to Birmingham was in the small town of Whistler, near Mobile, where the young priest was an immediate success.

During his time at St. Paul's, the congregation grew rapidly, and Father O'Reilly supervised the construction of St. Paul's noted gothic cathedral. In addition to being a driving force in the founding of St. Vincent's, Father O'Reilly also worked with the Daughters of Charity to found the East Lake Atheneum Orphans Home in 1903.

Newspaper accounts called Father O'Reilly "public spirited" and "broadminded" and said he was not only "esteemed by every class" but also "in many respects the foremost citizen of Jefferson County."

And conditions were worst among the poor.

Charity Hospital had opened in 1890, funded by a private trust and supplemented by public funds. Having seen more than 400 patients in 1892, the hospital burned in December 1894. The continuing economic depression prevented its being rebuilt. Although an infirmary continued to operate in a portion of a private physician's practice, for four years Birmingham was without a hospital.

Health care was scarce, and for the poor it was usually unattainable.

A Call for Help

Bishop Edward P. Allen of Mobile wrote Mother Mariana at the Mother House in Emmitsburg on December 28, 1897 and formally asked the Daughters to establish a hospital in Birmingham:

> *The city is a growing one, and bids fair to be the Pittsburg [sic] of the South. In all of north Alabama...there is not a hospital worthy of the name. The number of accident cases around the mines and railroads in that district is truly appalling, and at present there is no place adequately equipped to provide for them.*

Mother Mariana's reply of January 4, 1898, was favorable, although she frankly hoped to put off the hospital for a year because of heavy demands on the Sisters at the time. Bishop Allen wrote back on January 28 that he would urge the citizens of Birmingham to prepare for the hospital and that he hoped to get work under way before the end of the year.

Throughout the spring, Birmingham's Father O'Reilly preached the idea to the community. The citizens' meeting he organized on June 8 in the Temperance Hall at St. Paul's was "largely attended." Those at the meeting formed an organizing committee to report in two days.

At the June 10 meeting, the group christened themselves the Sisters of Charity Hospital Association and established a governing body that would include a cross-section of the city's population. The president was H. H. Sinnige; Father O'Reilly was named first vice president, Robert Jemison second vice president and W. P. McCrossin secretary.

The first "subscription" was Bishop Allen's for $100. By the end of the meeting, $1,040 had been committed. More contributions and commitments of services came during the next few weeks, including $500 each from the City of Birmingham and from Jefferson County.

Within a month, Bishop Allen purchased, for a reported $4,000, an oak tree-covered lot in Fountain Heights, which he touted in a letter to Father Lennon as being "as good as could be secured anywhere in the city limits." He underscored that the land would be transferred to the Sisters free of charge as soon as they would accept it.

This location was convenient to the city's industrial activity, six miles from Pratt City, 12 miles from Bessemer and "near the proposed location of the new million-dollar steel plant at Ensley."

Bishop Allen also relayed the commitments of the majority of the railroad, mining and manufacturing companies to send their patients to the new hospital.

Mother Mariana's only condition in accepting the land was that if it were ever sold, the money must be used to purchase and build elsewhere.

The Hospital Association met weekly during the summer, but not until September 8 did Father O'Reilly report the purchase of the 10 acres in Fountain Heights.

Also, at this meeting, Father O'Reilly announced the lease with Henry DeBardeleben for the use of his former home as a temporary hospital.

The stage was set. St. Vincent's Hospital was nearing reality.

Archives, Birmingham Public Library

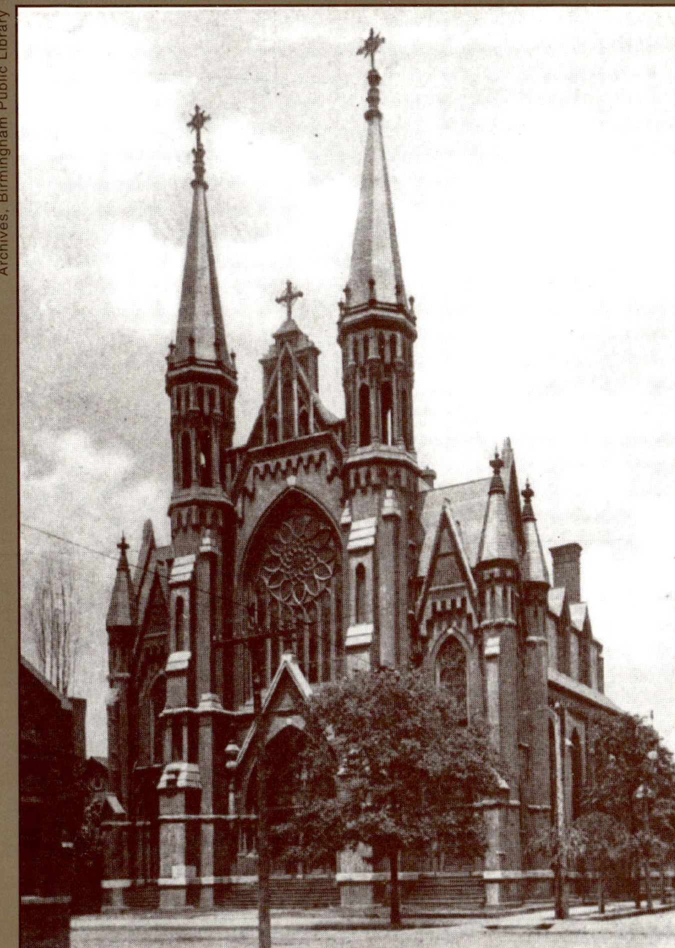

The Cathedral of St. Paul

The first congregation of St. Paul's met in a 30-foot by 60-foot wooden structure built in 1870.

In 1880 the Diocese purchased new land for the church at its present site and built a frame rectory there. The next year, St. Paul's first priest, Father J. J. Browne, arranged to have the original building moved to this location, 22nd Street and Third Avenue North, and enlarged.

By 1886, St. Paul's had a congregation of more than 1,000.

Construction of the present gothic cathedral was planned by Father O'Reilly. The cornerstone was laid in 1890, and the building was dedicated in 1893.

First Offerings

The Sisters accepted their first patients before they had a chance to complete the "repairs" to the mansion. On November 29 a young boy, Willie A. Alidge, "was received," as was a Mrs. Jungeman the next day. Alidge was in "an advanced stage of consumption." The Sisters' Diaries are not specific about Mrs. Jungeman, except that she, like Alidge, "received treatment during illness." Young Alidge soon asked to be baptized, and the Sisters gave him instruction. On December 8, the same day he blessed the hospital, Father O'Reilly baptized the boy. "Wasn't this a nice offering of a soul?" Sister Benedicta wrote to Mother Mariana on December 11.

Sister Benedicta mentioned a third patient in that letter, although not by name. Also in the letter she asks Mother Mariana for a watch, having observed Sister Placida, a graduate of pharmacy training with 14 years' experience, having to take the pulse of a patient with a clock. "I thought you might have a watch you could send me for her, one that has a second hand on the face. I never saw a nurse holding a clock" to take a patient's pulse.

St. Vincent's formally opened on December 20, 1898, according to the Diaries, "for inspection and the reception of patients," and that same day a Dr. Rodgers performed the hospital's first operation. On December 24 Father O'Reilly celebrated the first Mass in the hospital chapel.

On December 27 the Sisters held a reception for the public, assisted by a reception committee that included a number of wives of Hospital Association members, including Mrs. Sinnige, Mrs. Jemison and Mrs. McCrossin.

A newspaper account called the temporary hospital "far superior to many permanent institutions of the kind" with an "atmosphere of orderly system and unceasing yet unobtrusive watchfulness." The same account also states that at the time of the reception, there were four male patients in the temporary hospital.

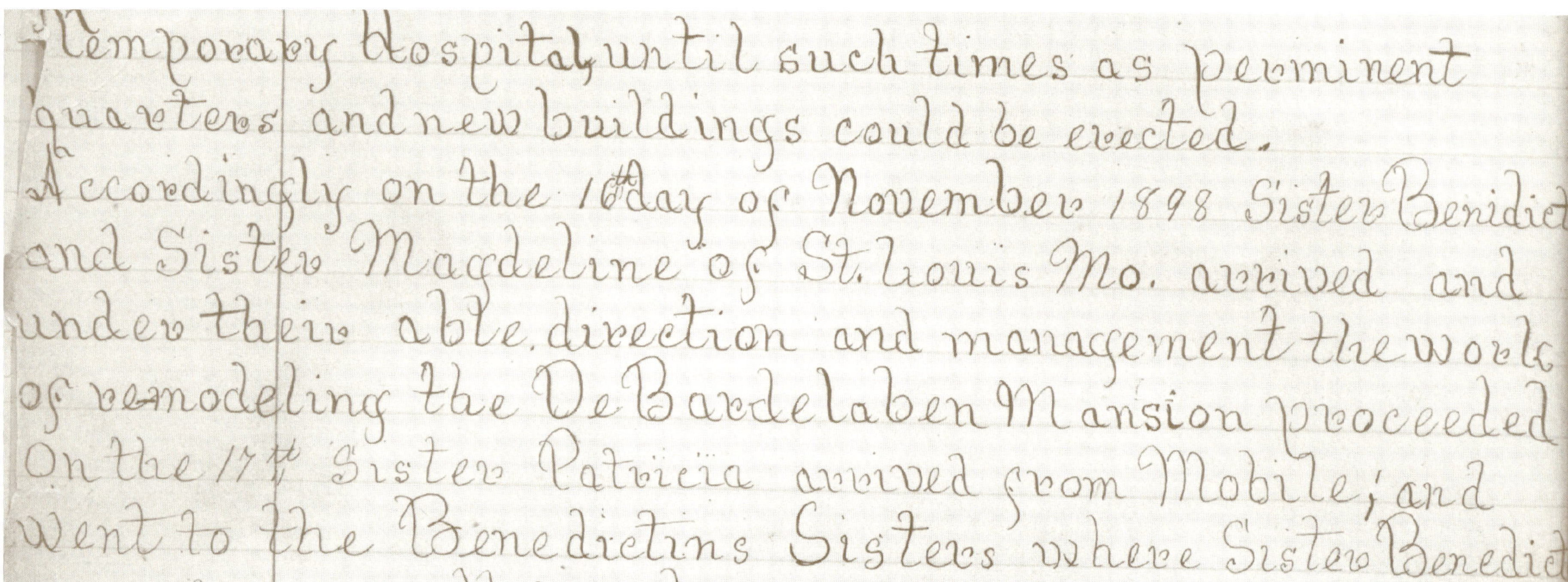
Temporary Hospital until such times as perminent
quarters and new buildings could be erected.
Accordingly on the 16th day of November 1898 Sister Benidict
and Sister Magdeline of St. Louis Mo. arrived and
under their able direction and management the work
of remodeling the DeBardelaben Mansion proceeded
On the 17th Sister Patricia arrived from Mobile; and
went to the Benedictins Sisters where Sister Benedict

Archives, St. Vincent's Hospital

In an elegant script, the Sisters at St. Vincent's recorded an account of events in the hospital. The originals of these Diaries, which document events through the late 1930s, are preserved in the St. Vincent's Archives.

In January 1899 Mother Mariana arrived for a short visit on her way to Mobile and left behind a new addition to the hospital staff, the young Sister Regina.

In January, with construction planned to begin in only a few months, the Fountain Heights location was abandoned in favor of a four-acre site at 27th Street and Avenue I (now Ninth Avenue South), a change probably made to prepare for the hospital's growth. Fountain Heights offered little room for expansion, while the new site in the South Highlands was in an area still sparsely populated.

Father Lennon described the new site (asking price: $6,000) as "just on the edge of the built up portion of the city within 10 minutes of the Union Station, and in a neighborhood whose character left no fears as to future developments." In February Father Lennon came to Birmingham, secured the new property and gave the construction bid to the Montgomery firm of Cook and Laurie for $67,939.

"With due ceremony and solemnity dirt was broken for the erection of St. Vincent's Hospital," the Diaries relate on March 11, "amidst a great concourse of people, of all creeds, and denominations."

Having launched a noble institution, Sister Benedicta then returned to Emmitsburg.

And on March 13, a new Sister Servant arrived to take the helm, one who would leave an indelible mark upon the hospital and upon Birmingham as well.

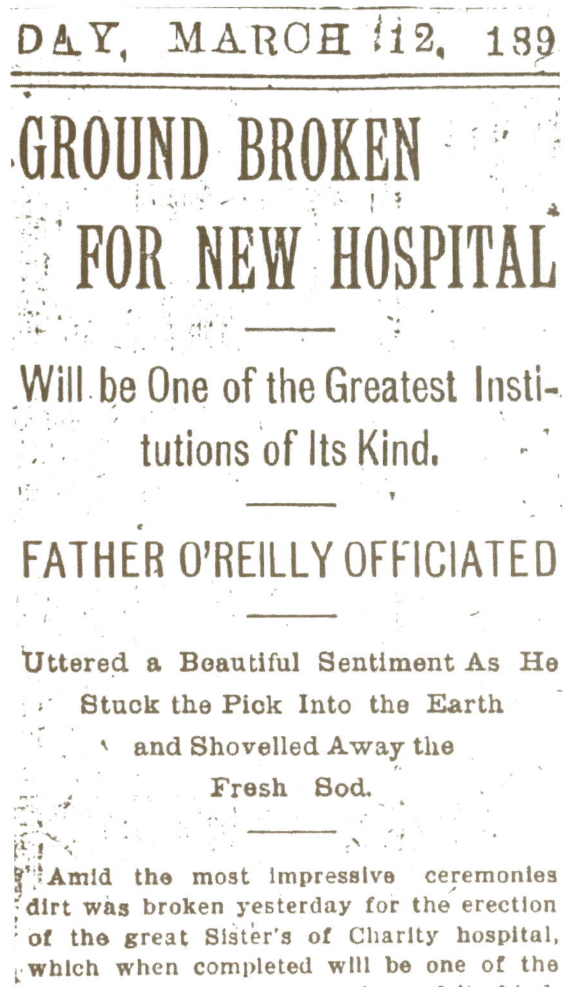

DAY, MARCH 12, 189

GROUND BROKEN FOR NEW HOSPITAL

Will be One of the Greatest Institutions of Its Kind.

FATHER O'REILLY OFFICIATED

Uttered a Beautiful Sentiment As He Stuck the Pick Into the Earth and Shovelled Away the Fresh Sod.

Amid the most impressive ceremonies dirt was broken yesterday for the erection of the great Sister's of Charity hospital, which when completed will be one of the

Excerpted from the Birmingham *Age-Herald*, March 12, 1899:

Amid the most impressive ceremonies dirt was broken yesterday for the erection of the great Sister's [sic] of Charity hospital, which when completed will be one of the greatest charitable institutions of its kind, not only in Birmingham, but in the entire south...

The ceremony of "breaking the ground" was begun yesterday morning at 10 o'clock, near the beautiful Walnut Grove where the building is to be situated. President Harry Sinnige, of the hospital association, called the gathering to order and he went over briefly the work which had been done to locate the hospital here. He spoke enthusiastically of the splendid services which had been rendered in this work by Father O'Reiley [sic]. His efforts have been untiring and have done the greatest amount of good. Mr. Sinnige refused to break the dirt for the building, saying that honor belonged to Father O'Reilly...

Father O'Reilly then took a pick and drove it into the ground, saying as he did so: "Up to this high eminence, 200 feet above the city, this noble building will be seen of all men, beckoning the afflicted of all degrees, high and low, rich and poor, into its comfortable walls...."

Chapter Two

Mount St. Vincent's

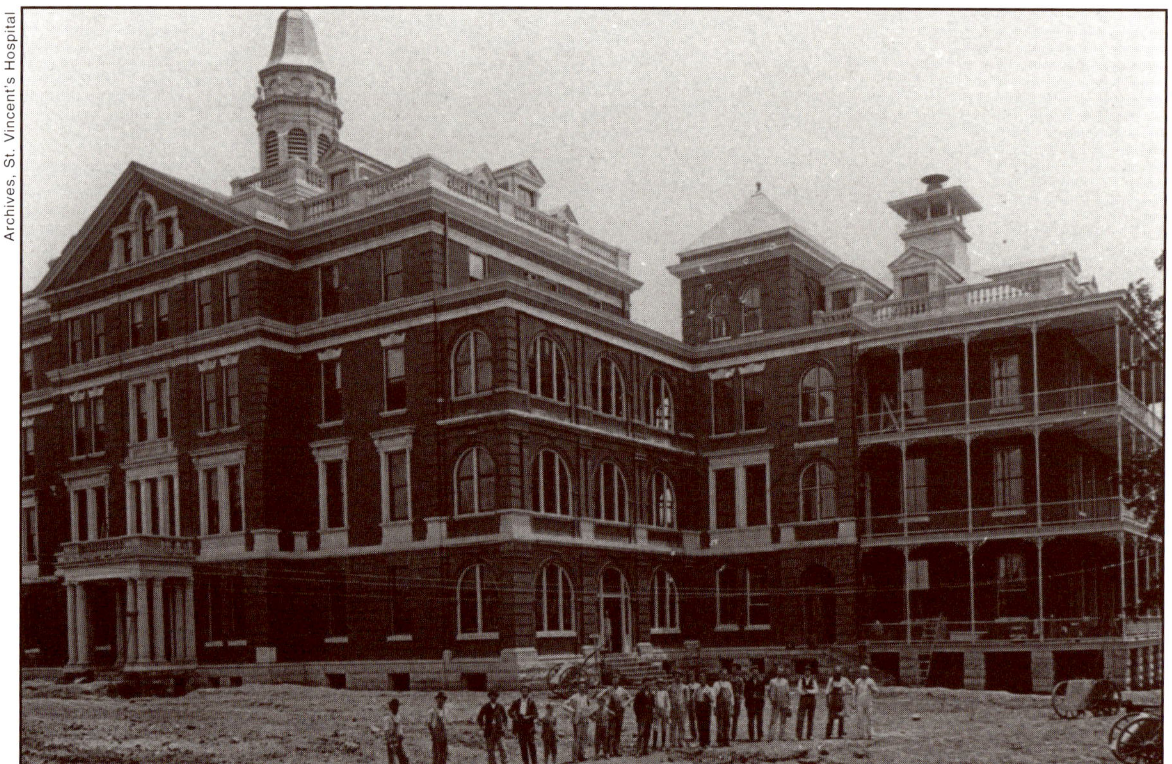

Archives, St. Vincent's Hospital

The "state-of-the-art" St. Vincent's, with construction crew, September 1900

The former Nora Moynahan was 35 years old when she arrived in Birmingham to take over responsibility of St. Vincent's.

Within her first week, Sister Chrysostom found the work-site of the new hospital idle from a shortage of bricks, the temporary hospital filled with patients and an overworked staff of Sisters without the traditional cornettes of the Daughters of Charity upon their heads. Some problems were solved more easily than others. After two unsuccessful attempts to "do up" the cornettes, they were sent to Evansville, and the ready-to-wear cornettes were returned in time for the celebration of Mass on March 25 (along with "the formula" for "how to do them up"). Sister Chrysostom delayed Sister Patricia's departure for her next mission until help was available, but, as resourceful as she was, Sister Chrysostom could not make construction begin until the first of June.

Born in Ireland and reared in Massachusetts, Sister Chrysostom was among the first nursing graduates at Boston's Carney Hospital in 1894. Early in her career, Sister Chrysostom's superiors noted her administrative ability. For most of the next two decades, she would hone this ability to near perfection as she struggled to maintain a charitable hospital in a city with an inadequate tax base and thousands of citizens engaged in dangerous occupations – a city known at the time as "the murder capital of the world."

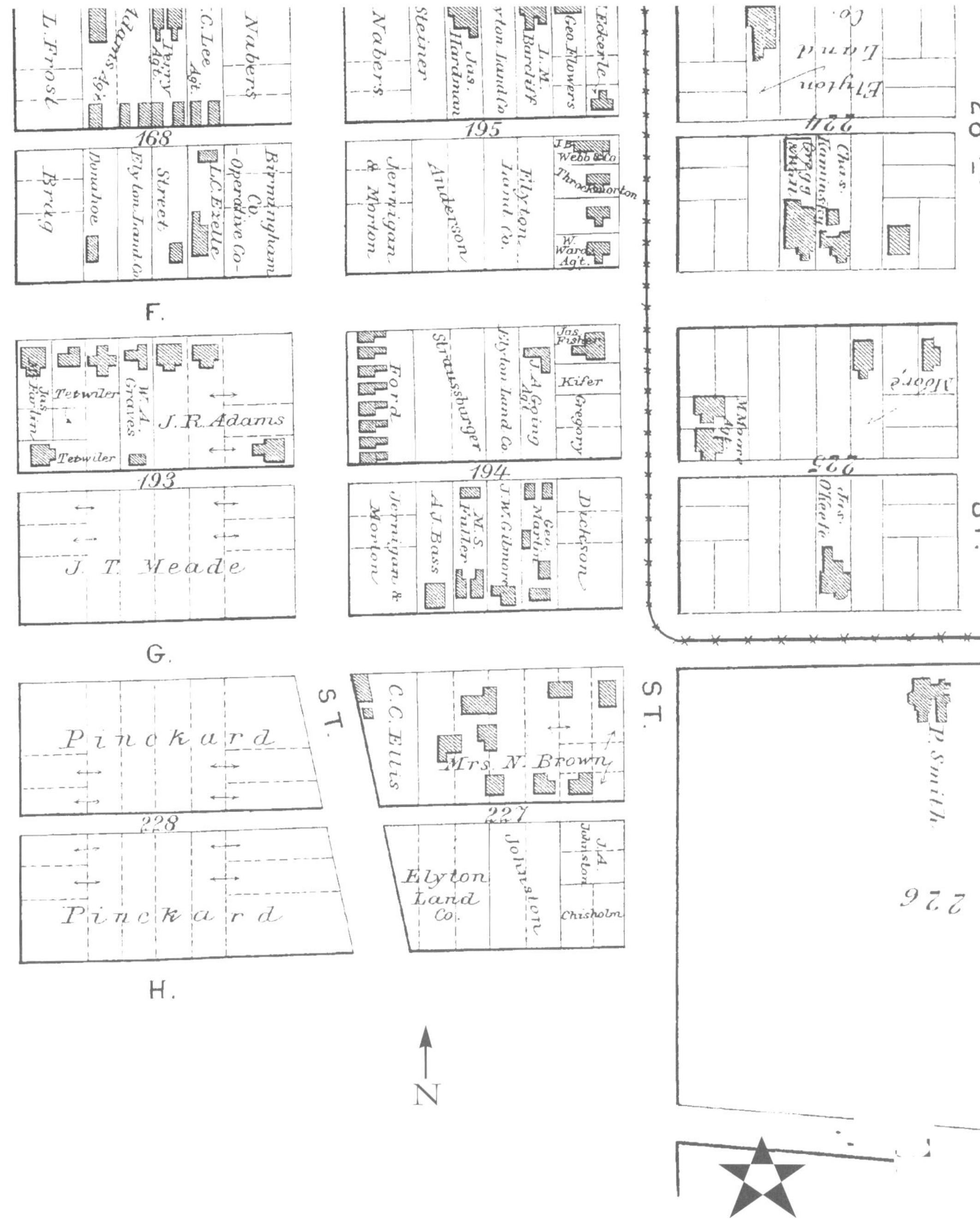

Archives, Birmingham Public Library

This 1888 city map shows the location of what would later be called "Mount St. Vincent's" (star at lower right). Although a number of houses were built during the next 11 years, as work began on the new hospital, the area was still considered to be "sparsely populated."

Sister Chrysostom Moynahan, an imposing woman with a keen mind and a serene smile, would become the first registered nurse in the state of Alabama, found the state's first school of nursing and open Birmingham's first outpatient clinic that accepted patients regardless of their ability to pay.

Born in 1863 in County Kerry, Ireland and reared in Massachusetts, the former Nora Moynahan made her vows in 1891. She arrived in Birmingham in 1899 and supervised the construction of the imposing new facility built that year. She quickly became one of the city's most prominent citizens, as she used her calm resolve to guide the hospital through its difficult early years, which included a devastating tornado and recurring financial struggles.

At a time when almost half of all patients admitted were unable to pay for health care, St. Vincent's turned no one away. "If we do not have enough money to meet all our bills at the end of the month," she once told the other Sisters, "we will just wait and hope for the next month to pay for itself and clear the back debts as well."

When newly levied taxes threatened to put the hospital on the auction block, Sister Chrysostom lobbied the mayor until he used city funds to purchase St. Vincent's and return ownership to the Daughters of Charity.

Sister Chrysostom opened the city's first charity outpatient clinic, using what she called her "$5 nest egg." The "Outdoor Clinic," as it was called, attracted local press attention, lauding Sister Chrysostom for the impressive work being done there. Her reply was a plea for expanded streetcar service to allow the poor greater access to the clinic.

During her years at St. Vincent's, Sister Chrysostom also established the Ladies of Charity in Birmingham, an organization of local Catholic women who acted as the hospital's first auxiliary to assist in its mission to serve the poor.

After 18 years as administrator of St. Vincent's, Sister Chrysostom led the only band of American Sisters to nurse the wounded in Europe during World War I. En route to Italy, Sister Chrysostom told a shipmate, "It will be the happiest moment of our lives when we are ministering to the sick and wounded soldiers in Italy."

After two hospital assignments in Missouri, Sister Chrysostom returned to Alabama in 1933 as administrator of Providence Hospital in Mobile. She served there until her death in 1941, after more than 50 years of service as a member of the Daughters of Charity.

Sister Chrysostom was inducted into the Alabama Women's Hall of Fame in 1982.

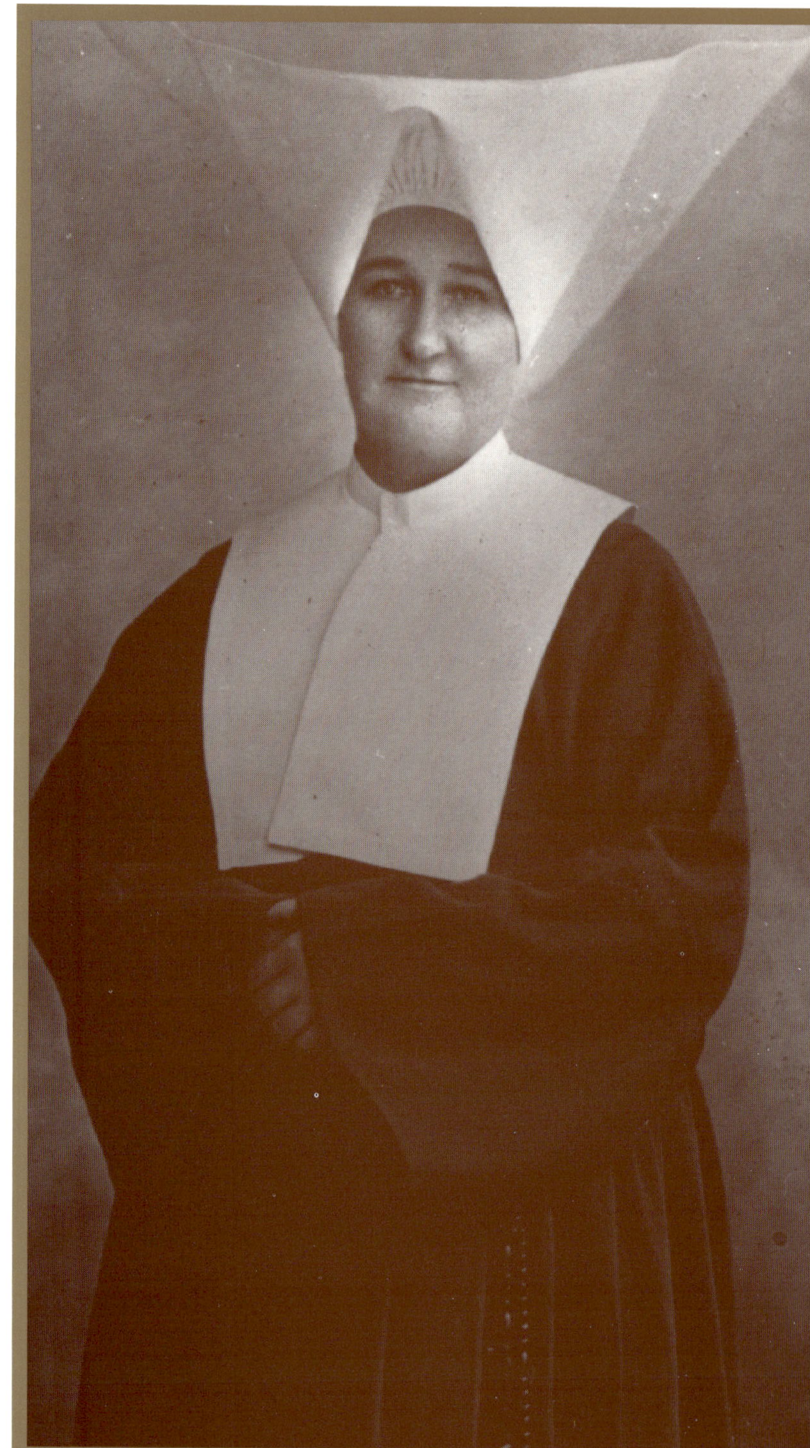

Archives, St. Vincent's Hospital

Sister Chrysostom Moynahan

Sister Chrysostom had begun the mission that would be her longest: ministering to the needs of the citizens of Birmingham from atop a high hill soon to be known as Mount St. Vincent's.

The Cornerstone of Brotherhood

The ceremony to lay the cornerstone took place the afternoon of May 30, 1899. The *Age-Herald* described Bishop Allen "in the full insignia of his office," addressing the "unusual spectacle of Jew and Gentile, Catholic and Protestant, standing together upon the strong platform of a universal brotherhood supported by the broad and sustaining principles of charity and humanity."

Mayor W. H. Drennen was unable to attend, and the city was represented by Alderman R. H. Kerr, who "eloquently expressed" a "hearty welcome" to the Sisters, "at whose coming...all would rejoice."

Father O'Reilly followed, and after marvelling at the growth of Birmingham during his years spent serving its citizens, he praised the Sisters for their work, which required "pure hearts, noble minds and strong intellects."

A number of prominent citizens spoke after Father O'Reilly finished, including Rufus S. Rhodes, followed by clergy from the First Methodist Church, St. Mary's-on-the-Highland and Temple Emanu-El, who "gave expression to the most beautiful sentiments."

Throughout the ceremony, Sisters Chrysostom, Antonia, Patricia and Regina stood close by, as did the two other priests of the Birmingham parish and six other priests from parishes across the state.

With the help of the other priests, Bishop Allen laid the stone with a specially made ceremonial trowel, more than 10 inches long, with a sterling silver blade, an onyx handle and gold appointments.

Before the cornerstone was sealed, W. P. McCrossin's young son Dixie inserted a copper box containing recent newspapers, a history of the Sisters of Charity Hospital Association, a Miraculous Medal and a number of other religious icons.

In the News

As construction was beginning on the the dramatic new St. Vincent's, a number of other dramas were taking place in Birmingham. From the May 1899 issues of the *Age-Herald*:

In the small mining town of Newcastle, just north of the city, a "drunken and infuriated" miner named Joe Pate got off the train on the Saturday afternoon of May 27 and "began firing at everything in sight." Pate, his pockets full of ammunition cartridges, then killed Henry Goldsweathersly, a "highly respected miner" who was "endeavoring to dissuade him from firing into a crowd." Pate, who had spent much of the day in Birmingham drinking "cheap booze," was then "overpowered by a crowd of determined citizens who were attracted to the scene."

Also that day, Captain W. P. Barker, "the engineer who laid off of the broad streets and avenues of the city," died at the age of 70 of sciatic rheumatism.

On May 29, more than 1,000 people attended the opening of the summer theatrical season in East Lake, with "up-to-date" vaudeville "specialties" that included Elise Du Barry, "the California nightingale."

On May 31 the Age-Herald *announced that Miss Ethel DuFre Houston, a "Birmingham girl who has adopted the operatic stage as a profession," had been chosen as the lead contralto of the International Grand Opera Company, which was described as "one of the best and most successful companies in America."*

The "grand opening" of a law against spitting on city sidewalks took effect on June 1, with the newspaper excitedly anticipating "the first man caught taking the sidewalk for a mark at which to aim his deposit of saliva will promptly be escorted to the police station." The minimum fine under the new ordinance was $1.

Dixie McCrossin would not live to see that copper box opened 73 years later, but one person would. Robert Jemison Jr., a member of one of Birmingham's most noted families who would eventually develop some of the city's most beautiful neighborhoods, was 20 years old the day he stood among the throngs to watch the first of three events of great importance to St. Vincent's. Later Jemison, whose family has continued to play a prominent role in the hospital's history, not only would witness Father O'Reilly's tragic fall from a horse five years from the laying of this cornerstone, but also would see the cornerstone of a new St. Vincent's laid in 1972.

A Tragic Anniversary

The time the Sisters spent in the DeBardeleben mansion – awaiting the permanent hospital's completion – began as a noble challenge and ended in tragedy.

Although daily operations went generally well, the hospital was usually overcrowded. In the first two years alone, 24 different local physicians are known to have admitted patients to St. Vincent's. Because of recent advances in turn-of-the-century medical technology and care, for the first time the well-to-do began to use the services of hospitals, instead of convalescing at home. The Sisters made room for as many patients as possible – patients often slept on pallets on the floor. The Sisters' Diaries record one day when there was not even floor space available, and six patients were turned away.

Although the mansion had adequate facilities for bathing at the time – a 30-gallon copper tub – the population of the temporary hospital waited in an all-day queue for a bath.

In August, Sister Elizabeth arrived from New Orleans to join the Sisters, although apparently the workload still was not eased enough to permit Sister Patricia to depart for her next mission.

In November 1899, however, as the Sisters' first anniversary in Birmingham approached, the challenging days at the mansion were to turn frightening. On November 12 Sister Patricia became ill, too ill to attend the Sisters' first retreat in Birmingham. Her condition was diagnosed the next day as walking typhoid. Before the retreat ended, Sister Regina also fell ill, and her condition quickly grew serious. Having been in bed for a week, Sister Patricia had not improved, and she was moved from the Sisters' quarters into the private ward.

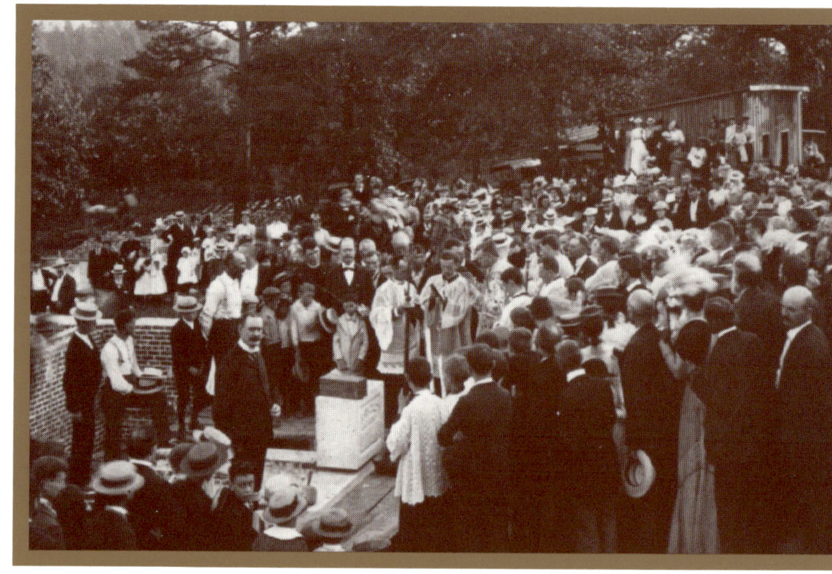

Archives, St. Vincent's Hospital

The laying of the cornerstone, May 30, 1899

Three days later, neither Sister had improved. Dr. Whelan, one of the first doctors to admit patients to the hospital, diagnosed Sister Regina's illness that day as confluent black smallpox.

At noon, the house was quarantined.

All the Sisters were vaccinated immediately, except for Sister Placida, who was quarantined with Sister Regina. All patients were quickly dismissed, except for a few who could not be moved.

Almost as quickly, Father O'Reilly tried to stop the traditional yellow flag of quarantine from flying over the temporary hospital. Apparently fearful of frightening the local populace and attaching a stigma to the hospital, Father O'Reilly brought over a pink flag marked "scarlet fever," but "Sister Chrysostom told him it would never do." The yellow flag went up, but Father O'Reilly "had it twisted around the post, so that it could not be seen."

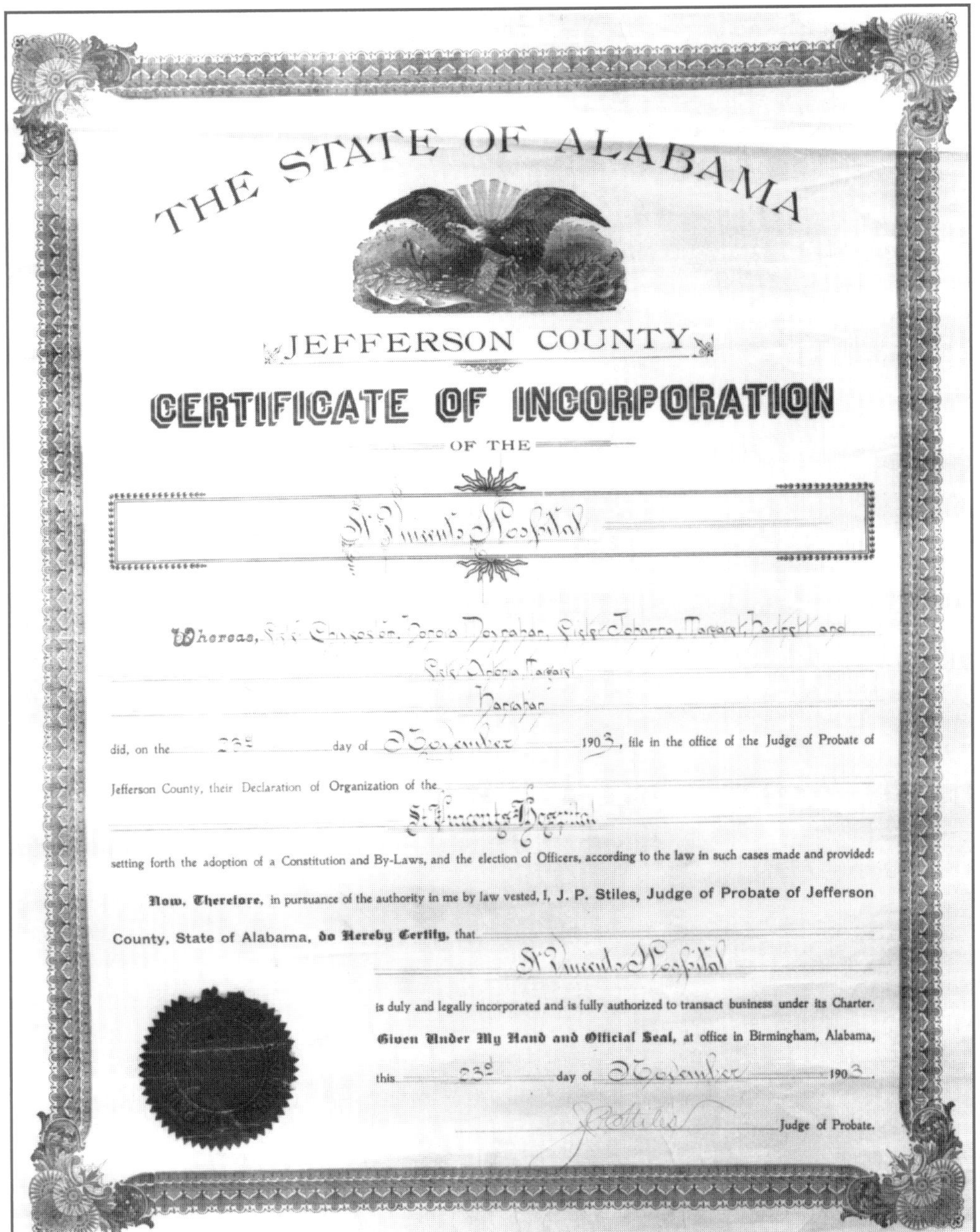

THE STATE OF ALABAMA

JEFFERSON COUNTY

CERTIFICATE OF INCORPORATION

OF THE

St. Vincent's Hospital

Whereas, [illegible]

did, on the 23d day of [illegible] 1903, file in the office of the Judge of Probate of Jefferson County, their Declaration of Organization of the St. Vincent's Hospital

setting forth the adoption of a Constitution and By-Laws, and the election of Officers, according to the law in such cases made and provided:

Now, Therefore, in pursuance of the authority in me by law vested, I, J. P. Stiles, Judge of Probate of Jefferson County, State of Alabama, do Hereby Certify, that St. Vincent's Hospital

is duly and legally incorporated and is fully authorized to transact business under its Charter.

Given Under My Hand and Official Seal, at office in Birmingham, Alabama, this 23d day of [illegible] 1903.

J. P. Stiles

Judge of Probate.

St. Vincent's Certificate of Incorporation

Archives, St. Vincent's Hospital

November 27 was Thanksgiving, and the remaining Sisters held "a sad and lonely feast." All the patients were now gone and neither Sister Patricia nor Sister Regina had improved. By the 29th, Sister Patricia was worse and Sister Regina was delirious. The next day the Sisters had a difficult time getting provisions because of the now widespread fear of visiting the house.

Sister Patricia showed no improvement over the next few days, and although Sister Regina initially improved enough for Dr. Whelan to offer hope for her recovery, she remained delirious. On December 4, Sister Regina was much worse and slipped into unconsciousness. Having received the last blessing from Father O'Reilly, she died at 9:30 that morning.

She was 20 years old.

The sexton was slow to dig the grave that afternoon, and Father O'Reilly and another of the parish priests helped him in the bitter cold. Since the undertaker refused to come near the sick room, Sisters Magdeline, Elizabeth and Placida placed the body of Sister Regina in her casket, which Father O'Reilly then helped lift over the veranda of the house.

While the others attended the funeral, Sisters Magdeline and Placida burned Sister Regina's bedding and clothing.

Sister Patricia recovered, and on December 24 Father O'Reilly was finally able to take down the yellow flag.

Finally, on January 1, 1900, the Sisters received the first patient since quarantine, an "accident case, colored male."

Dedication Day

The first months of 1900 passed with few outstanding mentions. Construction of the new hospital went slowly. Two new Sisters began missions at St. Vincent's: Sister Anna arrived in February and Sister Leo in August. Perhaps because Sister Anna was ill with typhoid during most of the months of June and July, Sister Patricia's departure for her next mission did not take place until September.

Possibly overeager, the Sisters began moving on September 27 into the wing, since the main building wasn't finished. It took three days to move the Sisters, partly because a traveling show was visiting town, and the movers took off to see it. The first patient in the new hospital, an L & N Railroad employee with multiple fractures, was brought in on September 29. Some of the working men were unaccustomed to seeing so much blood, and one of them was so frightened that "he ran off and did not return."

But because most of the equipment did not arrive immediately, the Sisters weren't prepared to accept every patient; in fact they regretfully turned 17 patients away the first week. The Sisters slept on the floor at first, then on cots from the armory. Finally their beds arrived October 16. There was no steam heat until November 15. And although the operating room was not ready, two operations were performed on November 22 in the basement.

Prior to the official opening, the hospital received a number of donations and contributions, including the Concordia Club's $300 to endow a bed, $100 from St. Paul's, sterilizers from a Dr. Brown and various furniture, as well as a "grand hall clock."

The completed hospital had cost far more than had been anticipated by anyone. Father O'Reilly had originally discussed with the Daughters of Charity a hospital costing about $40,000, of which $10,000 would be local contributions. The final cost, including property and furnishings, was estimated to be $250,000, and only about $30,000 of that came from the people of Birmingham.

Noble Sisters of Charity Throw Open the Doors of St. Vincent's Hospital---A Fine Institution

"The Sisters know no creeds here—they serve humanity in its widest sense," declared the Rt. Rev. Bishop Allen of Mobile as he stood in the grand stairway of the magnificent new St. Vincent's Hospital yesterday afternoon and talked to the assembled people who crowded the great halls. ple visited the hospital between 2 o'clock and 7 o'clock, and not one amongst them all was not amazed and delighted with the unsurpassable splendor of the general effect and the marvellous thoroughness of detail in the hospital's furnishings and appointments. Words of astonishment, exclamations of wonder and delight, sprung

Calling it a "palatial home of widest human charity," the Birmingham *Age-Herald* quoted Mayor Drennen as calling St. Vincent's opening "a real Thanksgiving Day for Birmingham and Alabama..."

The large crowd that toured St. Vincent's that day marveled at "the thoroughness of detail in the hospital's furnishings and appointments. Words of astonishment, exclamations of wonder and delight, sprung from every lip, and the good [S]isters, bright in their great happiness, were fairly overwhelmed with congratulations..."

"...[T]housands of visitors could scarcely believe what they saw. The dozens of magnificent rooms furnished by private or individual charity, some of them memorials to beloved dead, cause the greatest astonishment and delight..."

In the typically purple prose of the day, the Age-Herald *took exaggerated delight in listing every luxurious and technological marvel, "the beautiful and dainty little chapel with its exquisite altar; the pharmacy, with its counter and pots and mortars all of clear glass; the amphitheatre, with its numerous seats and "operating" tables; the perfect water arrangements; the succession of white-bedded wards, including the dainty wards for children; the model laundry...the engine room, with the largest boiler in Birmingham...*

"And the thousands are prepared to believe now that there is perhaps not now in existence a more complete, a more perfectly appointed hospital than St. Vincent's at Birmingham..."

A breakdown one year later detailed the expense as $172,829.71 for the buildings and about $50,000 for furnishings, of which Birmingham citizens donated $11,000 in cash and about $25,000 in furnishings.

This money, however, gave Birmingham possibly the best hospital in the Southeast. The hospital could comfortably accommodate 200 patients. One of the local newspapers bragged that the hospital's three operating rooms were "equipped with everything known to medical science to aid surgeons in their work." (The same paper also optimistically called the new building "fire proof.")

November 29 was Thanksgiving, but more importantly for St. Vincent's, it was Dedication Day of the new building. "This Thanksgiving is one to be remembered," the Diaries read. The ceremonies began at 9 o'clock that morning, with Bishop Allen, accompanied by a "procession of altar boys and priests," blessing each room of the building. The public exercises took place in the afternoon, with more than a thousand in attendance.

As the *Age-Herald* described the event, "At last, after all the struggles and trials, the toils and the hopes, the delays and the disappointments…and one of the most

Archives, St. Vincent's Hospital

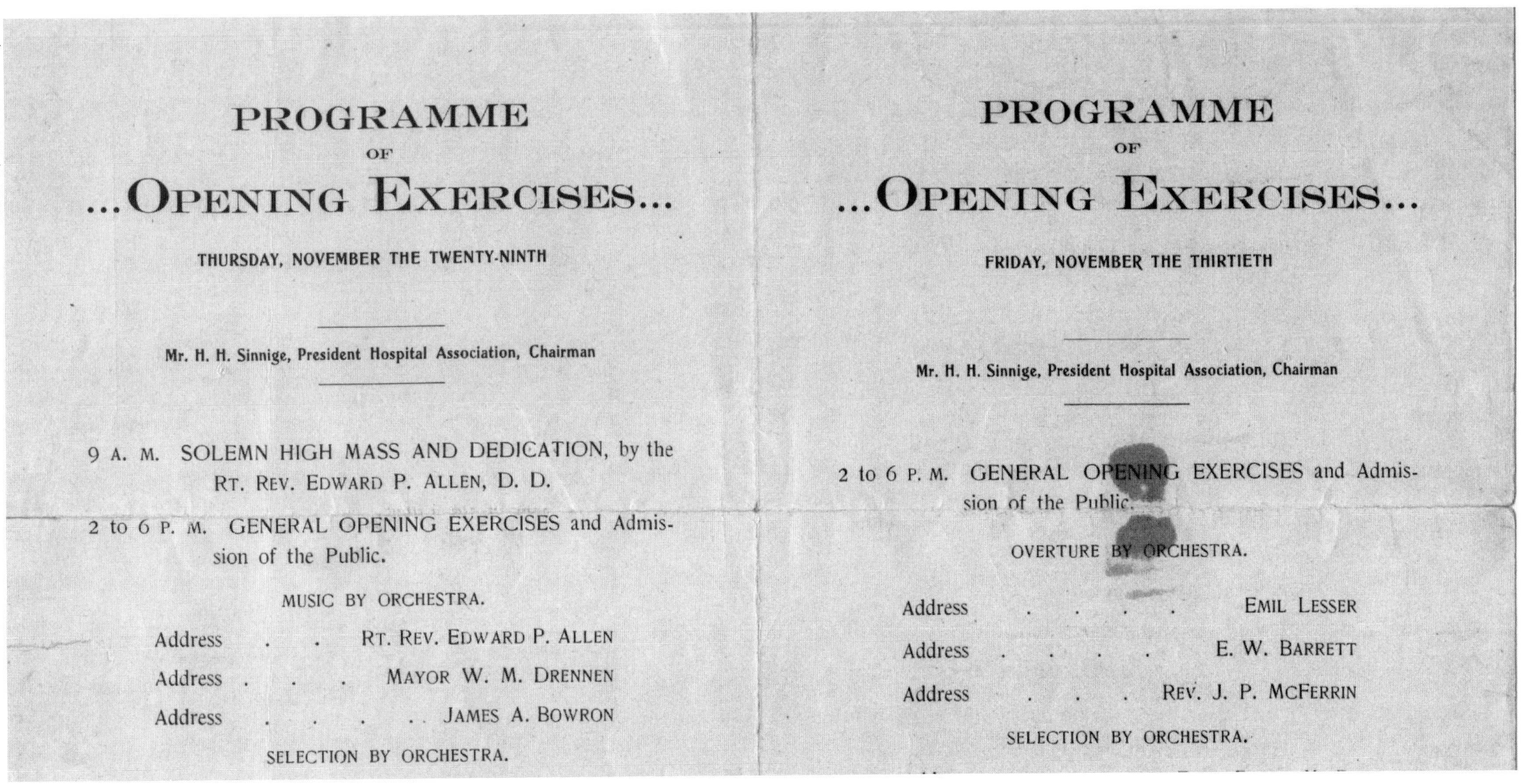

PROGRAMME

OF

...OPENING EXERCISES...

THURSDAY, NOVEMBER THE TWENTY-NINTH

Mr. H. H. Sinnige, President Hospital Association, Chairman

9 A. M. SOLEMN HIGH MASS AND DEDICATION, by the RT. REV. EDWARD P. ALLEN, D. D.

2 to 6 P. M. GENERAL OPENING EXERCISES and Admission of the Public.

MUSIC BY ORCHESTRA.

Address . . RT. REV. EDWARD P. ALLEN

Address . . . MAYOR W. M. DRENNEN

Address . . . . . . JAMES A. BOWRON

SELECTION BY ORCHESTRA.

PROGRAMME

OF

...OPENING EXERCISES...

FRIDAY, NOVEMBER THE THIRTIETH

Mr. H. H. Sinnige, President Hospital Association, Chairman

2 to 6 P. M. GENERAL OPENING EXERCISES and Admission of the Public.

OVERTURE BY ORCHESTRA.

Address . . . . . EMIL LESSER

Address . . . . . E. W. BARRETT

Address . . . . REV. J. P. MCFERRIN

SELECTION BY ORCHESTRA.

The original program for the opening of the new hospital

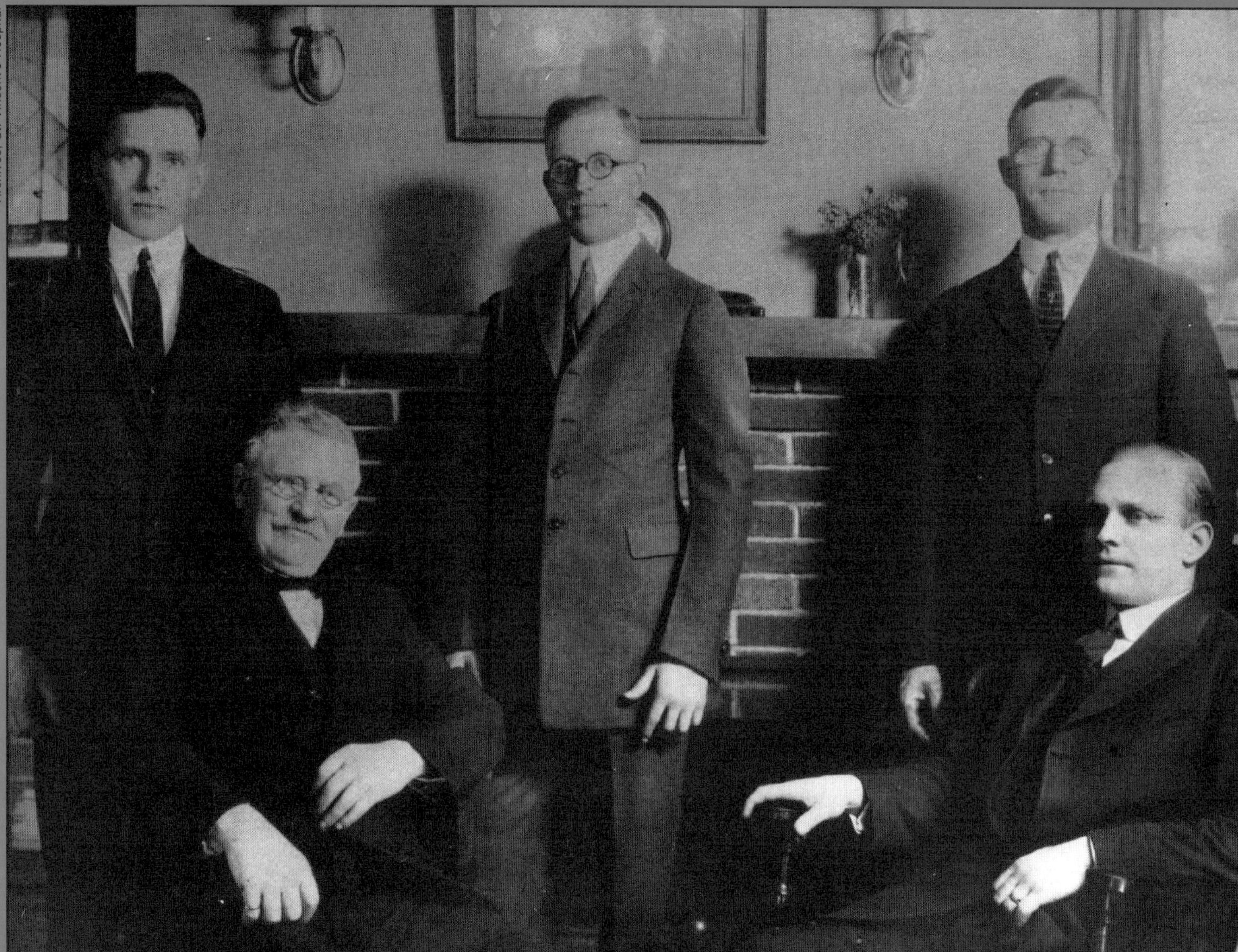

Archives, St. Vincent's Hospital

An early St. Vincent's medical staff: Dr. R. C. McQuiddy (standing left), Dr. Benedict (seated left), Dr. S. L. Ledbetter (standing center), Dr. Cowls (standing right) and Dr. E. P. Solomon (seated right) perfectly appointed hospitals in the world stood ready for the work of mercy…"

A huge crowd came the next day as well to the new hospital, a "palatial home of widest human charity," according to Mayor Drennen, and the music and speeches of the day before continued.

A Deadly Storm

As the hospital became fully functional, the Sisters began to settle into it, although circumstances were not to allow them to immediately slip into any form of routine. The hospital filled quickly to near-capacity, and the day-to-day operations of the crowded hospital were interrupted frequently with change and innovation, and then, in early Spring, with great tragedy.

The first months of 1901 brought a number of new Sisters to the hospital, as well as many "firsts" for St. Vincent's. The first resident, Dr. Carl Fox, arrived January 2; the first clinic in the operating room amphitheater took place on January 9; and the first lecture for nursing students took place February 13. On March 9, for the first time, doctors injected cocaine into the spinal cord of a patient for use as an anesthetic in an amputation.

On the cloudy morning of March 25, the young hospital was to face its harshest test so far. At about 9 a.m., a tornado struck from the west and proceeded to rip a path of death and destruction 150 feet wide "through the entire southern section," beginning at the "extreme southwest corner of the city" and moving eastward through Green Springs, Southside and Avondale. The tornado continued through the southeast area of the city, sparsely populated at the time, and then on to Irondale.

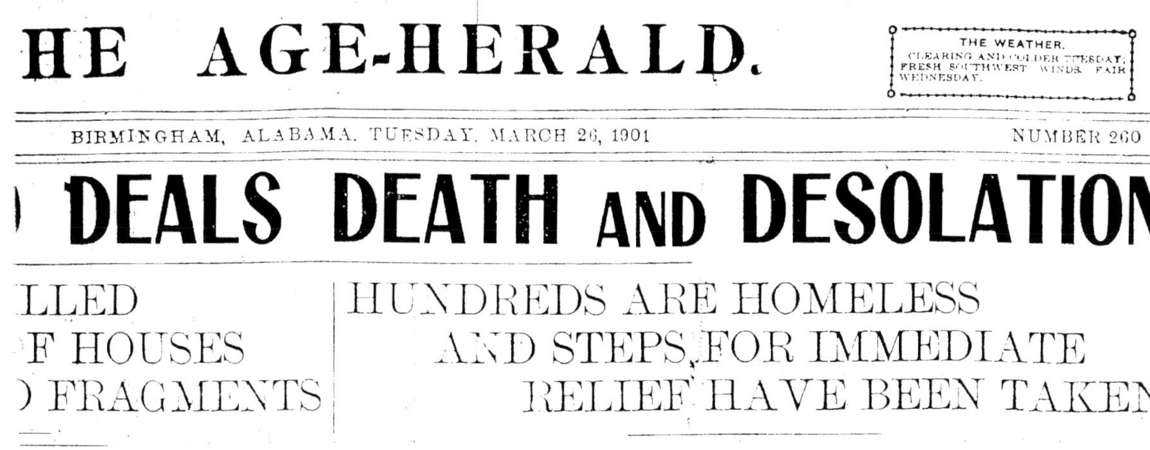

HE AGE-HERALD.

THE WEATHER. CLEARING AND COLDER TUESDAY; FRESH SOUTHWEST WINDS. FAIR WEDNESDAY.

BIRMINGHAM, ALABAMA, TUESDAY, MARCH 26, 1901 NUMBER 260

DEALS DEATH AND DESOLATION

LLED
F HOUSES
) FRAGMENTS

HUNDREDS ARE HOMELESS
AND STEPS FOR IMMEDIATE
RELIEF HAVE BEEN TAKEN

The tornado that struck Birmingham on March 25, 1901 was the worst disaster the city had faced since the cholera epidemic of 1873.

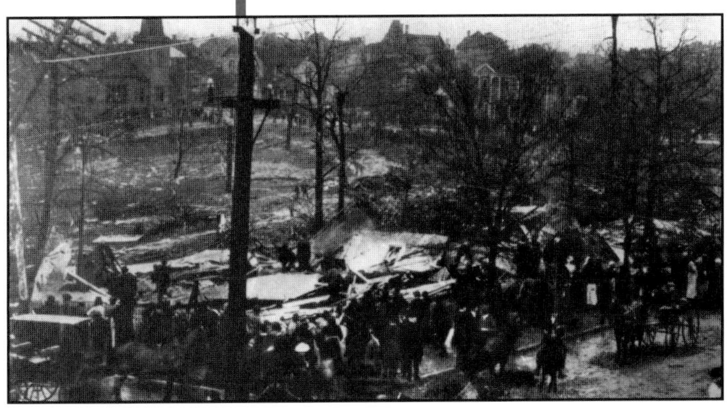

The morning following the tornado

Twenty people were killed and dozens injured. More than 1,000 were left homeless as an estimated 500 residences were destroyed. Property damage was estimated as high as $500,000.

Most of the injured were taken to St. Vincent's, where at least 22 remained the next day. Father Lennon sent this telegraph from Emmitsburg: "I praise God you have fared so well. Give every possible assistance to the sufferers!"

Although the tornado's path came within a block of the hospital, the newspaper reported two days later that "not one brick of that splendid edifice was disturbed," except for the northeast corner ward of the fourth floor, where "two massive pieces of lumber" struck, damaging the roof and smashing the plate glass windows and heavy oak window sashes. This being a ward for "paying" patients, it was unoccupied at the time, and all 200 patients of the hospital were uninjured.

However, "a heavy plate iron cornice was broken and twisted into rolls that looked not unlike huge twists of tobacco leaves."

The escape of one St. Vincent's patient was indeed, as the Age-Herald *described it, "almost miraculous." In preparation for a planned surgery, Major Frank Y. Anderson, accompanied by his wife, was hurriedly en route to the hospital from his home on 21st Street at the same time the tornado approached from the west. With his passengers oblivious to the approaching destruction, the coachman drove the horses "furiously," and then "seeing the roofs of houses in the air and appreciating the awful danger, he dashed into an alley and the tornado passed by."*

Twenty people were killed in Birmingham, four were killed in Irondale, and dozens more were injured. At least 1,000 people were left homeless as more than 500 homes were destroyed by the storm. The telephone poles on 20th Street were thrown into the busy street. Railway cars from downtown could go no further than Avenue G (now Seventh Avenue South), and hundreds of downtown businessmen spent much of the day not knowing if their families to the south were among the dead or injured.

Mercifully, St. Vincent's received little damage, and most of the injured were brought there for attention. Almost every private clinic received injured as well, including the infirmary where Dr. G. C. Chapman practiced. Sadly and ironically, Dr. Chapman was killed by the tornado as he returned from a house call near Five Points South.

Much of the tornado's destruction took place in the immediate vicinity of St. Vincent's. In a neighborhood slightly northwest of the hospital, called Brown's Hill at the time, nearly 100 homes, "mostly one-story cottages," were reported destroyed in a radius of only a few blocks. To the east of the hospital, much larger homes were damaged or destroyed, accompanied by a number of injuries and fatalities.

The huge trees on the hillside of St. Vincent's were "torn up by the roots, and large masses of stone were twisted out of the ground and broken and scattered all over the driveways of the entrance to the institution..." None of the 200 patients in residence at St. Vincent's that morning were injured.

The *Age-Herald* reported two days later that the "structure stood as solid as the hill it crowned, and yet it stood the fullest force and fury of the tornado."

Money Troubles and Other Routine Woes

By the end of 1901 the hospital had become a part of the city's fiber, but meeting the city's needs made finances a constant concern for much of the hospital's first decade. As many as 15 patients were admitted each day, with slightly fewer than half being charity patients.

A non-charity patient in 1901 paid from $7 to $25 a week for care, and most maladies required a week's stay. Even though almost as many paid little or nothing, all received identical care.

The hospital was well-staffed. There were 14 Sisters, 18 nurses, six orderlies, six "men nurses," and about 20 "servants." There were five to 10 doctors in the

Archives, St. Vincent's Hospital

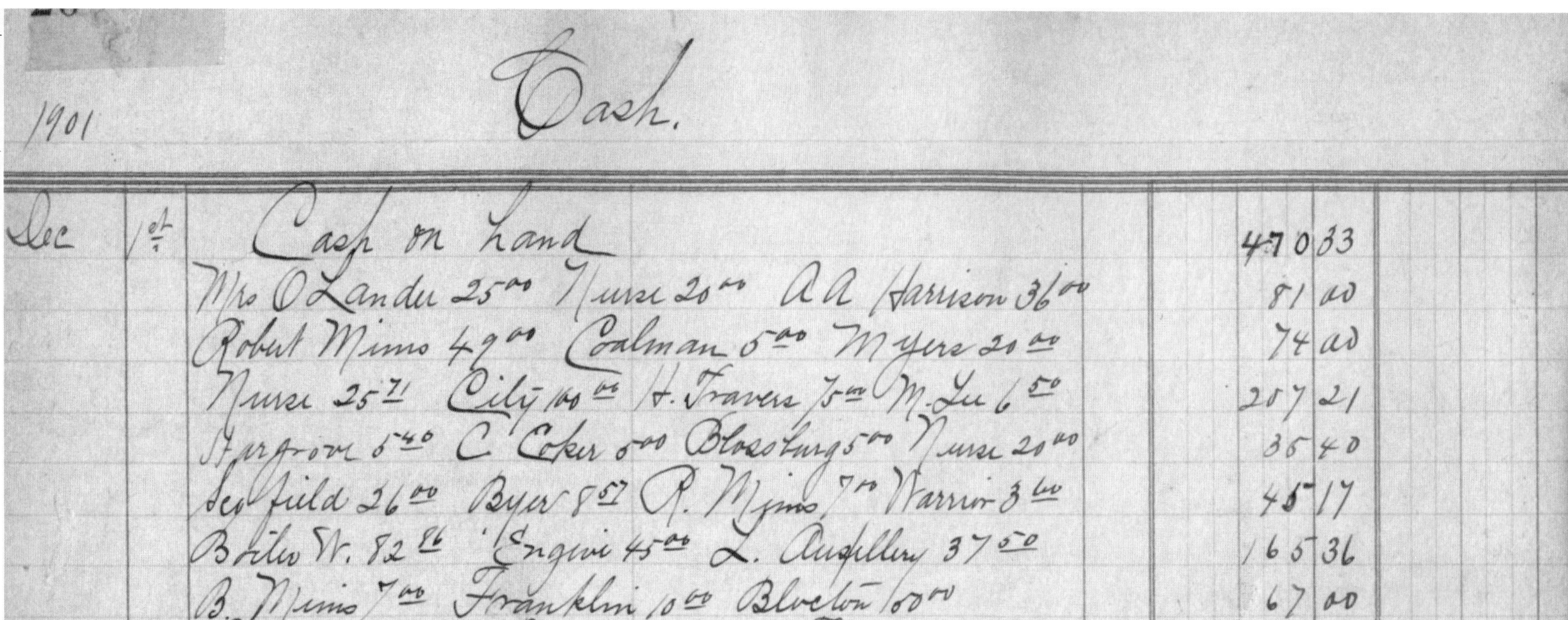

During the early 1900s, St. Vincent's had frequent financial problems.

hospital at all hours of the day. (Local physicians alternated as chief of surgery, each serving a term of three months.)

Even though the number of charity cases was high, because the hospital operated frugally, the quality of care was equally high. The nursing students were given only room and board, plus $5 each month for incidental needs. The Sisters, of course, received no pay, although they were furnished with "the necessities of life."

The annual report of patients received from November 1, 1901, to November 1, 1902, listed a total of 1,254 patients, with 572 being entirely free and 185 on a company medical plan. (Members of United Mine Workers contributed 10 cents each per month and employees of the Birmingham Rolling Mill contributed 25 cents each, which entitled them to one free treatment and hospital stay.)

While financial insecurity persisted, Sister Chrysostom's faith didn't waiver. "If we do not have enough money to meet all our bills at the end of the month," she is quoted as saying, "we will just wait and hope for the next month to pay for itself and clear the back debts as well."

Thanksgiving was the anniversary of Dedication Day, which established the holiday as a focal point for donations to the hospital. Five hundred dollars of donations came in on Thanksgiving of 1901 and a similar amount the next year.

The hospital faced uncertainty on a regular basis, but a routine was slowly being established. The nurses began classes each first week in September and had their first clinic in the middle of each October. Nursing exams would take place the next May and coincide with an all-day outing to East Lake, which became an annual tradition.

The Ladies of Charity auxiliary had their first meeting November 7, 1901, which began many decades of service to the poor through aid to the hospital.

As the days passed, the daily incidents at St. Vincent's came to resemble a poignant drama. In 1901 another Daughter of Charity, Sister Antoinette, died at St. Vincent's and was buried next to Sister Regina. Shortly afterward a nurse died of typhoid fever. A train wreck injured seven in November of that year, and another train wreck two weeks later injured seven more. A panic in a crowd at an unspecified "colored church during their convention" killed one and injured seven more.

On September 4, 1902, a man named Date Dozier was brought in after being shot in the abdomen. The shot left two perforations in his stomach and three in

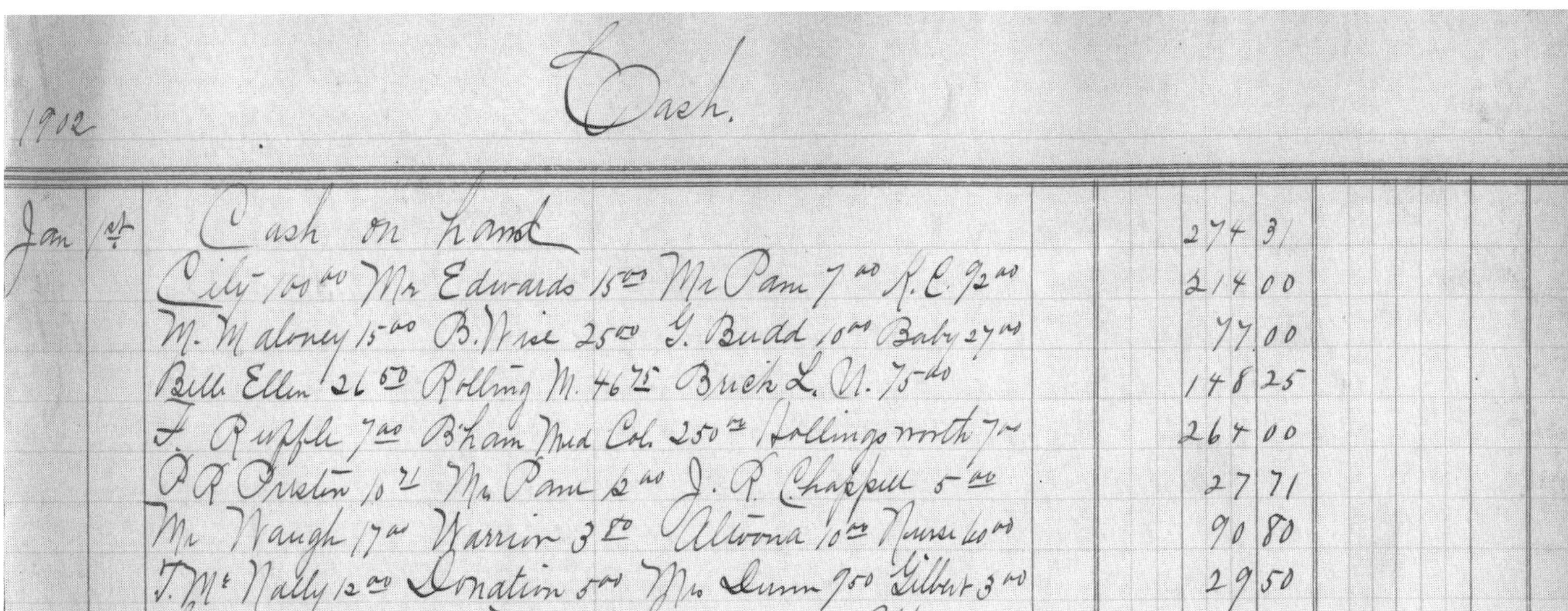

1902 Cash.

Jan	1st	Cash on hand	274	31
		City 100.00 Mr Edwards 15.00 Mr Pam 7.00 R.E. 92.00	214	00
		M. Maloney 15.00 B. Wise 25.00 G. Budd 10.00 Baby 27.00	77	00
		Belle Ellen 26.50 Rolling M. 46.75 Brick L. U. 75.00	148	25
		F. Ruffle 7.00 B'ham Med Col. 250.00 Hollingsworth 7.00	264	00
		P.R. Preston 10.71 Mr Pam 12.00 J. R. Chappell 5.00	27	71
		Mr Waugh 17.00 Warrior 3.80 Altoona 10.00 Nurse 60.00	90	80
		T. McNally 12.00 Donation 5.00 Mr Dunn 9.50 Gilbert 3.00	29	50

his intestines. After an operation, "one of the first successful operations of that kind performed in this city," the patient was doing well.

Other days, however, more closely mirrored a soap opera. During a November 1901 operation, it was discovered that the man being treated was in fact a woman dressed in men's clothing. Mayor Drennen made an appearance as a patient in October 1902, and in March 1903 Dr. Presley sent over an "Esquimaux" (Eskimo) patient, who was considered quite an oddity. Later, in 1905, Dr. Riggs removed a fibroid tumor weighing more than 37 pounds. The patient recovered.

Another remarkable episode during the hospital's first decade involved a freak accident that necessitated one of the first-ever operations involving the heart. Irene Johns, a 16-year-old "nurse," was playing with the three children for whom she was employed to care. One of the children, playing in a swing, accidentally bumped into the young black girl, which forced a hat pin that was sticking in her clothes to be driven into her chest. Although at first uncertain about the best course of action, doctors at St. Vincent's performed what one local newspaper called "one of the few operations on the heart that has ever been successful, not more than two dozen of them being included in medical annals." A 2-inch piece of the hat pin was removed from young Irene's chest, and the doctors expected her to recover completely.

On May 26, 1903, St. Vincent's graduated "the first class of trained nurses that Alabama has ever known." The three young ladies, Lucy Catherine Maguire, Mary Agnes Thompson and Annie Loretta Leahy, had completed three years of lectures and practical work. Dr. Cunningham Wilson was master of ceremonies for the event, which was held in the amphitheater and began with a piano and violin duet by two nursing students. Bishop Allen came from Mobile for the momentous event.

Sister Chrysostom fell ill with typhoid three weeks later, and her condition quickly became serious. She not only had been shouldering the strain of St. Vincent's, but also had been in charge of establishing a charity hospital in Montgomery. After two weeks, her condition was still serious enough for Mayor Drennen to send a concerned telegram from his vacation home in Blount Springs, 35 miles away.

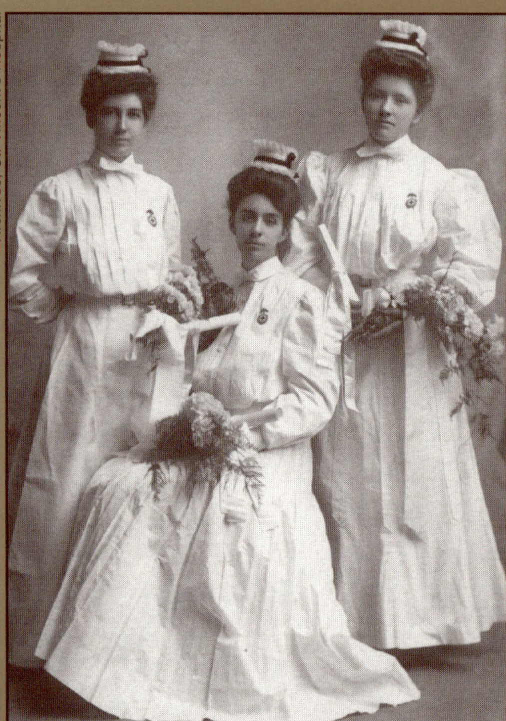

Archives, St. Vincent's Hospital

In 1903 St. Vincent's Hospital School of Nursing graduated the first three nurses trained in the State of Alabama. These three, Mary Agnes Thompson, Lucy Catherine Maguire and Annie Loretta Leahy, were the first of 1,836 that would graduate during the next 84 years from the hospital's nursing school.

At right, Miss Thompson's diploma

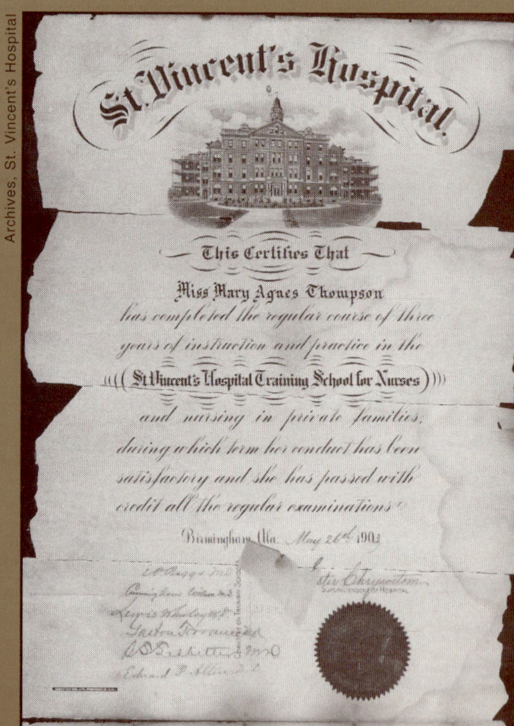

St. Vincent's Hospital

This Certifies That

Miss Mary Agnes Thompson

has completed the regular course of three years of instruction and practice in the

St. Vincent's Hospital Training School for Nurses

and nursing in private families, during which term her conduct has been satisfactory and she has passed with credit all the regular examinations.

Birmingham, Ala. May 26th 1903

Archives, St. Vincent's Hospital

For a week the citizens of Birmingham kept vigil for the wounded Father O'Reilly through daily updates on his condition. The death of *"the most popular citizen of Birmingham"* was front-page news, and his funeral was called *"the greatest funeral on record in the South."*

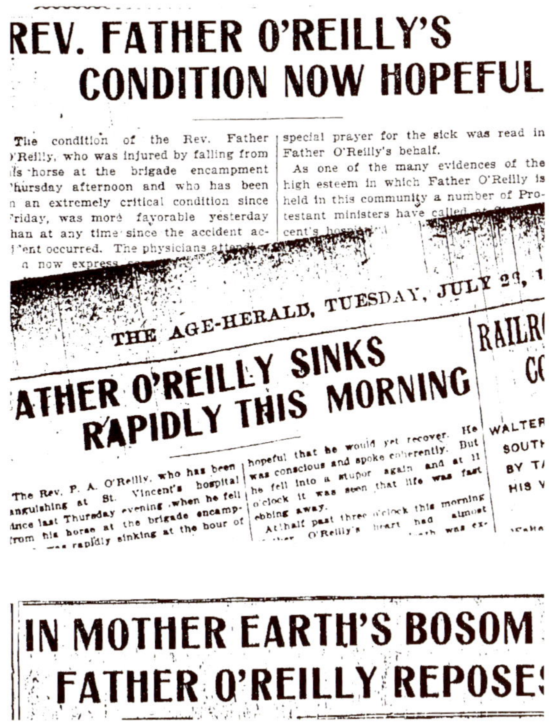
REV. FATHER O'REILLY'S CONDITION NOW HOPEFUL

THE AGE-HERALD, TUESDAY, JULY 2

ATHER O'REILLY SINKS RAPIDLY THIS MORNING

IN MOTHER EARTH'S BOSOM FATHER O'REILLY REPOSES

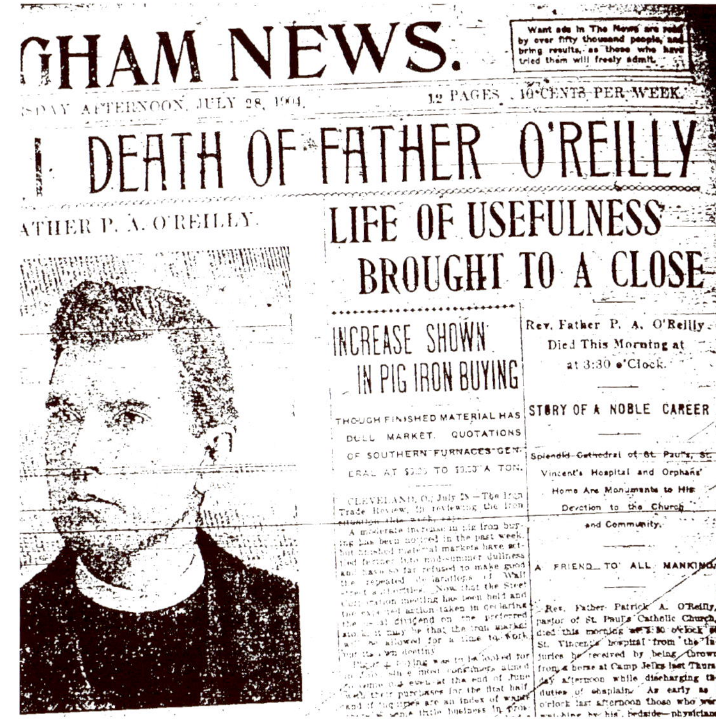
GHAM NEWS.

DEATH OF FATHER O'REILLY

LIFE OF USEFULNESS BROUGHT TO A CLOSE

INCREASE SHOWN IN PIG IRON BUYING

Rev. Father P. A. O'Reilly Died This Morning at 3:30 o'Clock.

STORY OF A NOBLE CAREER

A FRIEND TO ALL MANKIND

Sister Chrysostom was still extremely ill when this entry was made into the Diaries on July 14, 1903: "Our opponent, the Hillman Hospital opened today." Her condition did not permit Sister Chrysostom to leave her room until August 6, and a relapse put her back in bed within two weeks. Eventually Father Lennon forced her to take a leave of absence, and she went to Virginia to rest until November 5.

Donations were slow on Thanksgiving 1903, and although the Sister Servant of St. Vincent's had recovered, money was still tight.

St. Vincent's was in the headlines in May of 1904 as the famous newspaper writer and political aide Julien Walker died there. Walker, whose federal government positions included serving as consul to Scotland, had left the service of Congressman J. H. Bankhead and returned to Birmingham to begin a newspaper of his own. He had been admitted to St. Vincent's in June of 1903, suffering from "violent delusions," and he lay there very ill for two weeks, then recovered enough to be released. He was equally delusional upon his return the next Spring, and he died two days later. He was 43 years old.

Newspaper headlines only weeks later signaled more bad news, as in June 1904, St. Vincent's increasing financial problems became a full-scale crisis. The hospital and grounds had been put up for sale for non-payment of taxes.

On June 20 Father O'Reilly visited the mayor to make a plea for the hospital. The outcome was probably an appropriate illustration not only of the persuasive powers of the charismatic priest, but also of the mayor's understanding that St. Vincent's must not be lost. Father O'Reilly left the mayor's office with a $100 donation and a sizeable reduction of the taxes, which would keep the financial wolf from the door of the hospital for almost two years.

Tragedy Strikes Again

Saving St. Vincent's from taxes proved to be Father O'Reilly's last public service to his church or his city.

On July 19, 1904, Father O'Reilly was named chaplain of the Alabama National Guard and requested to take part in a review of the troops two days later.

Before leaving for the brigade's encampment in Owenton, Father O'Reilly, "full of life and vim and activity," dropped by the offices of the Birmingham *Ledger* "to give some information whose publication would tend to keep alive in the community the interests of a great charity."

If not in support of St. Vincent's, this last act of community service by Father O'Reilly was most likely on behalf of the East Lake Atheneum Orphans Home,

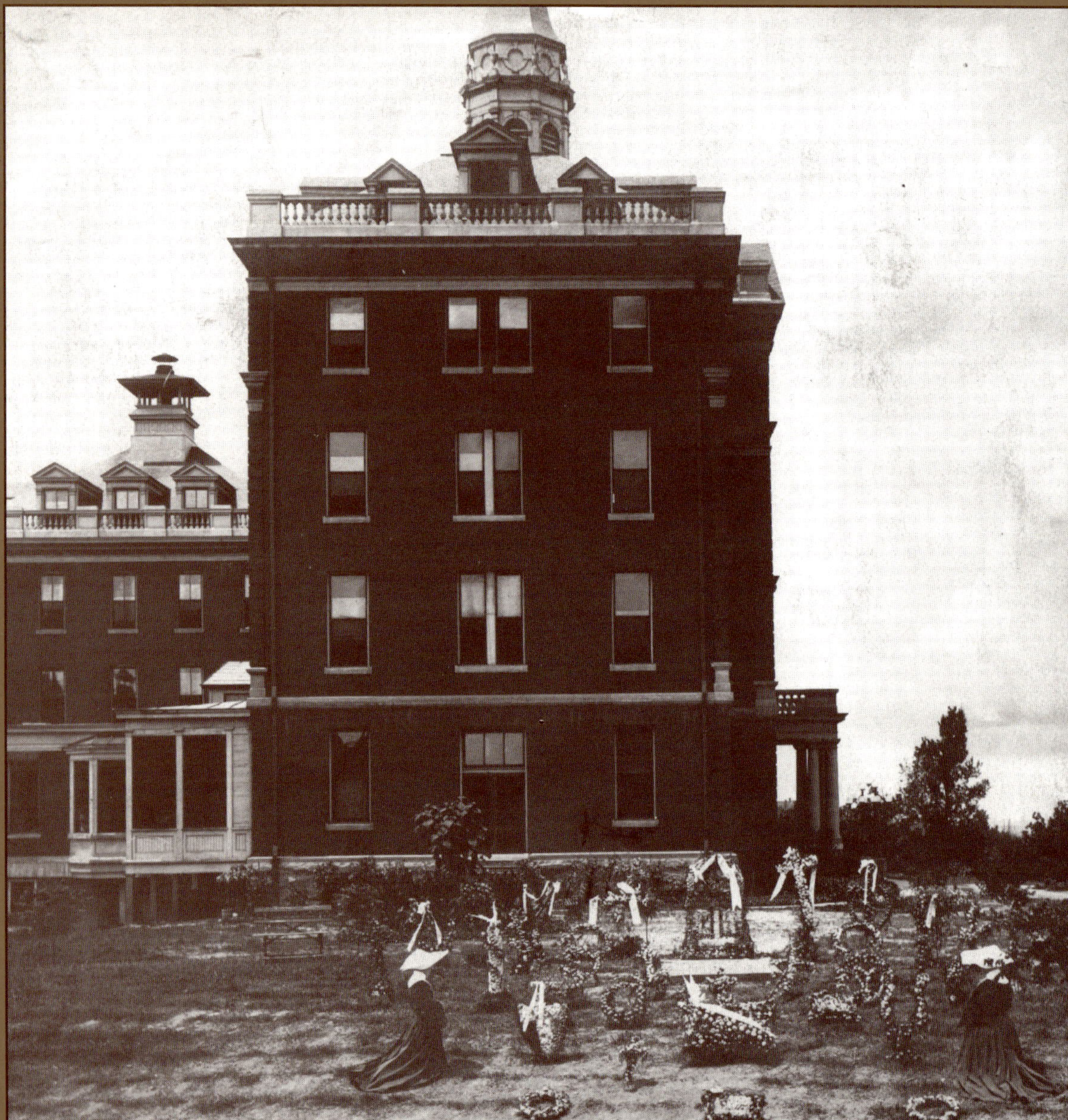
Archives, St. Vincent's Hospital

Two Sisters pray over Father O'Reilly's grave following his burial on the grounds of Mount St. Vincent's, east of the hospital.

which Father O'Reilly had helped found in 1903. The home, which cared for more than 100 orphans each month, was operated by the Daughters of Charity until 1948 under this name and as St. Thomas Home-on-the-Hill until 1971.

Two hours later, following the review of troops with the governor and his staff, Father O'Reilly was thrown by his horse. His skull was fractured, and immediately upon his arrival at St. Vincent's, it was apparent that his life was in danger.

Fearing a blood clot in Father O'Reilly's brain, Dr. Wilson operated the next morning, and although the surgery was inconclusive, there was hope that the priest would recover.

For a week, Father O'Reilly's condition was erratic, at times lucid and at times "at the point of death." The Sisters and staff, along with the citizens of Birmingham, waited with anxiety and hope. The phone at St. Vincent's rang "constantly," according to one newspaper account, and a flood of well-wishers came to the hospital in person, although few were allowed to see him. Telegrams arrived from all over the country. Every newspaper in Birmingham ran stories each day with details of Father O'Reilly's condition at press time.

At 3:30 a.m., Thursday, July 28, Father O'Reilly died. The news was the lead story in newspapers, and Father O'Reilly was called "the most popular citizen in Birmingham." As the priest lay in state at St. Paul's, "hundreds came by the hour" to pay their last respects, "fully 1,000" on Thursday night and thousands more on Friday. The mourning drapery was provided for free by the

Loveman, Joseph & Loeb department store, with assistance in the draping by members of the hook and ladder company of the fire department headquarters.

The funeral on Saturday morning was described as the largest in attendance the city had ever seen, and as the "greatest funeral on record in the South."

The procession, which included the governor, Mayor Drennen and the city aldermen, was so large that it was thought to require every public and private carriage and every horse in the city. Flags at City Hall and the Capitol in Montgomery flew at half mast during the funeral. Mayor Drennen closed City Hall the morning of the funeral.

In response to "popular sentiment" that Father O'Reilly be buried on the hospital grounds, the city attorney had quickly drafted a resolution, which the city aldermen immediately signed, allowing Father O'Reilly to be laid to rest on a knoll to the east of St. Vincent's. Mrs. Rufus Rhodes, one of the ladies who acted as hostess when the hospital opened in 1898, was the first to place flowers on Father O'Reilly's grave.

Almost immediately a popular movement began to build a monument for Father O'Reilly. At the first meeting to solicit subscriptions for the monument, which took place the Friday afternoon following the funeral, 131 people made donations totalling $925 to the monument fund.

The monument, a likeness of Father O'Reilly sculpted by Guiseppi Moretti, who created the Vulcan statue, would eventually cost $4,000. It was unveiled on the third anniversary of Father O'Reilly's death.

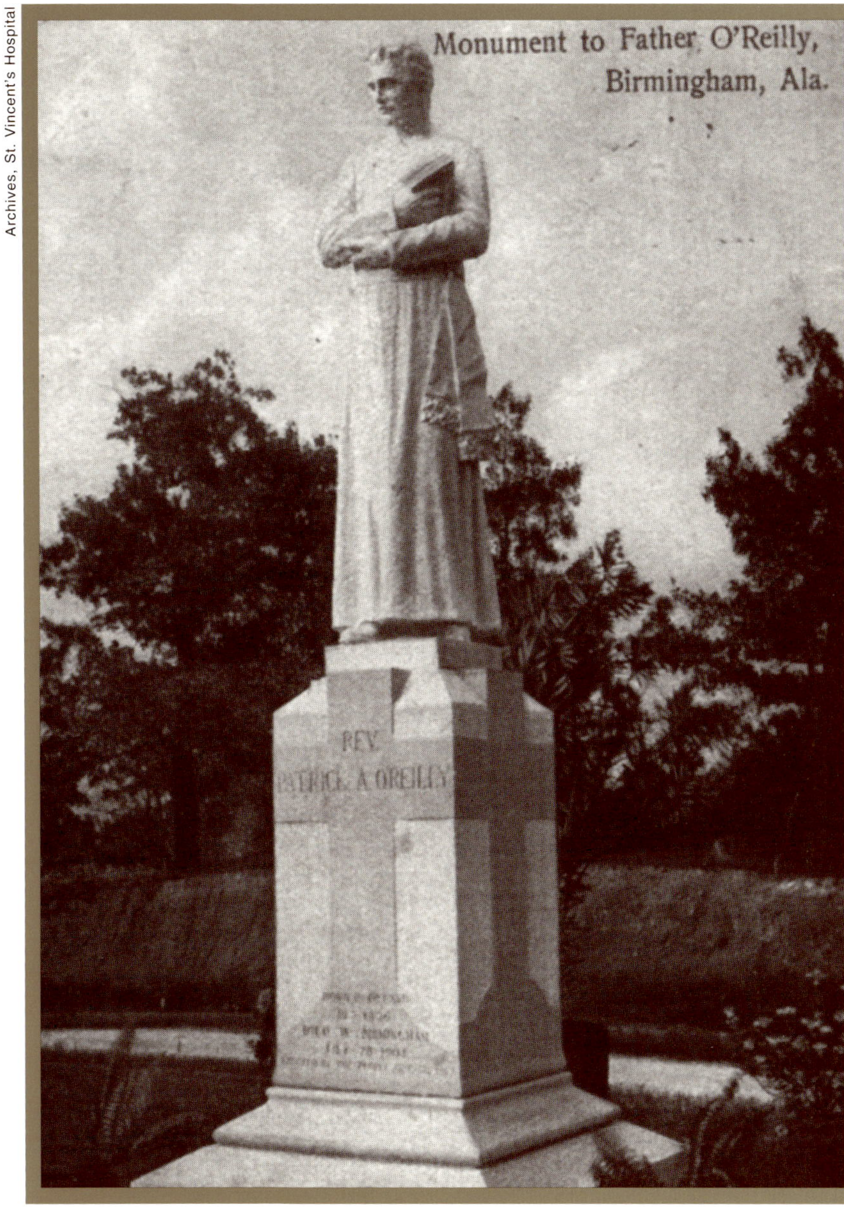

Monument to Father O'Reilly,
Birmingham, Ala.
REV.
PATRICK A. O'REILLY

Archives, St. Vincent's Hospital

The monument that Guiseppi Moretti, creator of the Vulcan statue, carved for Father O'Reilly's grave was of white Alabama marble from Talledega County, the same marble used for the Lincoln Memorial. Moretti felt it compared favorably with the Italian marble used by Michelangelo. On the third anniversary of Father O'Reilly's death, two little girls dressed in white pulled the cord for the unveiling of the statue, which stood on a pedestal six feet high. This souvenir postcard illustrating the monument was printed about 1910.

The Sisters' Life

Excerpts from the Diaries of St. Vincent's

September 7, 1903 "Picnic on the grounds. Mr. Sullivan played the fiddle."

June 12, 1907 A nurse is dismissed for "entertaining a dentist and other gentlemen while on night duty."

May 11, 1908 A heated discussion. "Snorers will have to leave the dormitory."

November 28, 1908 Dr. Carl Fox sent each Sister a rooster for Thanksgiving.

December 24, 1909 "Big Christmas party in the amphitheatre. Drs. Watkins and Young sick for three days afterward."

For Sale: Charity Hospital

The Diaries were somewhat correct in 1903 when they called Hillman Hospital "the competition." The Hillman was actually a revival of the charity hospital in Smithfield that burned in 1894. For three years beginning in 1896, the money that had funded that hospital was used to treat patients in a wing of a physician's clinic and beginning in 1899, in a rented house. The Hillman opened in its permanent facility in July of 1903.

While both hospitals were struggling to offer care to everyone who needed it, they were also competing for the same donations from individuals. At St. Vincent's, the number of charity patients was steadily increasing, and the city's monthly payment of $100 was soon not enough.

In October of 1904, Jefferson County began giving St. Vincent's $200 each month for the care of charity patients, but three months later the county cut this appropriation in half. In the summer of 1905 the city assessed St. Vincent's $2,000 for street improvements. Sister Chrysostom visited the new mayor, George Ward, but the two did not resolve the issue.

By 1906 it was obvious that funds were not available to care for the number of charity cases in the area. The city was spending only $2,400 annually at the time to support the charity hospitals, while Chattanooga appropriated $7,200 annually and Atlanta and Memphis each appropriated $45,000.

It was probably no surprise that in February of that year, both St. Vincent's and Hillman went on the auction block for non-payment of taxes. The newspaper coverage of the incident was considerable, and the city council, at Mayor Ward's urging, voted to remit the assessments against the hospitals. The mayor wrote the management at each institution a business-like letter officially informing them of the vote. It wasn't until March 22 that the Diaries note: "Mayor Ward sent the deed over. The assessments due have been erased from the books."

A Thriving City, A Thriving Hospital

During the first decade of the century, Birmingham grew considerably, about 20 percent. The consolidation of the suburbs into "Greater Birmingham" that had been debated for more than 10 years would finally take place in 1910, doubling the population to more than 120,000. Four downtown skyscrapers created a formidable skyline.

Archives, St. Vincent's Hospital

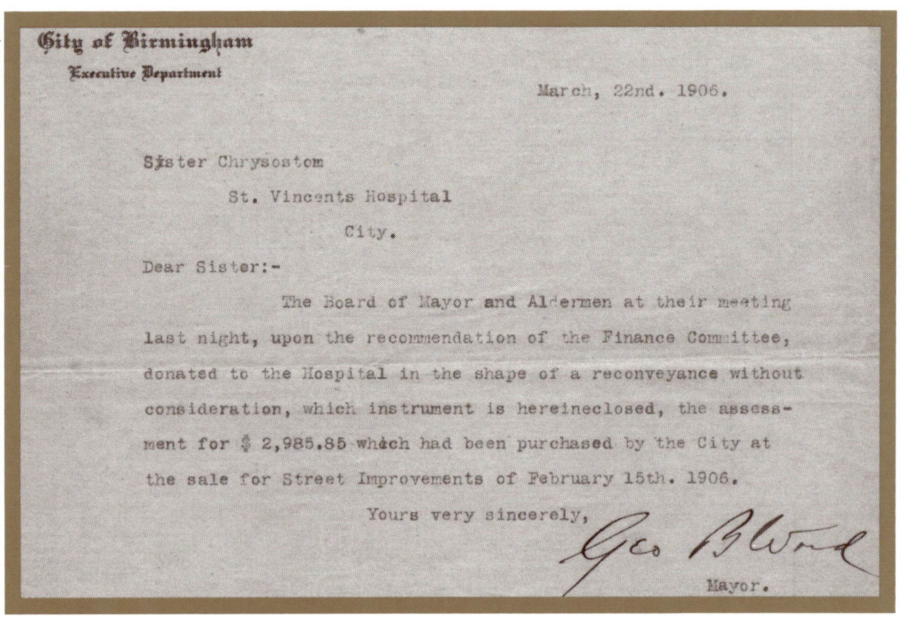

City of Birmingham
Executive Department

March, 22nd. 1906.

Sister Chrysostom
St. Vincents Hospital
City.

Dear Sister:-

The Board of Mayor and Aldermen at their meeting last night, upon the recommendation of the Finance Committee, donated to the Hospital in the shape of a reconveyance without consideration, which instrument is hereinclosed, the assessment for $ 2,985.85 which had been purchased by the City at the sale for Street Improvements of February 15th. 1906.

Yours very sincerely,
Geo B Ward
Mayor.

In 1906, Mayor George Ward saved St. Vincent's from the auction block.

Archives, St. Vincent's Hospital

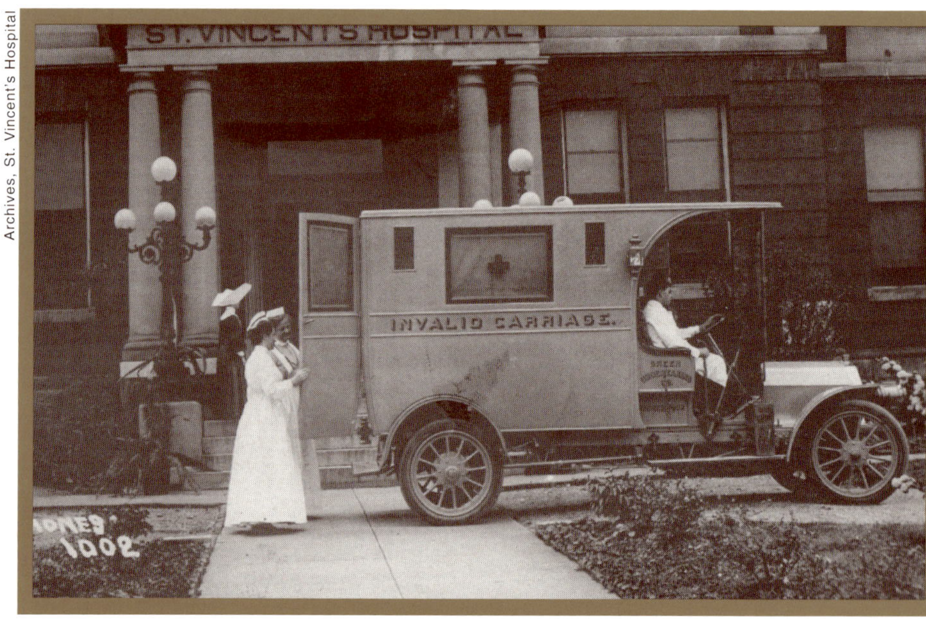

Nurses with ambulance, 1909

On a hill overlooking this skyline from the south, St. Vincent's was growing as well.

Hillman had become the county hospital in 1907, to be operated by Jefferson County as a public charity. (An intriguing Diaries entry on May 20, 1907, states that "the majority" of the doctors wanted the Daughters of Charity to assume management of Hillman.)

St. Vincent's financial situation, however, was improving. Donations continued to be generous and broad-based, including many from a number of companies and private organizations. But the hospital continued to be crowded, to the degree that one night in June of 1907 saw some patients sleeping on the porch.

It was no coincidence, perhaps, that the next week the Diaries record the first discussion of a new patient wing. By the unveiling ceremony for the monument to Father O'Reilly on July 28, the first money had already been donated.

The hospital's annual report on November 1, 1907, included a plea for help in building a new wing that could accommodate an additional 100 patients. "When the fact is considered that St. Vincent's is conducted on...the lowest possible running expenses...Can the charitable people of Birmingham afford to let that wing go unbuilt?" (That report tallied 1,254 patients for the prior year, 572 being charity patients.)

The plan for a new wing began to take shape in 1908, a wing that would house 150 patients and cost about $50,000 to build and furnish. The Daughters of Charity committed to contributing half of that figure, and local contributions were expected to cover the other half. Donations trickled in throughout the year, possibly the most crowded year the hospital had seen.

There was an increase in patients of more than 40 percent the year ending October 31, 1908, 1799 total. And even though Hillman was now the county's charity hospital, the 419 charity patients that came to St. Vincent's that year attested to the growing need of the fast-growing community.

The Ladies of Charity auxiliary had become an effective fundraising organization, donating large sums every few months to the hospital. But funds to build the new wing were only trickling in. In October the Ladies of Charity, in addition to their other work, began to raise money specifically for the wing, first with a series of "card parties" held in the homes of a number of prominent ladies, followed by plans for a Bazaar.

The Bazaar took place from November 18 through November 28 in "the spacious room on 20th Street across from the Woodward Building."

St. Vincent's First Baby

On November 15, 1909, John S. Donovan became the first child born at St. Vincent's Hospital. Donovan later became president of Red Diamond Coffee.

Archives, St. Vincent's Hospital

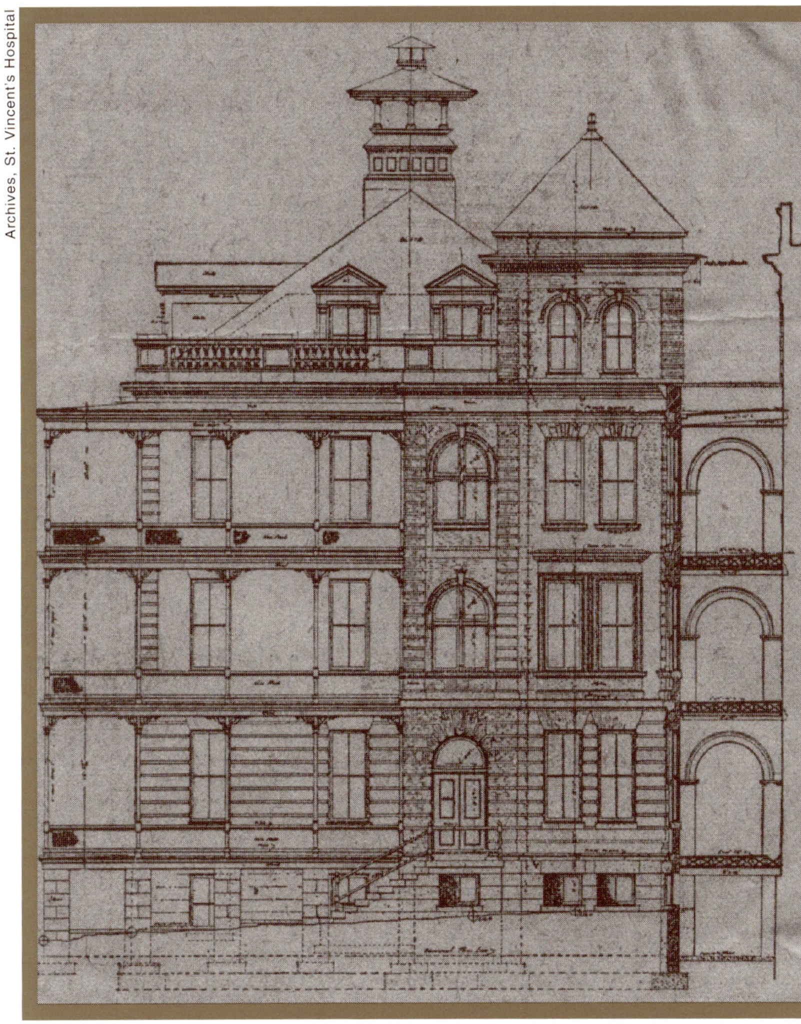

Architect Harry F. Wheelock's original drawing of the East Wing, which opened in 1911

The numerous booths at the Bazaar contained pillows, dolls, aprons and "fancy work." Lunch and dinner were sold every day of the Bazaar.

Contests were held in a number of categories, the winner being the one who collected the most money, including everything from "most popular nurse," to "most popular railroad superintendent" to "most popular undertaker." The "baby contest" included 100 contestants in four categories.

The Bazaar ended with a large auction of glassware, silverware, furniture and toys, followed by the contest for "most popular physician's daughter."

A resounding success, the Bazaar netted more than $2,600.

But the drive for funds for the new wing lost momentum again after the Bazaar. Sister Chrysostom was undaunted, however, and had plans drawn up by famed local architect Harry F. Wheelock, who had designed the DeBardeleben mansion where the Sisters had first opened St. Vincent's. Finally, in May of 1909, 50 Birmingham businessmen met on a Sunday afternoon to spearhead a fundraising drive that would make the wing a reality. The Sisters had about $7,000 in cash on hand for the wing, with about $4,000 more pledged to it. At the meeting, with Dr. Wilson presiding, the group named a committee to collect a list of 100 men who would each pledge to raise $150. After the meeting, the Sisters served ginger ale.

When ground was broken in June of 1910, the committee had already raised about $10,000. Newspaper stories quoted Sister Chrysostom as inviting all of Birmingham to the event.

The central figure at the ceremony was toddler Archibald Irving Grubb, representing his father, Judge W. I. Grubb, who was away. The junior Grubb, described by a newspaper as being 18 months old (although the Diaries describe him as

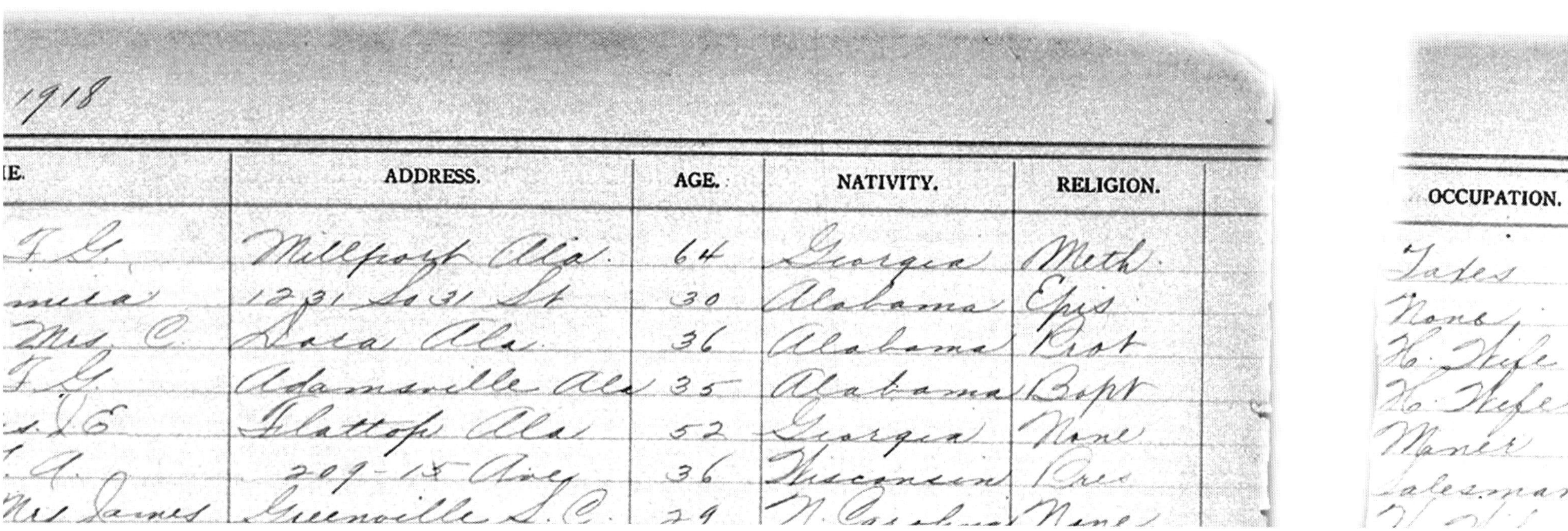

1918

[illegible]E.	ADDRESS.	AGE.	NATIVITY.	RELIGION.	OCCUPATION.
F. G.	Millport Ala.	64	Georgia	Meth.	Tates
[illegible]mela	1231 So 31 St	30	Alabama	Epis	None
Mrs. C.	Dola Ala	36	Alabama	Prot	H. Wife
F. G.	Adamsville Ala	35	Alabama	Bapt	H. Wife
[illegible]s. J. E.	Flattop Ala	52	Georgia	None	Manes
[illegible] A.	209-15 Ave	36	Wisconsin	Pres	Salesman
Mrs James	Greenville S. C.	29	N. Carolina	None	[illegible]

Archives, St. Vincent's Hospital

Some representative cases from the 1917-18 patient register:

• *A 30-year-old housewife from Eutaw was admitted on June 2, 1918, for a "confinement" of 15 days. The fee was $4.*

• *A 26-year-old waiter from Fifth Avenue North, of no religious affiliation, was admitted on July 10, 1918, with hemorrhoids. He was released two days later, and his bill was $1.50.*

"aged one year and two weeks"), posed for photos with a tiny hand on a decorated spade almost twice his height.

In May of 1911, the East Wing opened, with Judge Grubb able to take part without benefit of proxy. On September 5, "with a little nest egg of $5," Sister Chrysostom opened her "outdoor clinic" in the first floor of the new wing. The first patient, the Diaries noted, was a "native of the Emerald Isle," Ireland, homeland of the parents of many of the Sisters at St. Vincent's.

The new out-patient department, which actually needed an additional donation of $15 and some money from the hospital to open, offered the poor an extensive list of treatments for illnesses that didn't require a hospital stay: skin diseases, surgery, "genito-urinary," gynecological, "orthopoedic," and "treatment of the eye, ear, nose and throat." The clinic also offered X-rays.

In a newspaper feature written a month after the clinic opened, Sister Chrysostom said the most important thing the clinic needed was a streetcar line that would increase access to the clinic by the poor.

A Picture of the City

The new wing quickly filled with patients, and as the number of patients increased, so did the staff at St. Vincent's. The first medical staff of the hospital had numbered only five. By 1916 St. Vincent's had 29 physicians and three interns, with 50 student nurses and three graduate nurses working alongside the 18 Sisters.

The reputation of St. Vincent's and other local hospitals made Birmingham a regional medical center at least as far back as 1918. That year St. Vincent's admitted

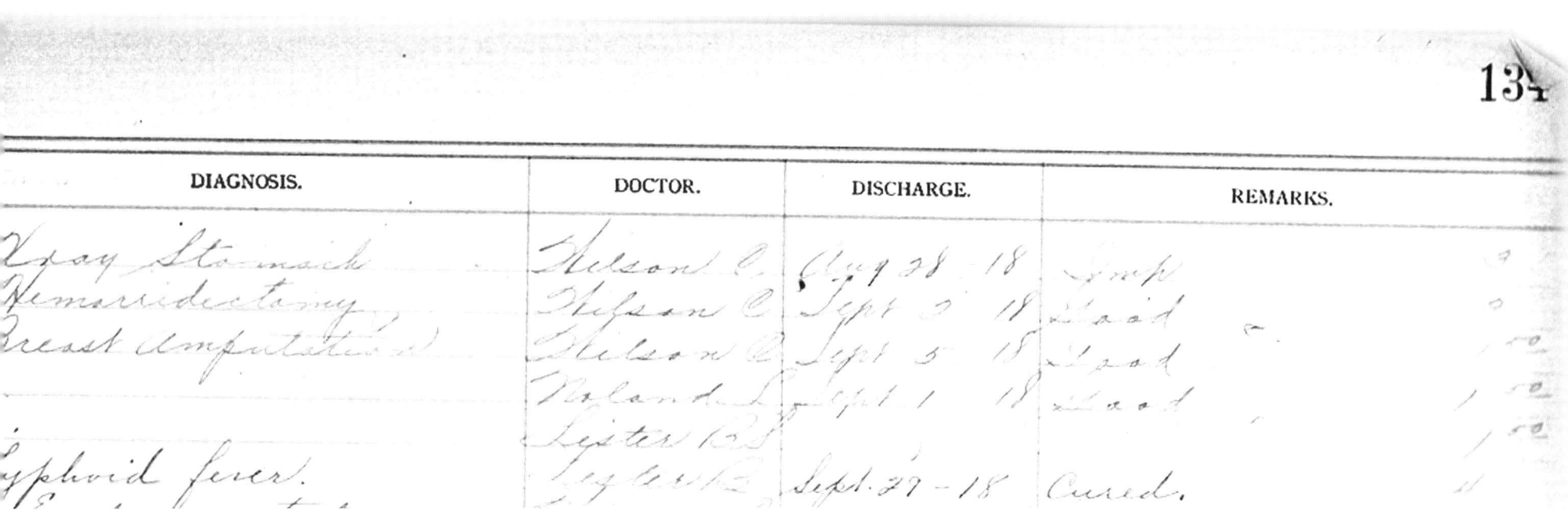
134

DIAGNOSIS.	DOCTOR.	DISCHARGE.	REMARKS.
X-ray Stomach	Wilson C.	Aug 28 18	Imp
Hemorrhoidectomy	Wilson C	Sept 5 18	Good
Breast Amputation	Wilson C	Sept 5 18	Good
	Noland L	Sept 1 18	Good
	Lester B.S.		
Typhoid fever.	[illegible]	Sept. 29 - 18	Cured.

• An employee of L & N Railroad (a "maulder"), 46 years old, was admitted August 5 with an injured eye. The eye was removed and he was released the next day!

• A Highland Park man was admitted May 26, 1918, with acute appendicitis. The 56-year-old Ohio native was treated by Dr. Cunningham Wilson. His condition was remarked "good," and he was released June 3. The fee was $6.

• In a possible case of domestic abuse, a "Mrs. Beaver" with an unknown address, unknown age, unknown birthplace, and identified only as a housewife, was treated for a dislocated right hip by Dr. W. B. Wilder on May 27, 1918. She was released "improved" on June 24. The fee was $1.50.

patients from towns within a few hours' travel, such as Sylacauga and Tuscaloosa, and from places of significant distance in that day: Florence, Fayette, Eutaw, Scottsboro, Boaz, Wetumpka and Troy.

The patient registers of the day listed a great deal of information about the hospital's patients, including address, age, "nativity," religion, occupation and diagnosis. Because St. Vincent's treated people of every race and economic level, this information provides an interesting snapshot of Birmingham at the time, as well as the relative sophistication of health care.

In the days of World War I, St. Vincent's admitted between 10 and 15 patients on a typical day. There was a surprisingly small number of deaths, most of them elderly, and these were recorded by the Sisters with the word "Death" in red ink.

A look at the patients admitted during the first seven days of June 1918:

Of the 70 patients admitted, only two died. The hospital stays ranged from one day (a tonsillectomy) to 56 days (a 43-year-old nurse from Avondale with a fractured skull and right clavicle).

These patients were born in a surprisingly varied number of places. Only two-thirds were born in Alabama, 11 were born in another Southern state and five more in other states.

Fully 10 percent of this patient sample was not native to the U.S., with the countries represented being Russia, Germany, Syria, England and Greece.

The number of religious backgrounds corresponded with this mix of varied birthplaces. Seventeen of the patients were Baptist, 13 were Methodist, eight were Catholic, seven were Presbyterian, six were Episcopal, three were Jewish and one was noted as "Greek," most likely Greek Orthodox. Two others were listed only as "Protestant," the religion of six of the patients was not known, and seven people – a surprising 10 percent – were noted to have no religion.

The largest number of patients were admitted for appendicitis and tonsillitis. Other common diagnoses and treatments of the day included pellagra, nephritis and typhoid, although many came to St. Vincent's for treatment of their hemorrhoids. A large number were admitted following falls and automobile accidents.

Other diagnoses reveal the dangerous life that existed for many, either in occupation or lifestyle. Several patients were admitted with "steele" in an eye, and many patients suffered from "multiple cuts" or "laceration of cervix."

The most expensive procedure was the delivery of a child, which cost $6. An appendectomy cost $5, a tonsillectomy $2.50. A two-week hospital stay was $4.

The patient register also reveals the extent of corporate insurance available to workers in that day. Patients employed by TCI, Sloss Furnaces, Alabama Power and the Birmingham Slag Co. (now a part of Vulcan Materials), among others, paid $1.50 regardless of diagnosis or treatment. Employees of A.R. Co. paid $2.

Archives, St. Vincent's Hospital

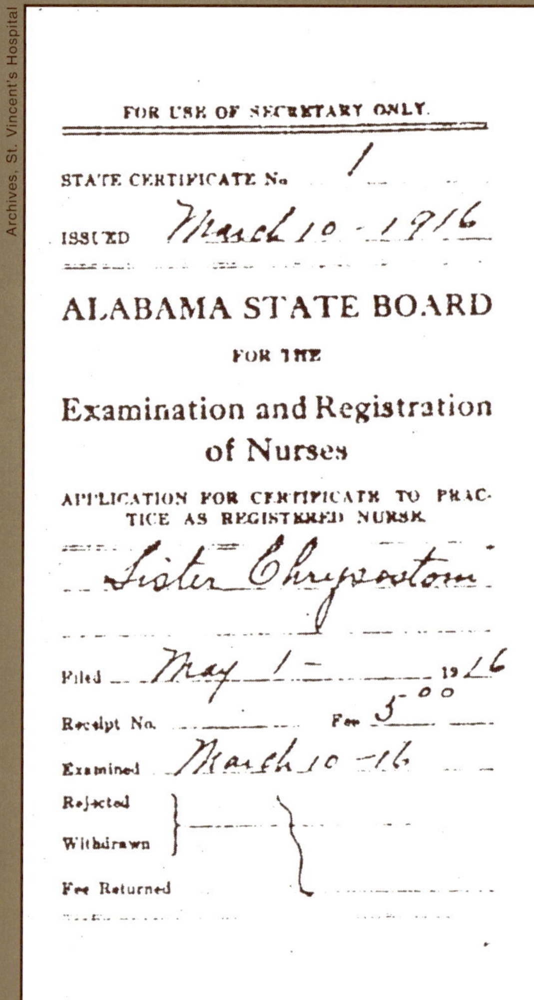

FOR USE OF SECRETARY ONLY.

STATE CERTIFICATE No. 1

ISSUED March 10 - 1916

ALABAMA STATE BOARD

FOR THE

Examination and Registration of Nurses

APPLICATION FOR CERTIFICATE TO PRACTICE AS REGISTERED NURSE

Sister Chrysostom

Filed May 1 – 1916

Receipt No. Fee 5.00

Examined March 10 – 16

Rejected

Withdrawn

Fee Returned

In 1916 Sister Chrysostom became the first registered nurse in the State of Alabama.

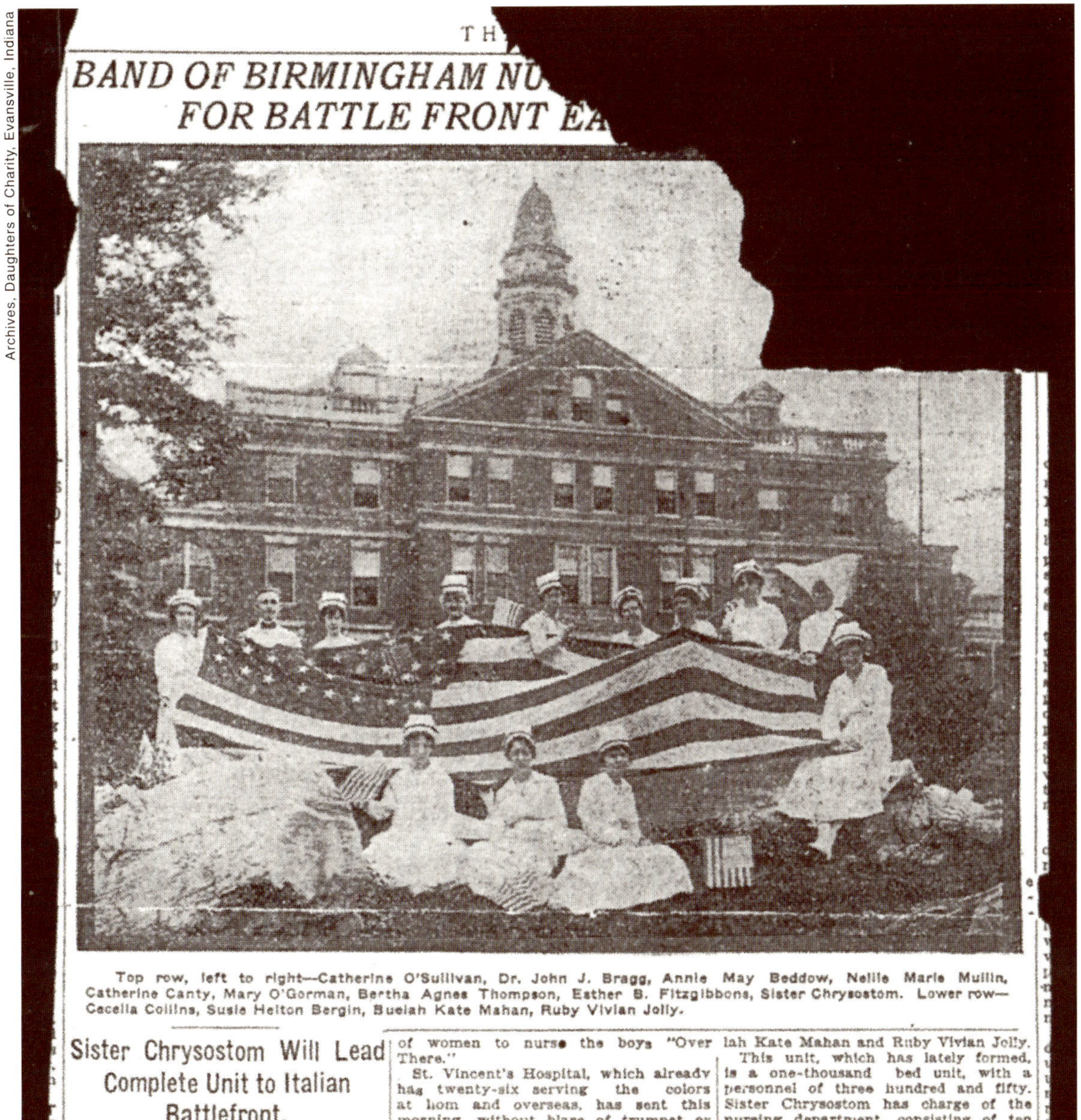

TH

BAND OF BIRMINGHAM NU
FOR BATTLE FRONT EA

Top row, left to right—Catherine O'Sullivan, Dr. John J. Bragg, Annie May Beddow, Nellie Marie Mullin, Catherine Canty, Mary O'Gorman, Bertha Agnes Thompson, Esther B. Fitzgibbons, Sister Chrysostom. Lower row—Cecelia Collins, Susie Helton Bergin, Buelah Kate Mahan, Ruby Vivian Jolly.

Sister Chrysostom Will Lead Complete Unit to Italian Battlefront.

of women to nurse the boys "Over There."

St. Vincent's Hospital, which already has twenty-six serving the colors at hom and overseas, has sent this morning, without blare of trumpet or

lah Kate Mahan and Ruby Vivian Jolly.

This unit, which has lately formed, is a one-thousand bed unit, with a personnel of three hundred and fifty. Sister Chrysostom has charge of the nursing department, consisting of ten

Archives, Daughters of Charity, Evansville, Indiana

Sister Chrysostom left St. Vincent's in 1917 to lead the only band of Sisters from the U.S. to serve in Europe during World War I. Pictured from left to right are the St. Vincent's nursing graduates who served with Sister Chrysostom:
(top row) Catherine O'Sullivan, Dr. John J. Bragg, Annie May Beddow, Nellie Marie Mullin, Catherine Canty, Mary O'Gorman, Bertha Agnes Thompson, Esther B. Fitzgibbons and Sister Chrysostom; (bottom row) Cecelia Collins, Susie Helton Bergin, Beulah Kate Mahan and Ruby Vivian Jolly.

Au Revoir, Sister Chrysostom

By the time the War Department accepted the Provincial Superior's offer of the services of the Daughters of Charity, St. Vincent's already had 26 nursing graduates serving in World War I. When Sister Chrysostom was chosen to head the nursing department – 10 Sisters and 90 graduate nurses – of a 1,000-bed base hospital being formed in Italy, she was characteristically eager to be of use.

"War makes its demands upon the women as well as the manpower of a nation," she said, "and all we can do, no matter what the sacrifice, should serve the interest of America's part in the war."

Birmingham was more hesitant to relinquish Sister Chrysostom – she who had guided the hospital through its hardest times, and who in 1916 had become Alabama's first registered nurse. A prominent local physician, Dr. Lewis C. Morris, even went so far as to write Bishop Allen to ask that Sister Chrysostom be ordered to stay at St. Vincent's.

After a period of training, Sister Chrysostom and 11 more graduate nurses from St. Vincent's sailed from Baltimore to Italy. She would serve the war effort under difficult circumstances, contract – and recover from – the Spanish influenza that killed millions, and be awarded the War Ribbon and the Golden Lion of Venice for her work.

She would eventually return to Alabama to serve as administrator of Providence Hospital in Mobile – in time being named as a member of the Alabama Woman's Hall of Fame – although she would never return to the service of St. Vincent's and the people of Birmingham.

Chapter Three

Soothing a Troubled City

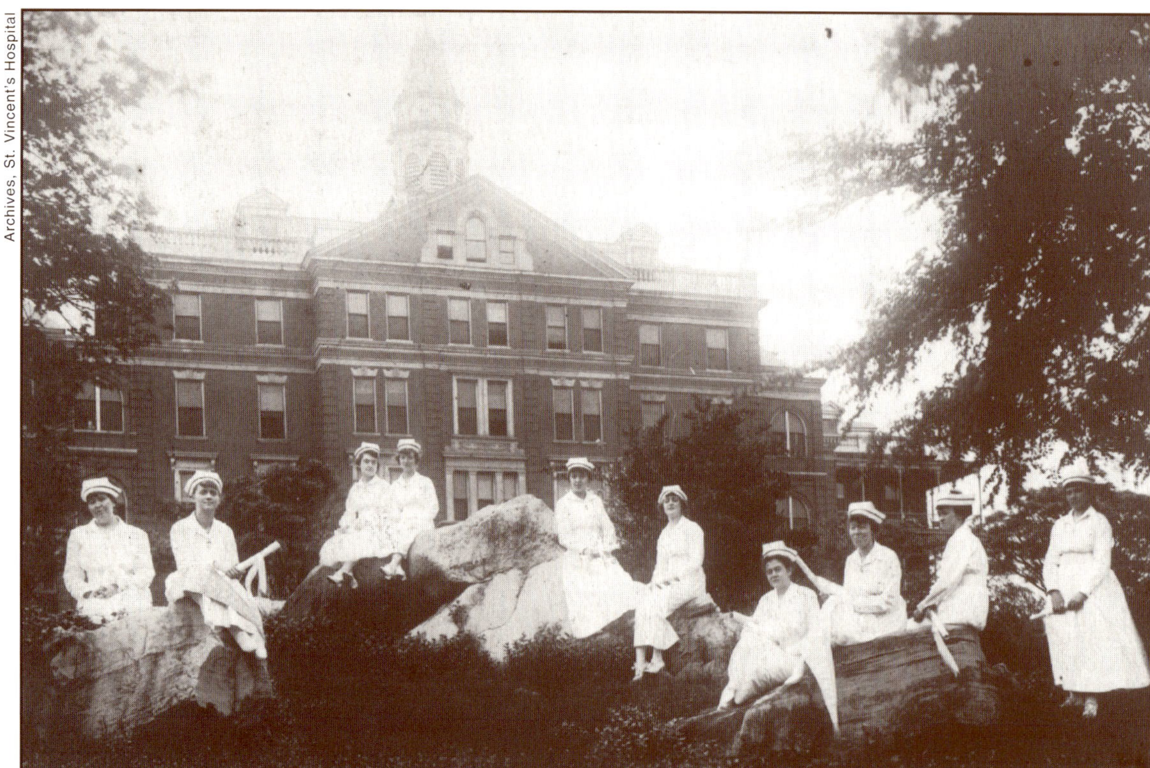
Archives, St. Vincent's Hospital

St. Vincent's Nursing School Graduating Class of 1920

As the 1920s began, greater Birmingham had swelled to a diverse population of more than 300,000.

Civic boosters bragged with some certainty that this would be the decade that Birmingham pushed Atlanta and New Orleans aside to the become the South's largest city.

But it was a decade of mixed fortunes. The upper class of the city began a migration onto and over Red Mountain, building massive Tudor-style estates in Redmont and Mountain Brook. The middle class also prospered, with many finding their own suburban escape in Edgewood, a middle-class community advertised as being "free of smoke and dust."

The working class and the poor had a rougher time. Birmingham didn't enjoy as great an economic boom as the rest of the country at the time. The migration of rural residents to urban centers, which began after World War I, swelled the numbers of unskilled laborers, and wage levels that were already depressed continued to languish. Demands for public services far outpaced the revenue needed to provide them.

A crowded Birmingham in the 1920s was suffering the same problems of every large city with a heterogenous population: tension between ethnic, religious and political extremists. The Ku Klux Klan gained strength, eventually gaining a strong wedge in city politics. Labor unrest and communist activism were common.

The widespread tolerance the city had enjoyed since its founding took a beating in the 1920s. For some time a vocal minority in Birmingham had expressed anti-Catholic sentiments that continued to escalate. A convent and Catholic school in Pratt City were burned, and St. Paul's was under armed guard at night on at least one occasion. This tension climaxed in 1921 with the murder of Father James E. Coyle, the rector at St. Paul's who had succeeded Father O'Reilly. After officiating at the wedding of a recent convert to a man of Puerto Rican descent, Father Coyle was shot by the girl's father, a lay Protestant minister, who was later found not guilty (by reason of temporary insanity) by an all-Protestant jury.

It was in this environment that St. Vincent's continued to minister without fail to the sick and injured of every race, creed and class. It was to these painful wounds that St. Vincent's tended, continuing to stand as an institution of love and charity that would help heal a city scarred by hate and prejudice.

And it was during the 1920s that the nursing school at St. Vincent's came into its prime as one of the hospital's strongest outreaches.

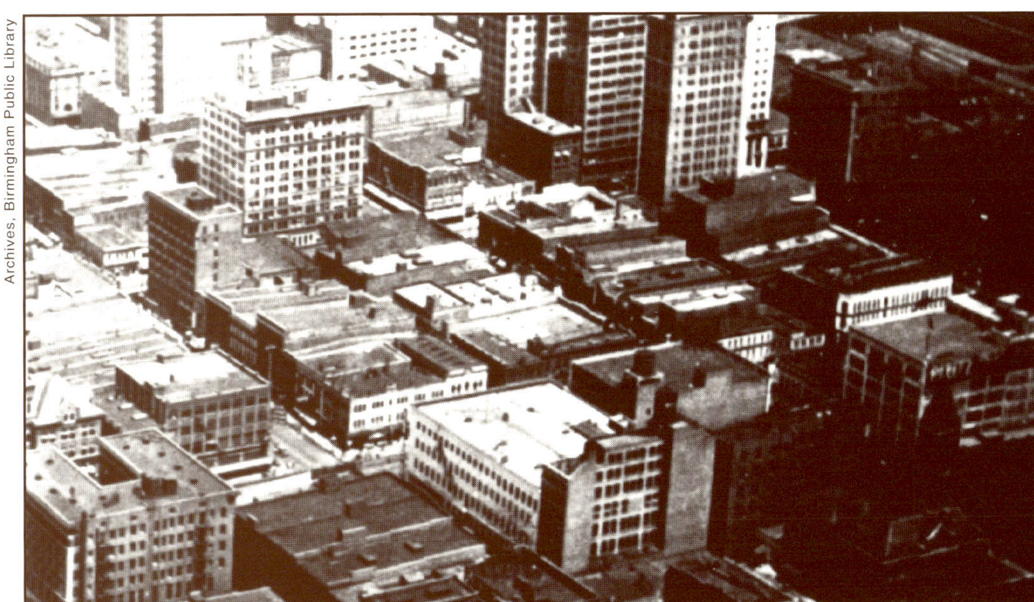

Archives, Birmingham Public Library

This 1920 aerial photograph illustrates the scope of the city's development more than 75 years ago.

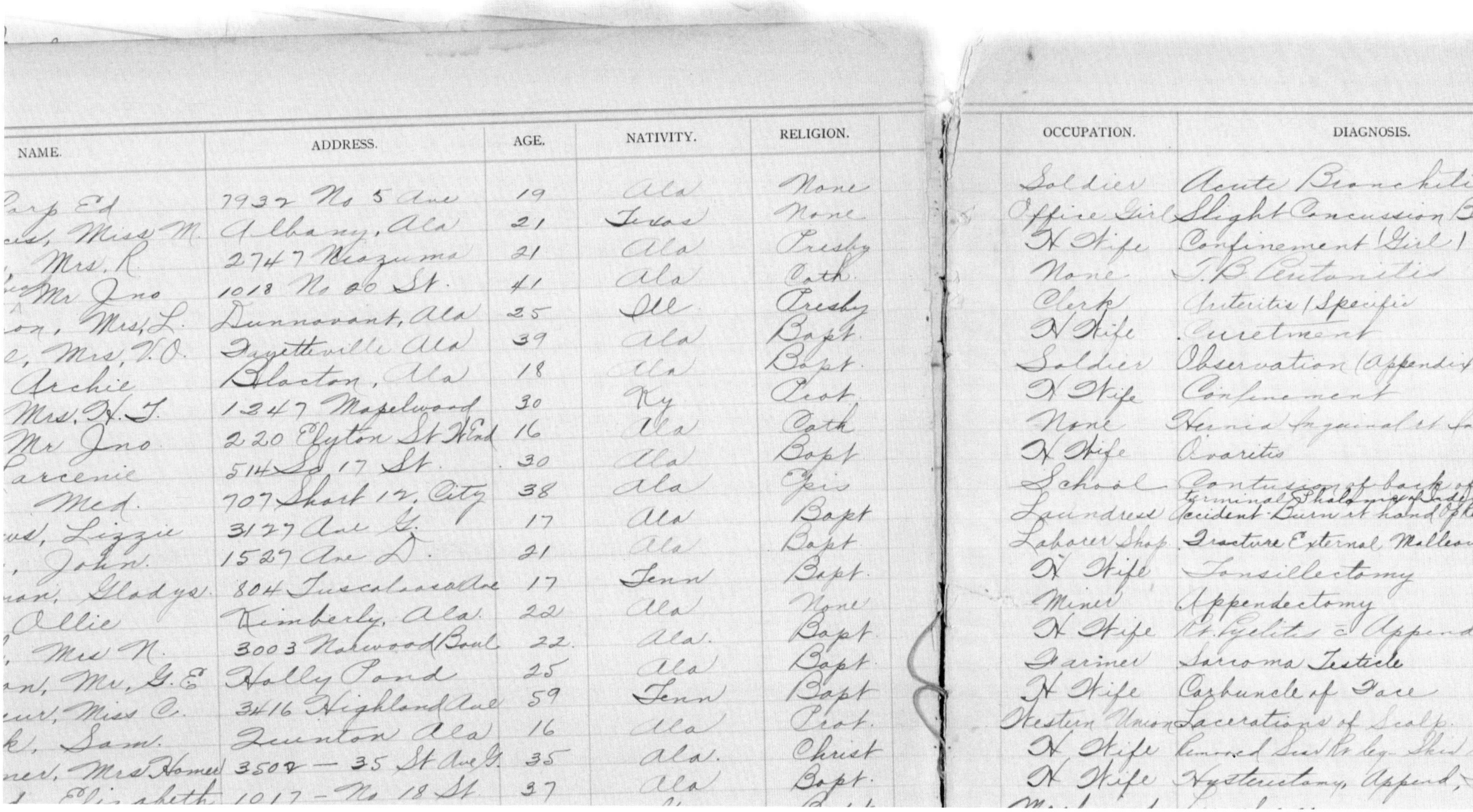

Archives, St. Vincent's Hospital

The diversity of the Birmingham population was more evident in the 1920s than ever before, as were the patients being treated at St. Vincent's. Some selected cases from this period:

- *A 24-year-old painter of North First Avenue, an Irish immigrant, was admitted January 6, 1923, with a complex skull fracture. He died the same day.*

- *A girl, age 6, was admitted December 24, 1921, with "empyema." She was not released to return to her Cliff Road home until January 30, 1922.*

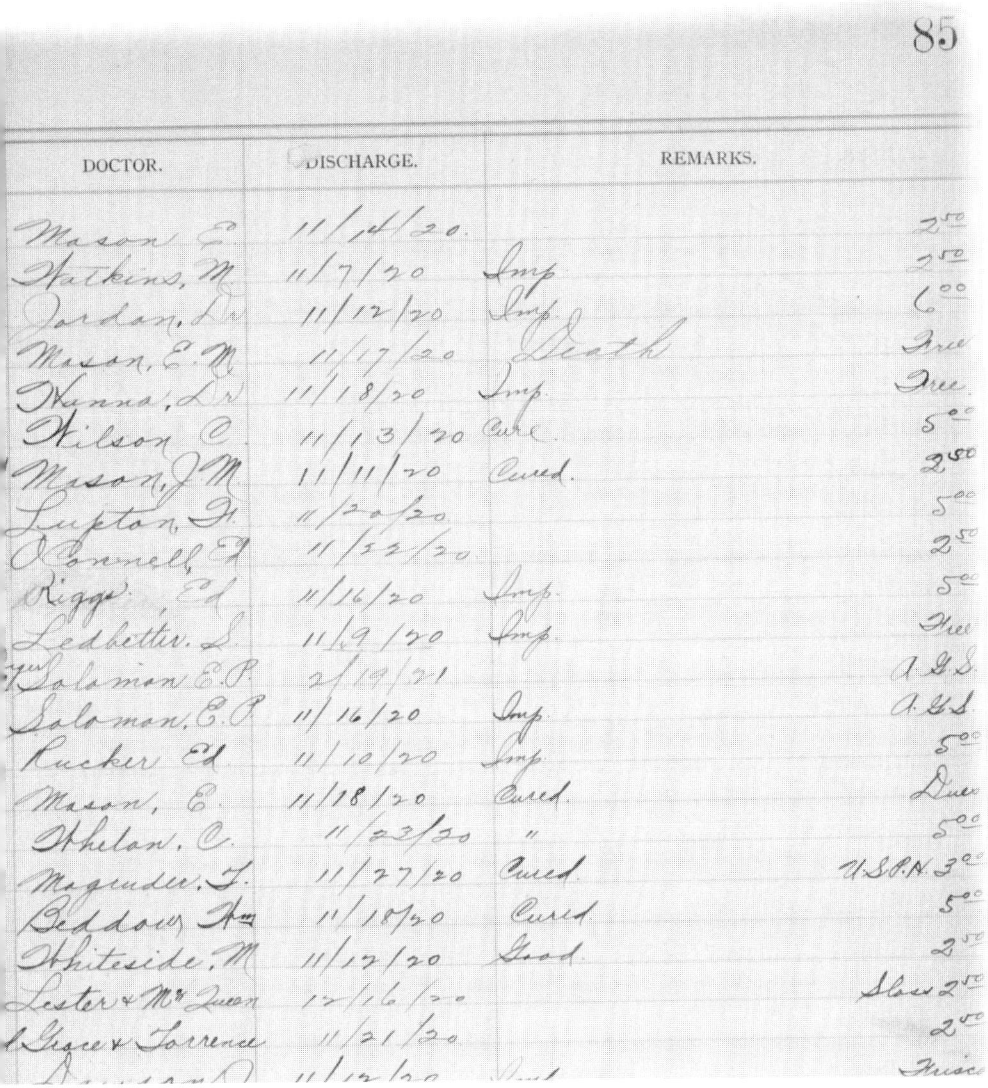

85

DOCTOR.	DISCHARGE.	REMARKS.	
Mason E.	11/4/20.		2^{50}
Watkins, M	11/7/20	Imp	2^{50}
Jordan, Dr	11/12/20	Imp.	6^{00}
Mason, E.M	11/17/20	Death	Free
Henna, Dr	11/18/20	Imp.	Free
Wilson C	11/13/20	Cure	5^{00}
Mason, J.M.	11/11/20	Cured.	2^{50}
Lupton, F.	11/20/20.		5^{00}
O'Connell Ed	11/22/20		2^{50}
Riggs Ed	11/16/20	Imp.	5^{00}
Ledbetter. L	11/19/20	Imp.	Free
Soloman E.P	2/19/21		A.G.S.
Soloman, E.P	11/16/20	Imp.	A.G.S.
Rucker Ed	11/10/20	Imp.	5^{00}
Mason, E.	11/18/20	Cured.	Dues
Whelan, C.	11/22/20	"	5^{00}
Magruder, F.	11/27/20	Cured	U.S.P.H. 3^{00}
Beddow, Wm	11/18/20	Cured.	5^{00}
Whiteside, M	11/17/20	Good.	2^{50}
Lester & McQueen	12/16/20		Slow 2^{50}
Grace & Torrence	11/21/20		2^{50}

• *A "coal operator" who lived on Highland Avenue, 67, was admitted May 17, 1922, with a tumor on his lower back. He was released "improved" the same day.*

Birmingham, the Smelting Pot

The migration of unskilled workers from all over the South – indeed, from all over the world – seeking jobs in the mines and furnaces reached its peak during the years of the "Jazz Age." As the demand for work soon surpassed the supply, Birmingham boiled over with people of all colors and backgrounds, and now with class distinctions the likes of which the city hadn't before seen.

As a hospital dedicated to the poor, St. Vincent's was frequently crowded with new arrivals, both the employed and the unemployed, although the middle class, many for whom poverty was not a completely distant memory, were equally well represented.

Perhaps surprising to some, the upper crust, the men who owned the industries that made the city glow at all hours of night and day, came to St. Vincent's as well. The neighborhood around the hospital had changed from sparsely populated hills into an upscale enclave of homes of the city's most prominent inhabitants. Many had emotional ties to the hospital, dating from the days of St. Vincent's founding, and many more found it a convenient and quality choice. Judge W. I. Grubb, long affiliated with the hospital, was treated for appendicitis at St. Vincent's, only blocks away from his impressive Highland Avenue home.

A sample from patient registers of the time underscores the hospital's dedication to service of all in need, as well as the increasing variety of people who comprised Birmingham's citizenry.

Of the first 100 people admitted to St. Vincent's in 1923, only 45 were born in Alabama, and 14 outside the South. Almost as many patients who were native to Alabama, 41 people, had moved to Birmingham from other Southern states.

The register also gives strong testimony to the quality of the care at St. Vincent's. Of these 100 patients, only one died.

Also, the fee structure at St. Vincent's had become more complex, although not a great deal more expensive. "Full-term labor" now cost $8. One serious case of chronic appendicitis cost $10, the most expensive treatment in surviving records of the early 1920s.

The administrative tenure of Sister Magdalen Welch, who had replaced Sister Chrysostom, lasted only until 1920, when she was replaced by Sister Angela O'Brien. Sister Angela supervised the hospital's efforts to accommodate the growing pool of patients and the rapid changes in the field of medicine.

Archives, St. Vincent's Hospital

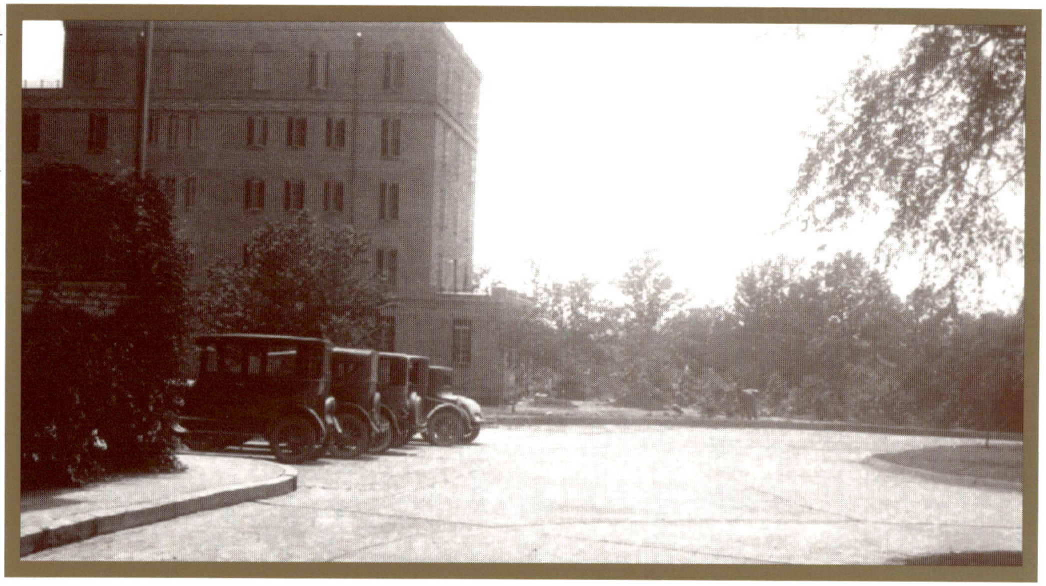

The new driveway, 1925

In 1923 St. Vincent's required an extensive renovation, in part to accommodate the new "X-ray" and Pathology Departments. At the time, certain lab tests required the red blood cells of a sheep, and the hospital kept sheep on the premises for this purpose. (The sheep also played at least a small role in keeping the grass on the grounds under control.)

Dr. Thomas V. Magruder Jr., grandson of Chief of Surgery Dr. Cunningham Wilson and son of St. Vincent's physician Dr. Thomas V. Magruder Sr., remembers the ram as a territorial beast. "The ram did not like us walking on the grass," the younger Dr. Magruder recalled. Once, as a young boy, Dr. Magruder and his nurse waited outside the hospital for his father, when the ram ran over and knocked them down. Fortunately, "no damage was incurred by me, the nurse – or the ram," he said.

Also, in response to the proliferation of automobiles, the hospital built a new parking area in 1925.

As the demand for nurses increased during the decade, so did the number of young women enrolling in the St. Vincent School of Nursing.

In the 1920s, nursing was still one of the few occupations available to women. And therefore, in an urban environment like Birmingham, it was one of the few means of support for any woman who did not marry immediately. Nursing was, at the time, a profession almost exclusively comprised of young single women. Most nurses who later married opted to quit work, and for those few who decided to continue to work, most doctors and hospitals gave unmarried nurses priority in employment.

The students rose each day at 6 a.m. and reported for roll call 30 minutes later. After

The Sisters' Life

Excerpts from the Diaries of St. Vincent's

December 24, 1925. "The new driveways are completed, everyone is charmed with this improvement, as it has provided a large parking space."

October, 1927. "Captain Beaty, at the request of Sister Antonia, wrote to 'Lindy' [Charles Lindbergh, who had recently gained fame for his solo flight across the Atlantic], asking him to fly over the Hospital on his trip to Birmingham...At the appointed time we were all on the 4th Main porches and fire escape, Mr. Downs up on the roof...Lindy came directly to the Hospital and circled round the cupola, stuck his head out and waved at us, while the people at Fairfield waited for him."

October 12, 1929. A Mr. and Mrs. Lovelle collected money and purchased a "lovely Ford sedan" for the Sisters so they might "be able to more easily visit the poor." The Lovelles' gift included a license for the car, a year's worth of gas and materials to build a garage.

November 14, 1929. Six of the Sisters returned from a visit to Mobile. "They had a wonderful time yesterday" and even "took a dip in the Bay."

prayers and breakfast, the students were on duty by 7 o'clock. They graduated, upon passing graduation exams, after about three years of training. There would not be a state test for licensing nurses until the 1930s.

As patient numbers continued to climb, so did the number of student nurses, who at the time, all lived in the hospital. In January of 1925, St. Vincent's broke ground on a building for the training and housing of the growing student population, a facility that Sister Chrysostom had envisioned building more than 10 years before.

The new nursing school, Laboure Hall, opened formally on March 19, 1926. As was typical of past expansions of the hospital, the community crowded into the building to see the dormitory, classrooms, gymnasium and library. Hundreds visited that day, and the Diaries remark, "It was late before the last ones departed."

A local landscaper, Mr. Woods, had worked for two weeks "beautifying the grounds." Woods also loaned the Sisters 50 palm trees for the open house, and dozens of flower arrangements arrived from well-wishers. A widow donated "a handsome clock in memory of her husband," and Johns Undertaking Company gave a Victrola for the entertainment room.

An Old Sister, A New Sister

On Friday, April 29, 1927, Sister Chrysostom arrived from St. Louis for her annual retreat. Many people of Birmingham came to the hospital to pay their respects. "Crowds flocked to see Sister Chrysostom," the Diaries record. "This continued until Sunday night," when Sister Chrysostom went into the seclusion of retreat. While her visit did not permit a great deal of time with the people she had previously worked alongside for many years, Sister Chrysostom's visit was emotionally charged until her departure on May 11. As darkness arrived at Mount St. Vincent's, the Sisters had such difficulty letting Sister Chrysostom leave, she almost missed her train. "Such kissing and hugging and goodbyes you never saw before, however, all reached the station on time."

In the summer came the departure of Sister Angela, and the Sisters at St. Vincent's were anxious and eager to hear the identity of the new Sister Servant. "After our dinner, we all assembled at the front door to await the arrival of our new Sister Servant," the Diaries read. "At 12:20 the car drove up…" and two sisters emerged, and then "our own dear Sister Alphonsine stepped out."

The Sisters' writings convey a sense of elation about the new arrival, but the nervousness of the new Sister Servant didn't pass as quickly. At dinner, "Sister Alphonsine was so nervous she spilled the chicken gravy all over her cloth apron." Her three years in charge of St. Vincent's, however, would be relatively uneventful, and when she departed in 1930, the city of Birmingham was suffering a months-old depression that had paralyzed the country and the Magic City.

St. Vincent's was needed now more than ever.

In the News

Birmingham during the Jazz Age suffered from a number of growing pains, many involving overcrowding and the shortage of public services in a city that had almost grown too big for its britches. From the pages of *The Birmingham News* and *Age-Herald*:

A 1921 letter to the editor from an East Lake resident derided a recent increase (to 8 cents) in streetcar fare: "…every time they raise the fare, they drive more people away from the line who would be glad to ride the cars."

A June 14, 1923 issue reported that about 25,000 "men, women and children" visited Pizitz's Annual June Celebration Sale. Eight uniformed policemen "undergoing every variety of bodily contortion" maintained order with the assistance of a number of firemen. As the doors opened for the sale, members of the crowd who "adopted football tactics and stormed the corner entrance" smashed two display cases, throwing shattered glass "right and left."

"Build Viaduct on 24th Now" read the front-page headline on September 3, 1924. Major General William S. Sibert, chairman of the State Docks Commission, reported that "all parties could and should agree to build now this viaduct, thus giving some immediate relief to an intolerable situation" downtown traffic was encountering with train crossings.

In 1927, zoning on Highland Avenue was changed from "residential" to "business" from 20th Street to the intersection where the "new" fire station is located. Lots that had gone for $100 per front foot in 1900 were now commanding five times that price.

An August 18, 1929 story detailed the high level of "interest in Birmingham motor circles" over the recently introduced "Hupmobile Six," sold by the Jefferson Motor Company.

Photos: Archives, St. Vincent's Hospital

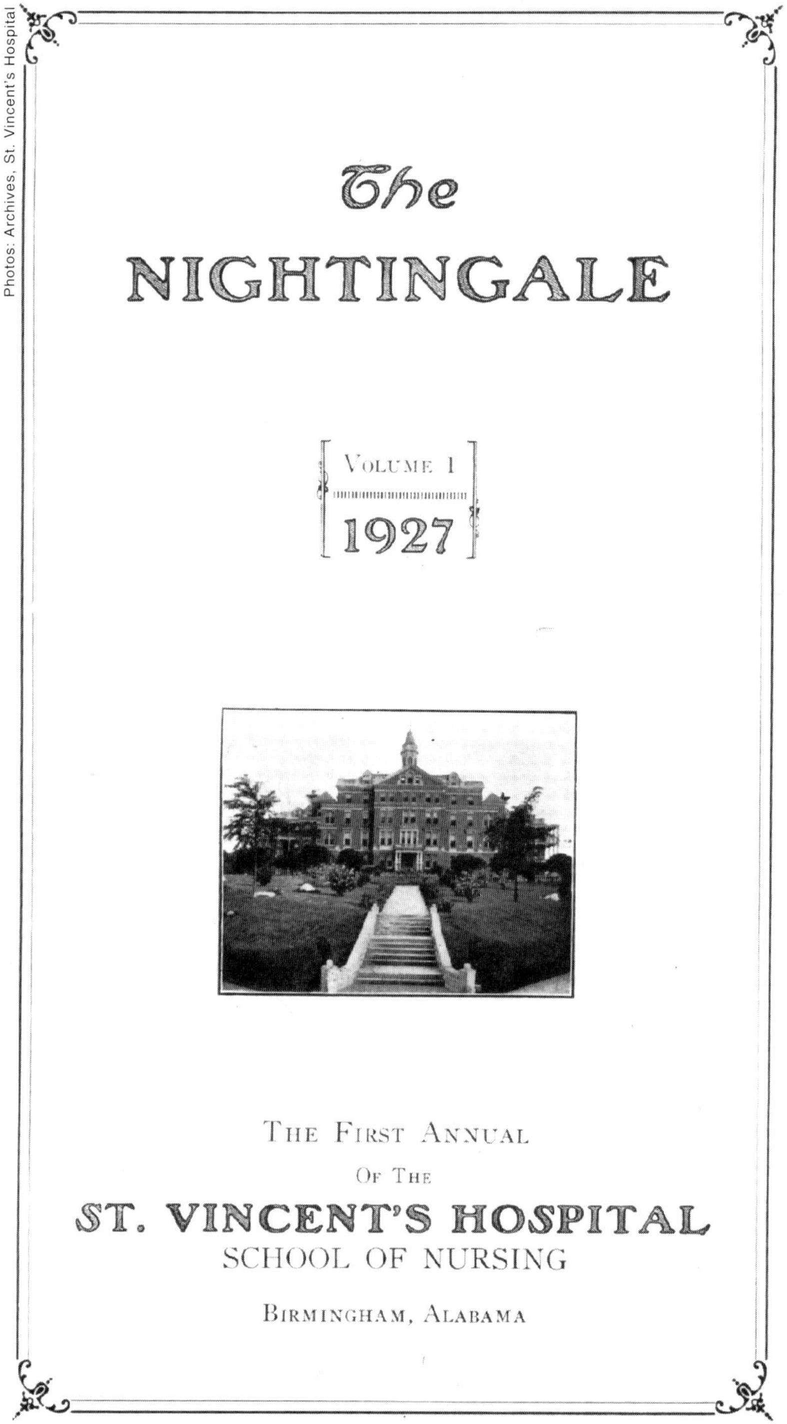

The Nightingale

Volume 1

1927

The First Annual
Of The
ST. VINCENT'S HOSPITAL
SCHOOL OF NURSING
Birmingham, Alabama

From the School of Nursing's first yearbook

The School of Nursing

One side effect of Birmingham's meteoric growth of the 1920s was a shortage of nurses. It was during the latter part of that decade that the St. Vincent School of Nursing came into its own. The completion of Laboure Hall and the increasingly large number of young women in the program created a more campus-like environment.

All nursing students were female and were not allowed to drink, smoke

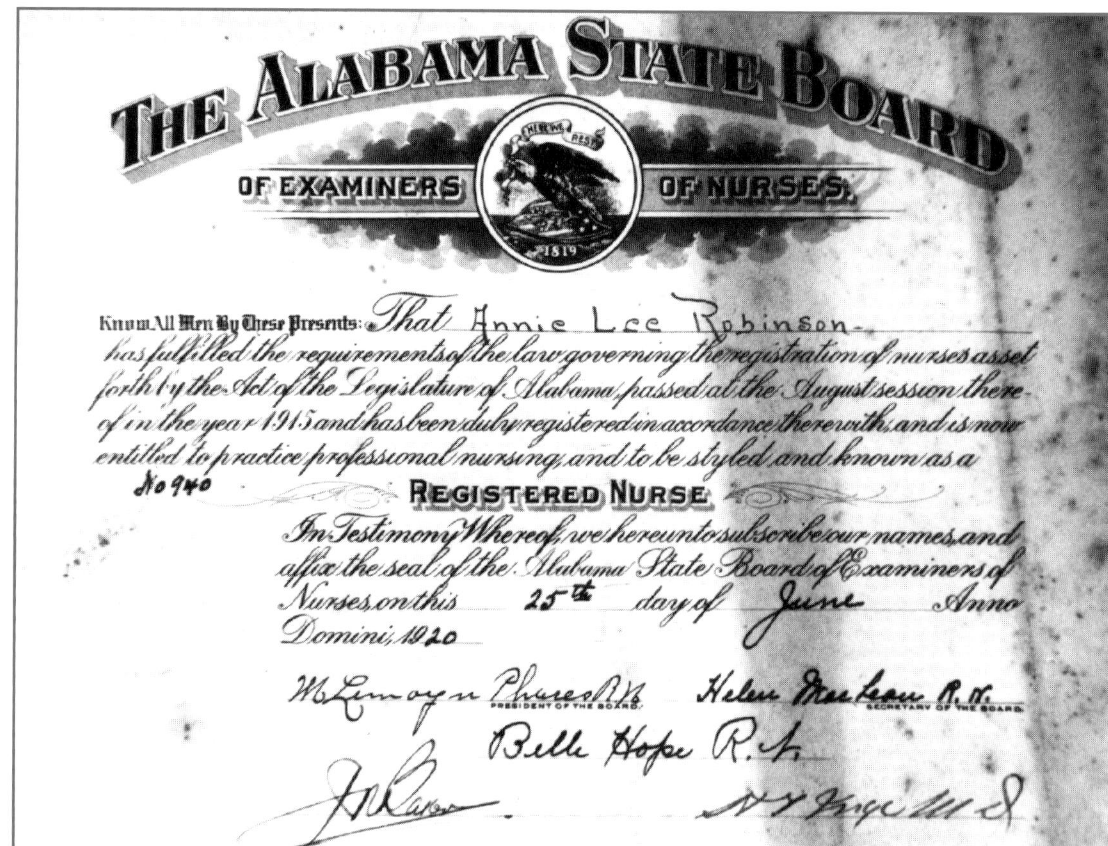

THE ALABAMA STATE BOARD OF EXAMINERS OF NURSES

1819

Know All Men By These Presents: That Annie Lee Robinson has fulfilled the requirements of the law governing the registration of nurses as set forth by the Act of the Legislature of Alabama, passed at the August session thereof in the year 1915 and has been duly registered in accordance therewith, and is now entitled to practice professional nursing, and to be styled and known as a

No 940 REGISTERED NURSE

In Testimony Whereof, we hereunto subscribe our names and affix the seal of the Alabama State Board of Examiners of Nurses on this 25th day of June Anno Domini, 1920

President of the Board

Secretary of the Board

The State of Alabama began registering nurses in 1916, with Sister Chrysostom being No. 1. By the time Annie Lee Robinson graduated from St. Vincent's in 1920, she was only number 940.

or marry. More than one student was dismissed for being secretly married.

Mary Kostick, a 1929 graduate, told *The Birmingham News,* "We had a Victrola in the entertainment room and the dorm, and a piano. I used to play it a lot, and we'd all sing and dance."

Elizabeth O'Roark Carroll, who also was a student in the late 1920s, recalled a demanding program of long hours.

"We worked seven to seven, and we got three hours off every day. Students went to school year-round," she said. "We started working with patients the day after we were accepted."

Mrs. Carroll also remembered the family-like atmosphere where the other students provided almost the only social life, which often included nearby Underwood Park.

"The park was real important to us," she said. "We played tennis and played on the swings."

"Men weren't allowed in the building, and if you had a date, all there was to it was a walk around Hanover Circle," she smiled. "We didn't have enough time off to go to a movie."

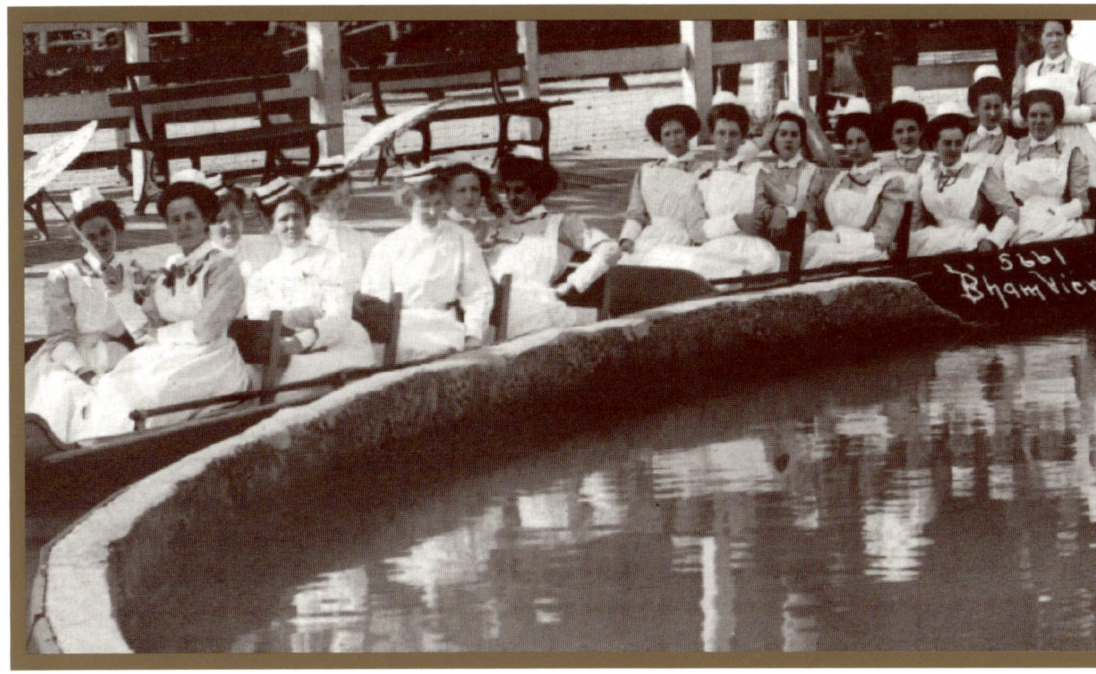

An outing to East Lake, one of the favorite excursions of the students in the 1920s

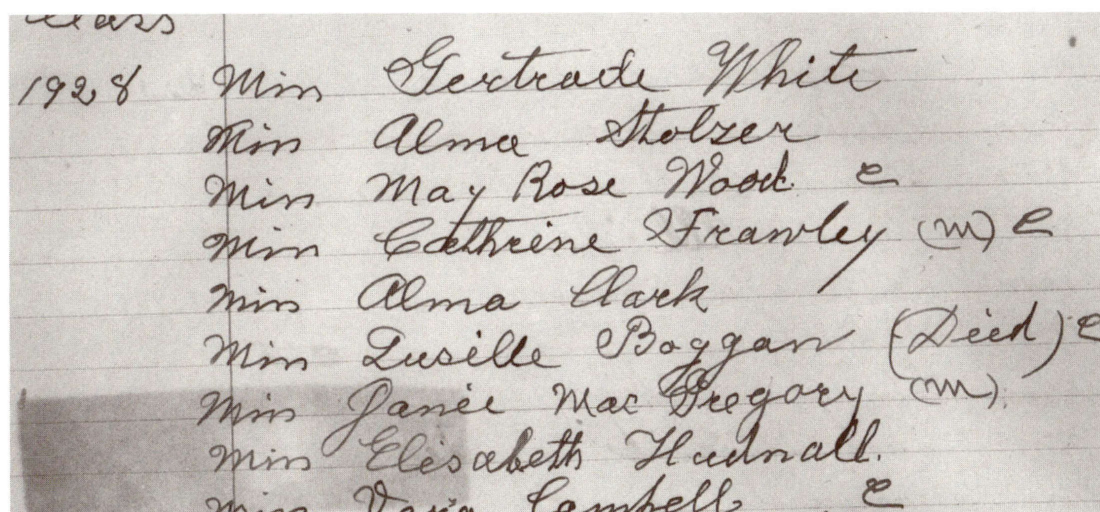

1928 Miss Gertrude White
Miss Alma Stolzer
Miss May Rose Wood e
Miss Cathreine Frawley (m) e
Miss Alma Clark
Miss Lucille Boggan (Died) e
Miss Janie MacGregory (m)
Miss Elisabeth Hudnall.
Miss Vera Campbell e

In a scrapbook begun in 1901, the nursing students recorded the names of each class, often noting marriages and deaths.

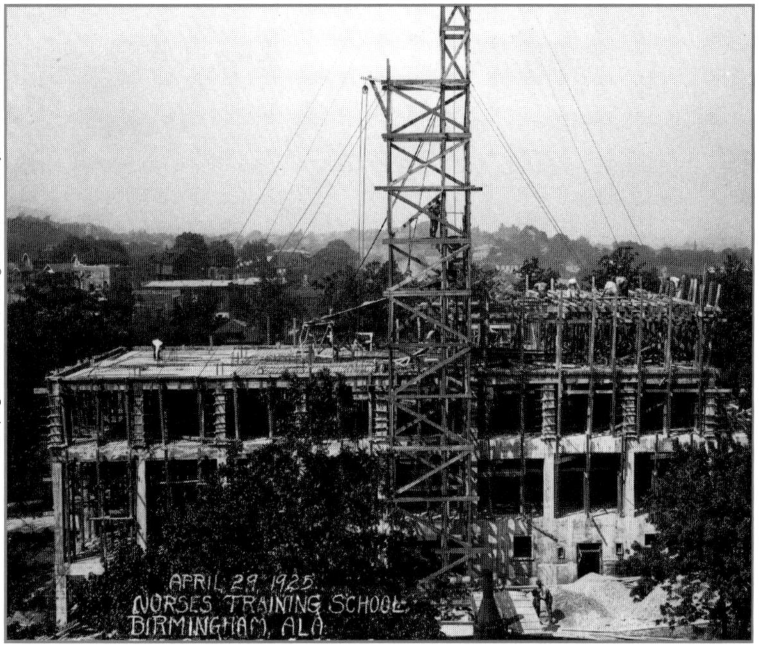

Laboure Hall under construction, April 29, 1925 (above), and after completion (below)

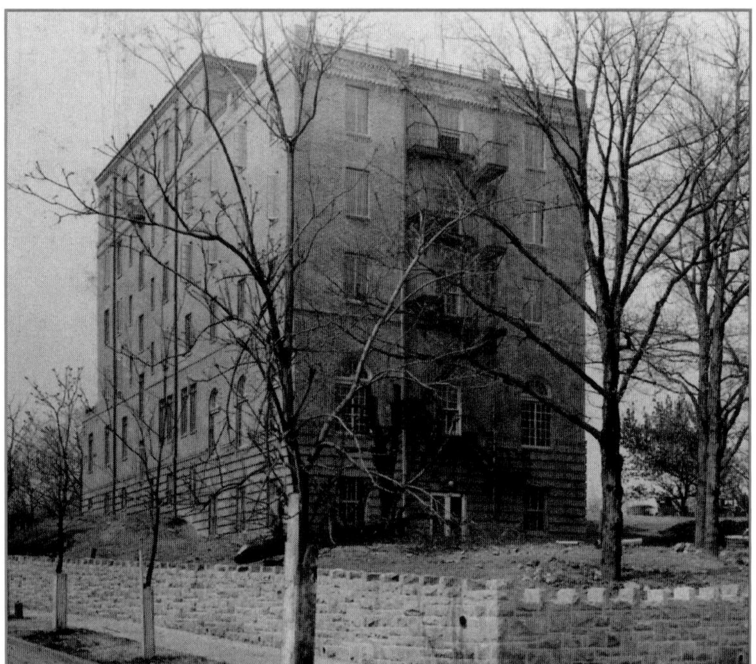

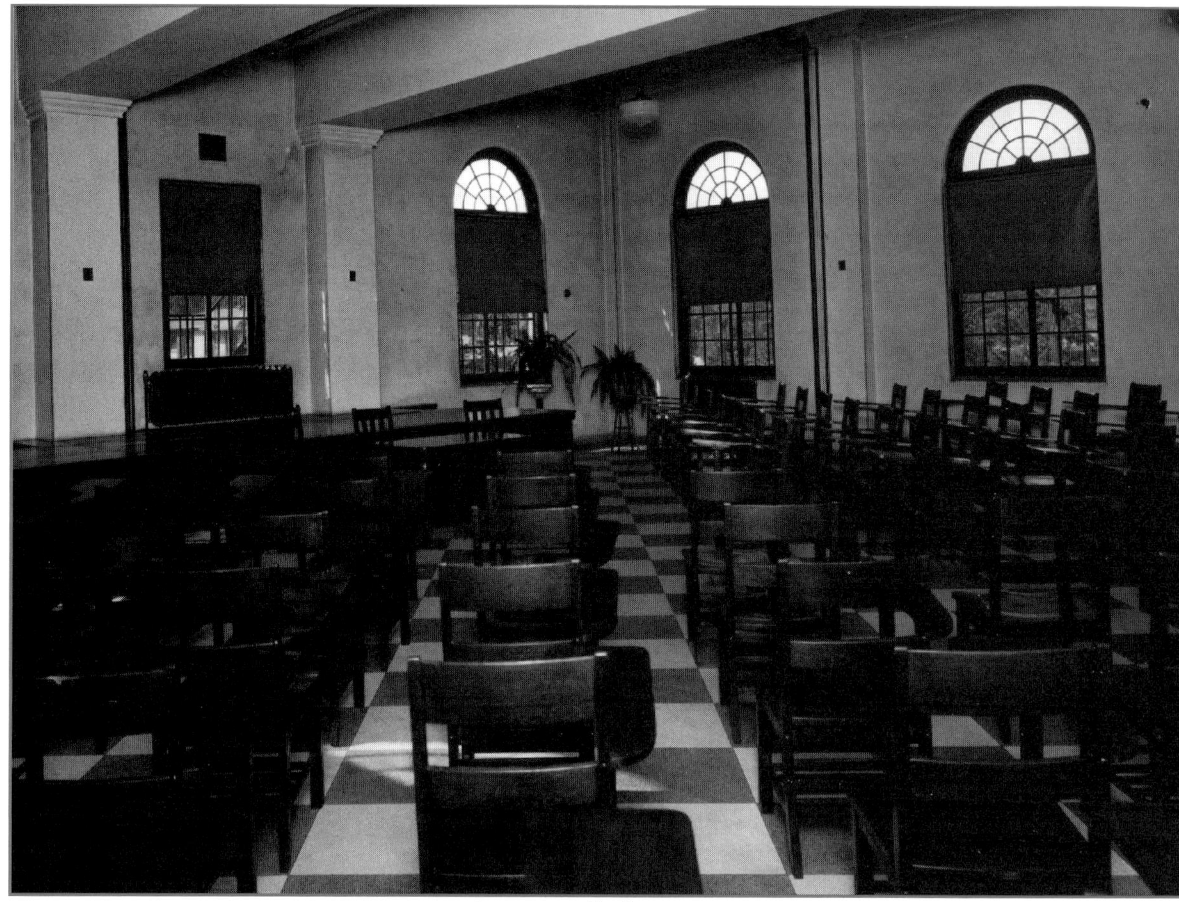

Laboure Hall classroom

Booming enrollment in the nursing program during the 1920s required the construction of Laboure Hall, completed in 1926, described as "beautiful and spacious" in a newspaper article.

Prior to the completion of Laboure, nursing students had lived in the hospital itself. In addition to dormitory rooms for the nursing students, Laboure Hall housed classrooms, a library, meeting rooms, a gymnasium and a roof garden.

For 30 years all students were required to live in Laboure, until enrollment in the program grew beyond the dormitory's capacity.

Laboure Hall was razed in 1982.

Archives, Birmingham Public Library

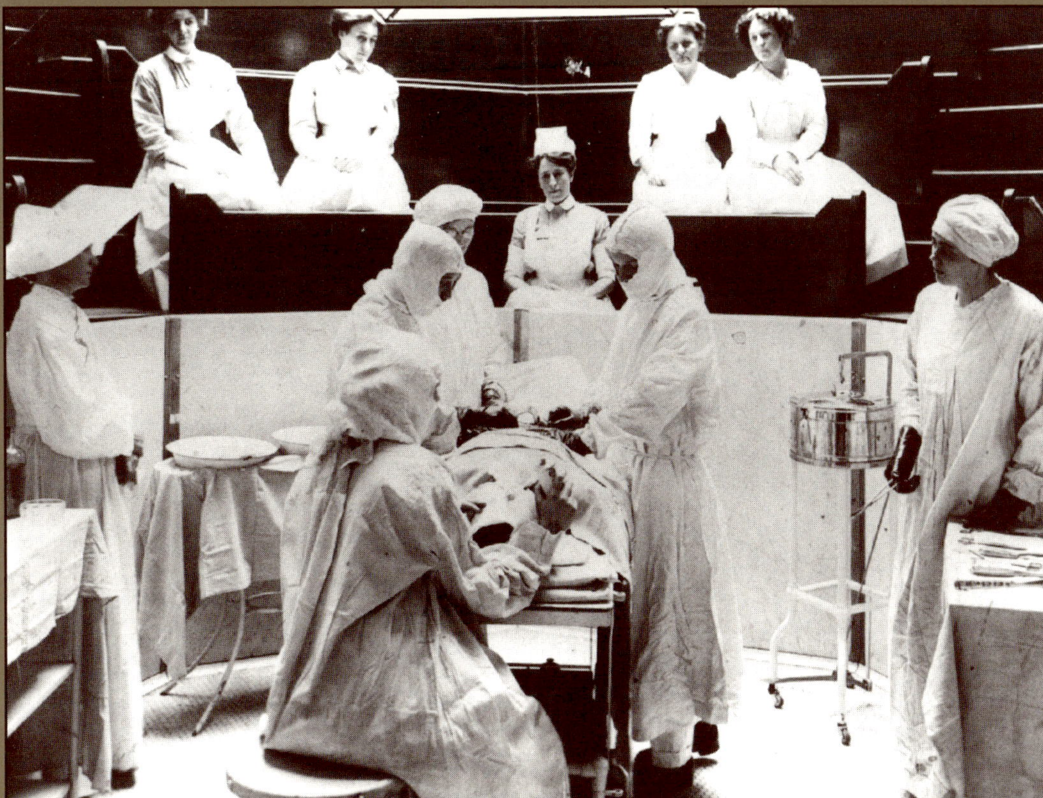

SURGERY AND ST. VINCENT'S

The original "state-of-the-art" St. Vincent's was an impressive facility that included an operating room with amphitheater for observation.

Surgery had only been routinely used as a medical tool for diagnosis and treatment since the turn of the century.

An anecdote by Dr. Cunningham Wilson, St. Vincent's first chief of surgery, illustrates the swiftness with which surgery came into prominence: "I saw only two abdominal operations in my student days and one in a year as an intern in a hospital...I had not seen an appendectomy."

Practically from the first days of the hospital's opening – only 20 years after the incidents Dr. Wilson described – surgery was a routine procedure at the hospital, and appendectomies were second only to tonsillectomies in the number of procedures performed.

Archives, St. Vincent's Hospital

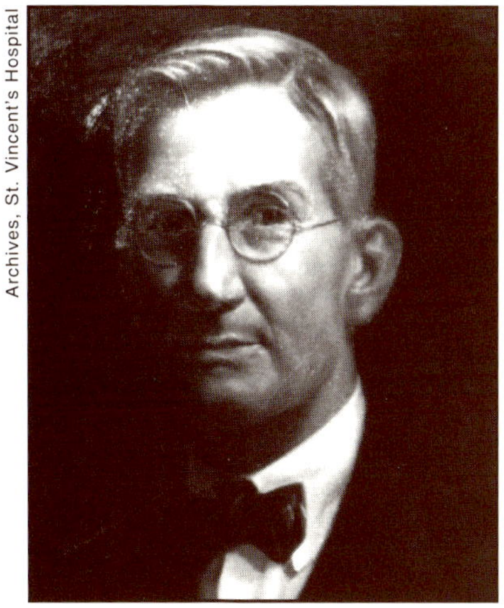

His Soul in His Work

Dr. Cunningham Wilson, one of the most devoted and dedicated members of St. Vincent's medical staff, was its first chief of surgery and the first president of its medical staff.

Born in 1860 on a farm in present-day Roebuck (the Roebuck Golf Course includes part of the farm), Dr. Wilson attended the country's first medical school, the University of Pennsylvania. He returned to Birmingham in 1885 and was part of one of St. Vincent's earliest medical staffs. Dr. Wilson served St. Vincent's as physician and benefactor for more than 40 years.

"A doctor's opportunity for helping his fellow man is unlimited," Dr. Wilson wrote in his book *A Fireside Story of Medicine in Birmingham*. "A doctor who puts his soul in his work has little time for anything else."

Dr. Wilson's tradition of commitment to St. Vincent's has been carried on by his son, Dr. Frank Wilson Sr. and his grandsons, Dr. Frank Wilson Jr., Dr. Thomas A. Wilson and Dr. Thomas Magruder.

The hospital's library is named for Dr. Wilson.

Chapter Four

Overcoming Hardships

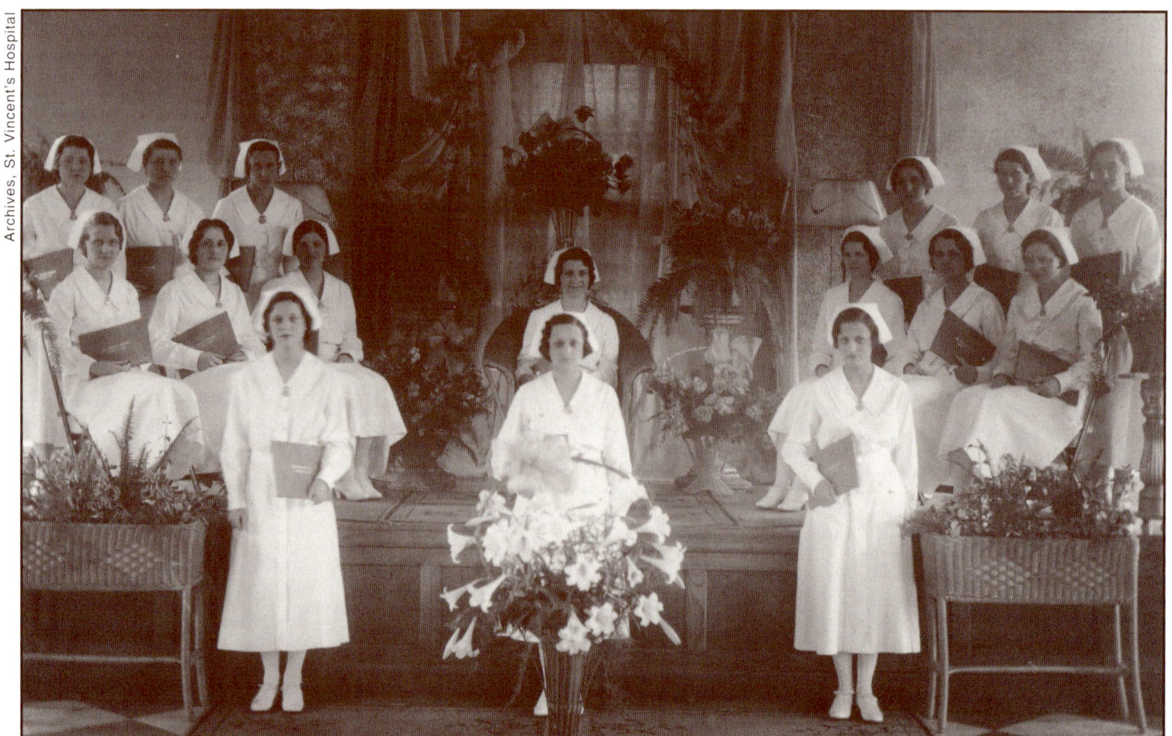

Archives, St. Vincent's Hospital

Graduation, Nursing Class of 1932

In late January 1930 Sister Alphonsine, the Sister Servant, received a letter that would signal the end of her mission at St. Vincent's. The telegram with this news arrived on February 4, and she left the city the next day.

All the Sisters except one went to the train station at noon to see her off. "She looked so sad and lonely sitting in the coach," the Diaries report. "May God bless and comfort her." The next entry, five days later, reads: "Sad days for us, no Sister Servant; [we are] anxiously waiting every day for news."

On Valentine's Day the phone call came, and within hours, the new administrator of St. Vincent's, Sister Alberta Sullivan, had arrived and been installed. The job she faced would be formidable, because not since the day St. Vincent's opened had the hospital been more needed.

"Hard Times Come Here First and Stay Longest"

The Great Depression hit Birmingham particularly hard. Though President Herbert Hoover's inauguration in 1929 had created "a thrill in the air" in Birmingham, it was not to last. More than 120,000 people in Jefferson County would lose their jobs. More than 1,000 mortgages would be foreclosed in the first three months of 1933 alone.

"Hard times come here first and stay longest" was a repeated Birmingham adage.

Within two years of the stock market crash, more than 60,000 people in Birmingham were living in crowded slums. Although constituting only 9 percent of the city's land area, almost 25 percent of the population was concentrated in these areas of substandard housing and poor living conditions. Forty-three percent of all cases of illness originated in the slums, as did 64 percent of the tuberculosis cases. Half of maternal mortality cases and 31 percent of infant mortality cases occurred here.

Following the gross overcrowding and shortage of public services that plagued much of the late 'teens and early 1920s, by the beginning of the Depression the city of Birmingham had a strong public health program. Death rates from communicable diseases had dropped sharply throughout the 1920s, reaching all-time lows in 1927, 1932 and, incredibly, in 1935.

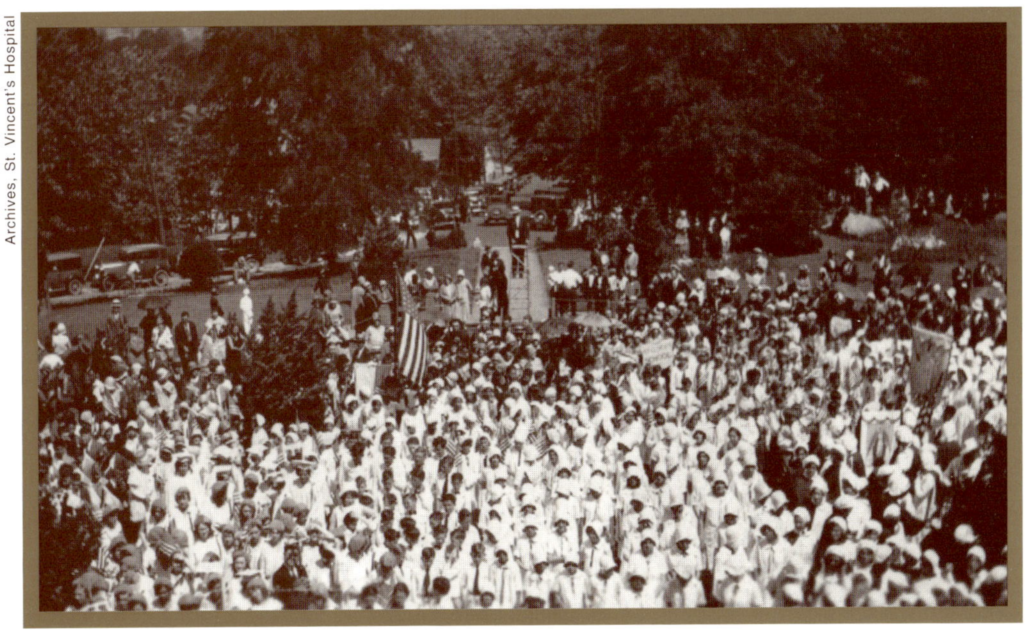

Archives, St. Vincent's Hospital

The first "Field Mass," or "Mass of the Angels," to take place in Birmingham was held in April 1930 on the lawn at the entrance to St. Vincent's. The service included a choir of 600 children, representing schools from across the city.

But the years of hardship and poverty wore down the people of the city. Infection and death rates in 1936 jumped dramatically, especially death rates from diphtheria, tuberculosis and childhood diseases. The infant mortality rate, "termed the best index of health condition" according to a Board of Health publication in 1936, rose sharply that year.

One of the biggest health problems of the Depression in Birmingham was pellagra. The number of cases reported in 1938 was two and one-half times that reported in 1929. Although not a communicable disease, the Board of Health studied it during these years because of the marked increase in the number of cases and because contraction of the disease is directly related to poor nutrition.

Pellagra typically affects adults. Only 1 percent of the cases in Birmingham during the Depression was in people younger than 15. Almost all of the areas of the city where pellagra was concentrated were poor areas. Although the incidence of pellagra increased throughout the Depression, the biggest increases came after 1935, the year that government assistance to the poor was paid in cash and not in groceries, as it had been prior to that year.

Lean Years and Hard Times

The Diaries note that on March 14, 1933, the "banks reopened." While this action was certainly a welcome sign, it didn't bring immediate prosperity. So, during the 1930s, the Sisters had to adjust to the changes the Depression forced on the people of Birmingham, and, therefore, on St. Vincent's.

Overall, fewer people sought the medical attention they needed during these years. Many were in a situation strange and unfamiliar to them: not having enough money for basic health emergencies. Many who could not afford medical help during the Depression did not feel comfortable accepting the charity of St. Vincent's. These people had not required charity before; indeed, before the Depression many of them had been involved in providing charity to the less fortunate, and their newly arrived financial straits were proudly denied in public situations.

Charity patients continued to come to St. Vincent's during the Depression, but the number of paying patients dropped dramatically.

The Sisters' Life

Excerpts from the Diaries of St. Vincent's

Wednesday, June 11, 1930. Tragedy for one of St. Vincent's physicians: "Dr. Constantine's 24-year-old boy lost his life on his way home from school. The excursion boat took fire, and many lives were lost. Only six weeks ago his 22-year-old boy was killed in an auto accident."

Tuesday, December 23, 1930. "We delivered Christmas baskets today. We had 12 cars at our disposal, everyone was anxious to help. Visited about 40 families."

Monday, April 20, 1931. "About 4 p.m. we were terrified by the arrival of several fire engines and two ambulances. Four other ambulances were on the way out to remove the patients. No one knew anything about the fire, or who sent in the alarm. Finally we discovered that a boy had crawled in the sewer after his top and got stuck. His mother called the fire department, then fainted. As it happened to be at our corner, she just said 'Come to St. Vincent's.'"

Sunday, August 6, 1931. "We are beginning to feel the effects of the Depression. Four Main closed."

Wednesday, January 29, 1936. "It snowed all day and night," ultimately 11 inches. On Thursday, the streetcars did not run and it was "impossible to use the auto." There was no change on Friday, "snow still on the ground, everything frozen." Although on Sunday rain had begun, the "ground is still covered with snow...The train is two and one-half hours late..."

Archives, St. Vincent's Hospital

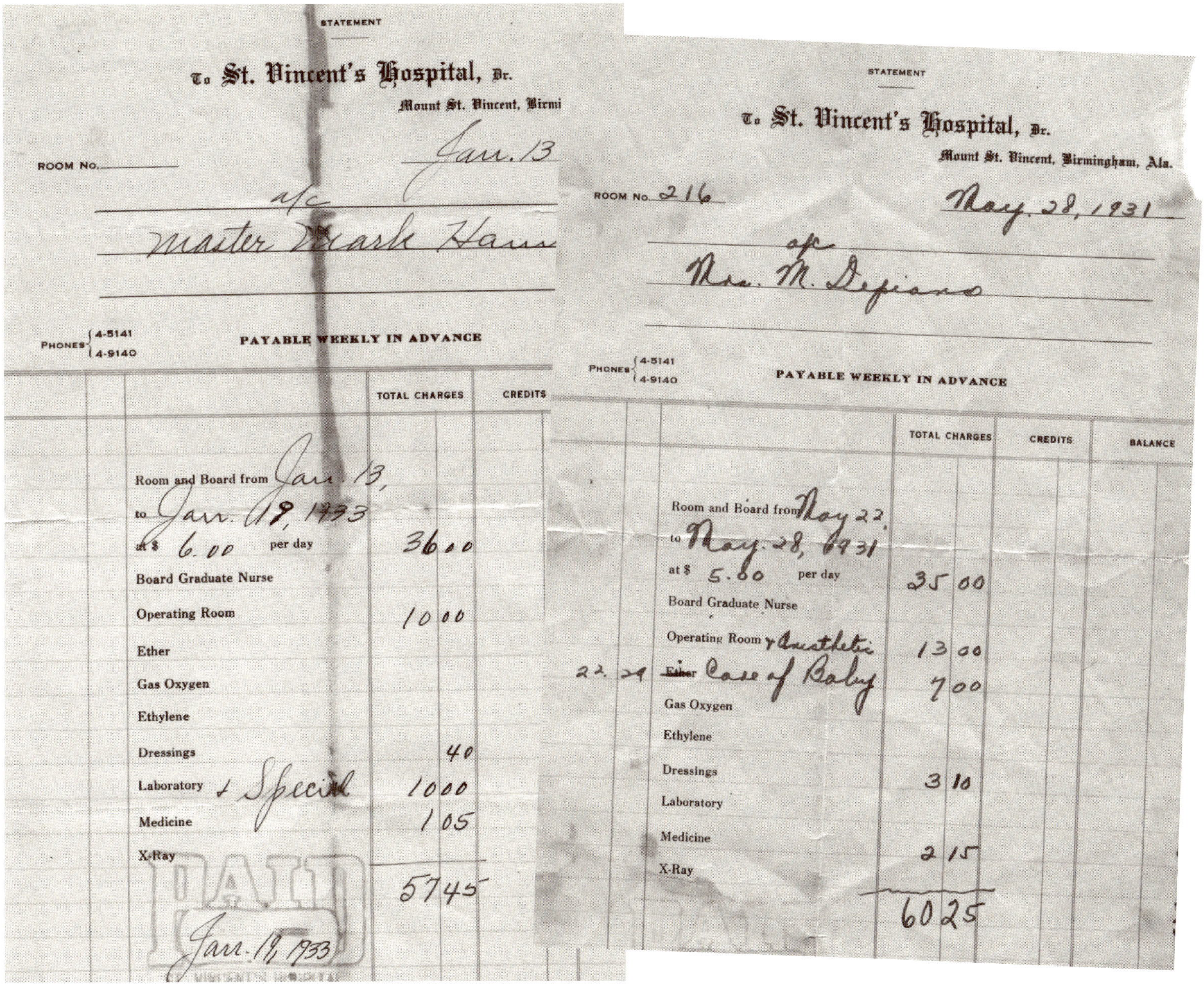

STATEMENT

To St. Vincent's Hospital, Dr.

Mount St. Vincent, Birmi

ROOM NO.

Jan. 13

a/c

Master Mark Ham

PHONES 4-5141 4-9140

PAYABLE WEEKLY IN ADVANCE

	TOTAL CHARGES	CREDITS
Room and Board from Jan. 13, to Jan. 19, 1933 at $ 6.00 per day	36 00	
Board Graduate Nurse		
Operating Room	10 00	
Ether		
Gas Oxygen		
Ethylene		
Dressings	40	
Laboratory + Special	10 00	
Medicine	1 05	
X-Ray		
	57 45	

PAID Jan. 19, 1933 ST. VINCENT'S HOSPITAL

STATEMENT

To St. Vincent's Hospital, Dr.

Mount St. Vincent, Birmingham, Ala.

ROOM NO. 216

May 28, 1931

a/c

Mrs. M. Defiano

PHONES 4-5141 4-9140

PAYABLE WEEKLY IN ADVANCE

	TOTAL CHARGES	CREDITS	BALANCE
Room and Board from May 22, to May 28, 1931 at $ 5.00 per day	35 00		
Board Graduate Nurse			
Operating Room + Anesthetic	13 00		
22. 29 ~~Ether~~ Care of Baby	7 00		
Gas Oxygen			
Ethylene			
Dressings	3 10		
Laboratory			
Medicine	2 15		
X-Ray			
	60 25		

PAID

A Depression-era surgery, complete with anesthesia and a six-day stay, cost $57.45.
The delivery of a baby during the Depression, including a week's room and board
for the mother and care for the baby, cost little more than $60.00.

“Miss Augusta Williams, daughter of a prominent lawyer, died in the O.R.,” the Diaries read in August 1931. The incident shot through the city.

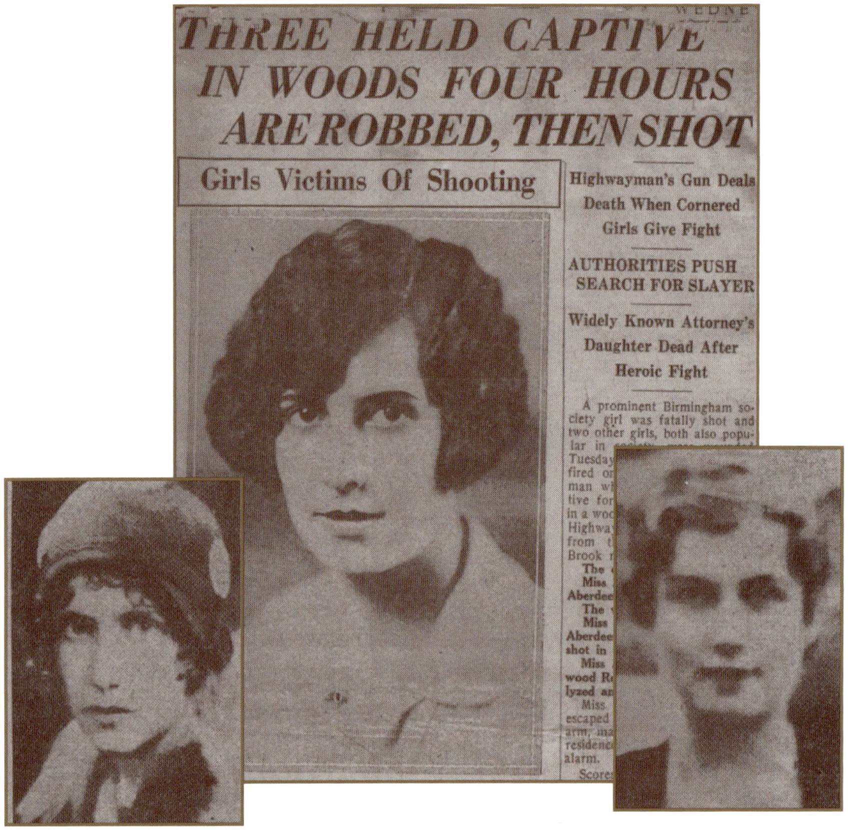

THREE HELD CAPTIVE IN WOODS FOUR HOURS ARE ROBBED, THEN SHOT

Girls Victims Of Shooting

Highwayman's Gun Deals Death When Cornered Girls Give Fight

AUTHORITIES PUSH SEARCH FOR SLAYER

Widely Known Attorney's Daughter Dead After Heroic Fight

A prominent Birmingham society girl was fatally shot and two other girls, both also popular in

Three prominent young society women on a late-afternoon drive were held captive for four hours and then shot by a “highwayman” on August 4, 1931. Nell Williams, shot in the arm, escaped to a nearby residence and summoned police. Her sister, 22-year-old Augusta Williams, and Jennie Wood, a 1928 graduate of Birmingham-Southern, were taken to St. Vincent’s. Augusta died shortly after her arrival at the hospital. Jennie died on August 6.

The three had been driving along Leeds Highway (now Old Leeds Road) about three miles from Mountain Brook when the armed man jumped onto the running board of their car and ordered them to turn off the highway. In a remote area about 100 yards from the highway, he took their money and held them captive until after dark. Eventually the girls attempted to escape, and the man shot all three, leaving after he decided they were dead. Before midnight, the entire area “was crowded with citizens, on foot and in automobiles” seeking the killer.

In The News

For 15 years beginning in 1930, there were two recurring news stories: the Great Depression and World War II. From the pages of *The Birmingham News* and *Age-Herald:*

With unemployment in Birmingham running high and “with the Jan. 1 deadline for receiving applications in Washington less than a month away...,” only three of 39 proposals for local Public Works Administration projects had been approved. According to a December 3, 1933, headline, “Not a man placed at work in state or shovel of dirt turned.”

In September 1936 local school authorities paid heed to a Health Department recommendation to delay the opening of school for one week “as a precaution against the possibility of the further spread of infantile paralysis.” The “epidemic has almost, if not quite, run its course,” according to health authorities, and “it would be a wise precaution to postpone school opening...”

Isolationism was prevalent in America during the Depression. “One out of every four boys at Birmingham-Southern College would refuse to be drafted into the U.S. Army should this nation become involved in the current European war,” reported a 1939 poll of students at Birmingham-Southern College.

A November 7, 1939, story reported encouraging news on the economy. “The upswing in industry, business and building operations that has been in progress several months will continue in 1940,” according to a government report. “The Birmingham-Atlanta area...led the country in consumer purchase gains in August...”

“If You Want to Beat the Jap Just Collect Your Iron Scrap” reads a headline on January 18, 1942. With the Pearl Harbor attack a recent, stinging memory, the upcoming Wednesday was to be “Scrap Day” in the city. “It takes steel to win the war,” the story goes on. “It takes scrap to make steel with which to stop the threat of invading hordes...”

Alongside the hospital, the Ladies of Charity increased their efforts on behalf of the poor of Birmingham. In 1931 alone, the Ladies administered 2,356 cases of relief.

In 1931 the low number of patients required Fourth Floor Main to be closed for three months. In early 1932 Fourth Floor West was closed indefinitely.

The number of requests for ward rooms increased during the Depression, and one by one the Sisters converted private rooms to ward rooms. For more than four years, from March 1931 to May 1935, the hospital had fewer than 100 patients each day.

After four years of precariousness and hardship, Sister Alberta left St. Vincent's in 1934, and Sister Lydia Hoffman took over the administration of the hospital.

More Bad News

Unfortunately, to compound the general feeling of despair in Birmingham, bad luck seemed to be omnipresent.

In 1931 three young girls, prominent "society" members on an afternoon drive, were abducted, robbed and shot. Two of the girls later died at St. Vincent's. The incident terrified the populace and prompted a manhunt involving hundreds of Shades Valley residents.

Archives, St. Vincent's Hospital

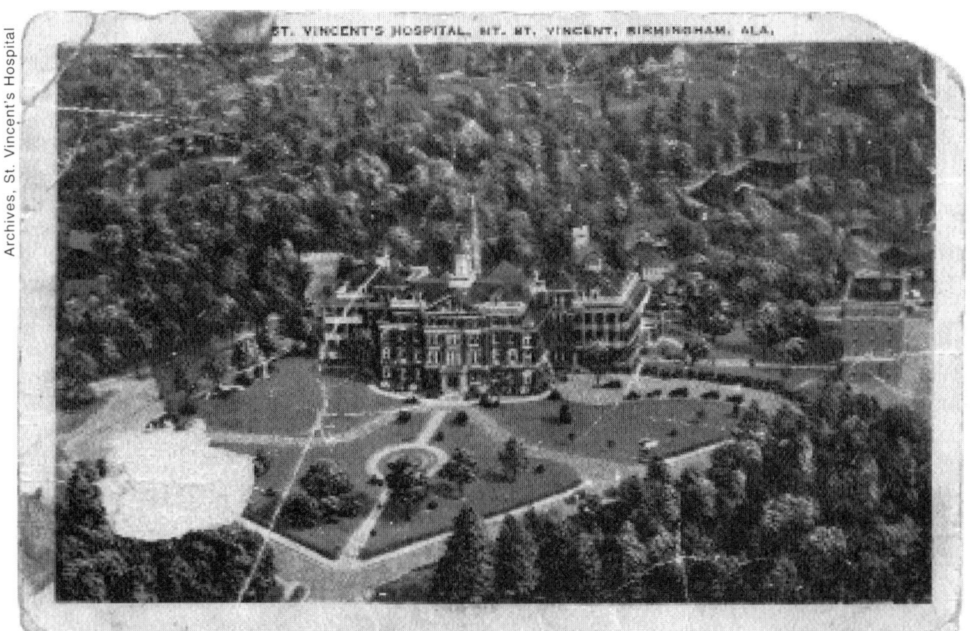

A mother from Cullman wrote on this postcard in April of 1937, "This leaves Hubert doing fine....Come down here and bring some more money. I paid $20 and you still owe $16.05 more, yet they took some more X-rays. I guess we can carry him out on Monday."

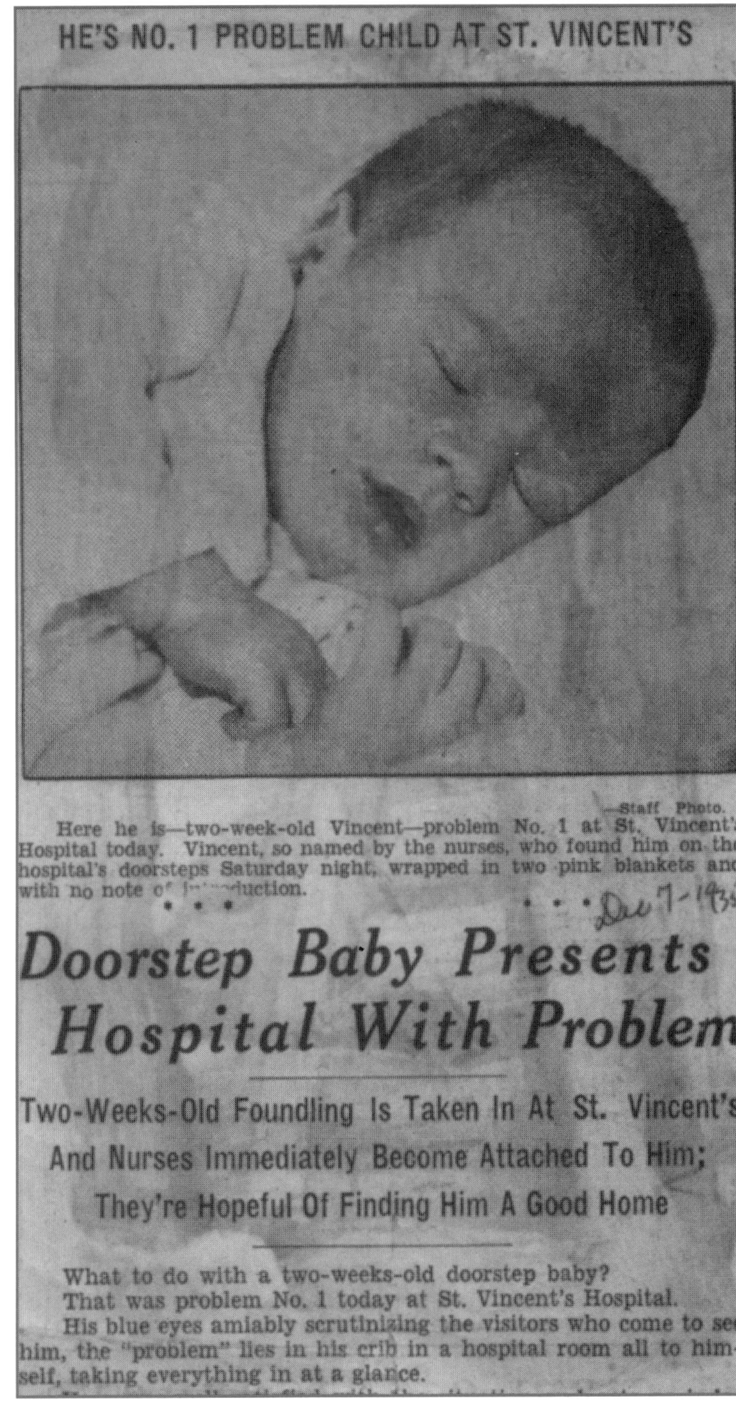

HE'S NO. 1 PROBLEM CHILD AT ST. VINCENT'S

—Staff Photo.

Here he is—two-week-old Vincent—problem No. 1 at St. Vincent's Hospital today. Vincent, so named by the nurses, who found him on the hospital's doorsteps Saturday night, wrapped in two pink blankets and with no note o[illegible]duction.

Dec 7-1935

Doorstep Baby Presents Hospital With Problem

Two-Weeks-Old Foundling Is Taken In At St. Vincent's And Nurses Immediately Become Attached To Him; They're Hopeful Of Finding Him A Good Home

What to do with a two-weeks-old doorstep baby?

That was problem No. 1 today at St. Vincent's Hospital.

His blue eyes amiably scrutinizing the visitors who come to see him, the "problem" lies in his crib in a hospital room all to himself, taking everything in at a glance.

Dubbed "Vincent" by the nurses at the hospital, this 7-pound, 2-week-old infant was abandoned on the doorstep of the hospital in 1935.

Shortly after noon on a busy Saturday in March of 1934, the huge Loveman, Joseph & Loeb department store caught fire. The fire raged out of control all afternoon, spreading to other buildings, including that of the Southern Bell Telephone and Telegraph building, which put 8,000 telephones out of service. Local radio stations broadcast continual updates from the scene, and these reports became the only source of information for the Sisters. Finally, with the hospital phone still out of service, they sent for additional doctors and nurses by messenger. The fire wasn't brought under control until nightfall.

That night 32 firemen were brought into St. Vincent's for treatment, including Fire Chief Hargrove, who was suffering from "injuries to his eyes, throat and lungs." On Monday, 10 firemen were still at St. Vincent's, including Hargrove. Fourteen more remained at South Highlands Infirmary.

All told, the damage from the worst fire in the city's history totalled $3 million, including some $500,000 to the Southern Bell building.

Another fire, in July of 1935, destroyed an Avondale lumber mill before spreading to nearby homes. A crowd of 35,000 gathered as the fire raged for three hours. Eighteen firemen, as well as one man who volunteered to help fight the flames, went to the hospital. Three of the injured came to St. Vincent's.

On October 27, 1935, Judge W. I. Grubb, longtime friend of St. Vincent's, died as he was preparing to go to Sunday Mass. His funeral two days later packed St. Paul's, with many who wished to attend not able to squeeze into the crowded cathedral.

Just after dark on December 6, 1935, nurses thought they were hearing the cries of a baby in the neighborhood, only to find a two-week-old boy, wrapped in two pink blankets, lying on the doorstep. The night supervisor said that in her 12 years at the hospital, this was the first baby abandoned there, "and I don't remember hearing of any such cases before."

The 7-pound infant, with dark hair and blue eyes, was clean and wearing an inexpensive white flannel dress. Becoming quickly attached to the child, the nurses called him "Vincent," and, to quote one newspaper, were "hopeful of finding him a good home."

A number of infantile paralysis cases were reported in the city during the summer of 1936. The epidemic reportedly covered all "Eastern and Middle West States," according to Jefferson County Health Department records. Eighty-five cases were reported, with 10 deaths. A 1937 outbreak of meningitis killed more than 100 in only two months, and two different outbreaks of typhus were traced to infected rats.

Of special sadness was the death of Sister Antonia shortly after Christmas in 1938. One of the original four Sisters who founded the hospital, Sister Antonia had been a nurse at St. Vincent's for all of the 40 years since. She was 77 years old.

St. Vincent's "Iron Lung Boys," as *The Birmingham News* dubbed them, made a Christmas Day radio appearance on WSGN in 1938. The boys, Charles "Buddy" Simms and Charles Boyd, thanked the audience for the many Christmas cards and gifts they had received during their illnesses, as well as WSGN and the *News* for contributing one of the iron lungs to St. Vincent's, and the Elks for donating the other.

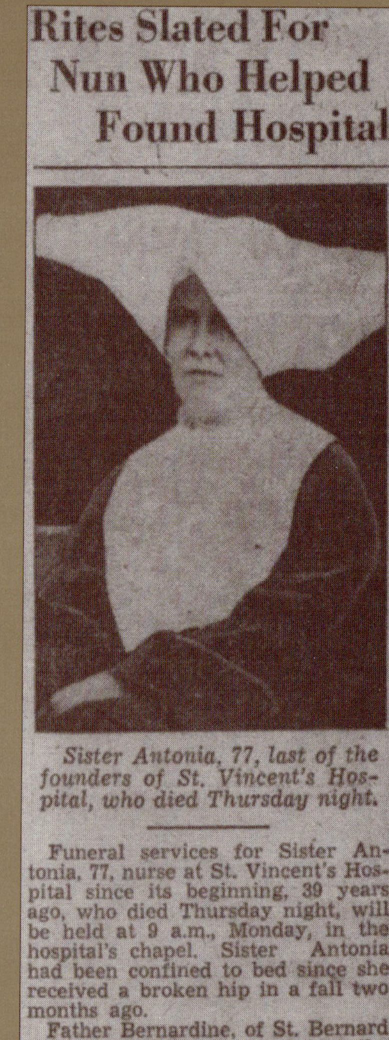

Rites Slated For Nun Who Helped Found Hospital

Sister Antonia, 77, last of the founders of St. Vincent's Hospital, who died Thursday night.

Funeral services for Sister Antonia, 77, nurse at St. Vincent's Hospital since its beginning, 39 years ago, who died Thursday night, will be held at 9 a.m., Monday, in the hospital's chapel. Sister Antonia had been confined to bed since she received a broken hip in a fall two months ago.

Father Bernardine, of St. Bernard

One of the last of the original Sisters of St. Vincent's died in 1938. Sister Antonia, nee Margaret Hanrahan, had nursed the sick and poor of Birmingham for 40 years. Born in Philadelphia in 1860, Sister Antonia served as a nurse in the Spanish-American War. She is buried at Elmwood Cemetery.

Hope and War

At St. Vincent's, no matter how lean the times, the quality of services was never sacrificed. The hospital continued to stand high on its hill as an ever-present symbol of hope.

As St. Vincent's celebrated its 39th anniversary, *The Birmingham News* said the hospital was "fully equipped in every department to meet any reasonable demand of modern medicine and surgery, and a constant effort is made to keep the hospital up to the highest standard in every way."

The situation of the nation slowly began to improve, but in Birmingham, the upswing was gradual. Eventually Works Progress Administration projects brought jobs to the city, pumping $361 million into Jefferson County in four years. In 1936 U.S. Steel began a $29 million expansion in the area.

The next years were slowly and increasingly better, but as a return to prosperity seemed possible, so did the probability of war. And when war came, nurses trained by St. Vincent's would go to all parts of the world to care for the sick and wounded.

In Birmingham, the war meant anxiety for the fate of the thousands of local men who were overseas, as well as sacrifice for those on the home front.

Dr. Joseph A. Cunningham said of those years, "Around town there was a noticeable absence of young men. And almost all of the remaining doctors were old."

Dr. Hiram Elliott recalls being with a fellow intern on a Birmingham streetcar when a woman tapped him on the shoulder demanding to know why he wasn't overseas. Although the men's service at the Tennessee Coal and Iron Hospital was recognized as vital to the war effort, "we felt the eyes of people on us," he said.

The war brought widespread rationing on the home front of many different items needed for the soldiers. Dr. Elliott remembers, "You couldn't get a Coca-Cola. They were all going overseas. But we didn't mind any of the shortages. Everybody's mind was on the American soldier and winning the war."

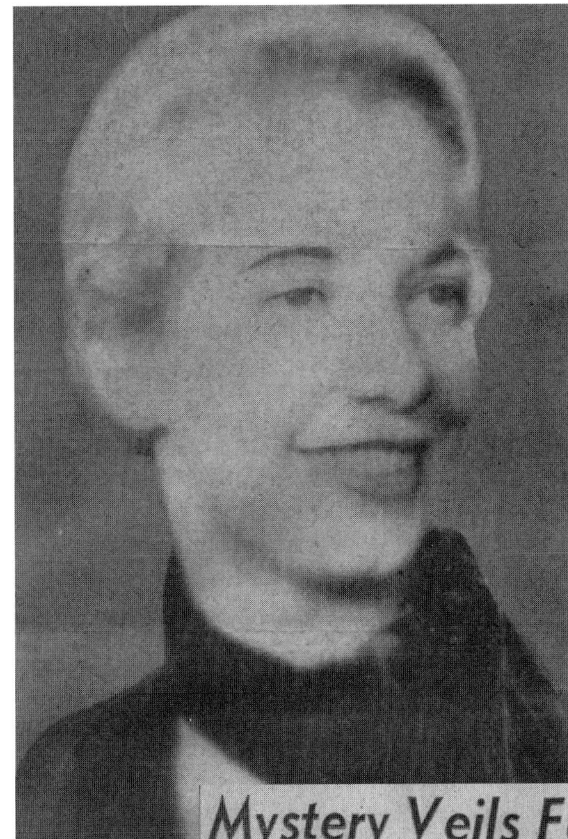

Nurse Of St. Vincent's Freed At Santo Tomas, Relatives Informed

Not since they received a letter dated Sept. 3, 1943, until they heard that her name was listed among the rescued prisoners from the Santo Tomas Prison Camp inside Manila, had the family of 1st Lt. Gladys Anne Mealer, chief nurse with the Army Air Forces at the time of the fall of Corregidor, had any word from her.

Informed by friends that his sister's name was called in a broadcast of the list of rescued prisoners, A. R. Mealer, 2417 39th Avenue, North, said that he at first thought it was just another rumor. "After what we have been through, I trusted no rumors so I called the radio station for verification."

* * *

Mystery Veils Fate Of Former St. Vincent's Hospital Attache

Miss Anne Mealer Is 'Missing In Action' On Corregidor As Her Adventures Are Climaxed

After 10 years as an army nurse, St. Vincent's graduate and former floor supervisor Ann Mealer would have been back in Birmingham on furlough. Instead, in 1943 she became a prisoner of war as Corregidor Island in the Philippines fell to the Japanese. She had been chief nurse at the army hospital on the island. Her family waited more than a year before learning she was among the prisoners rescued from the Santo Tomas Prison Camp in Manila.

CHAPTER FIVE

The Human Touch of St. Vincent's

Archives, St. Vincent's Hospital

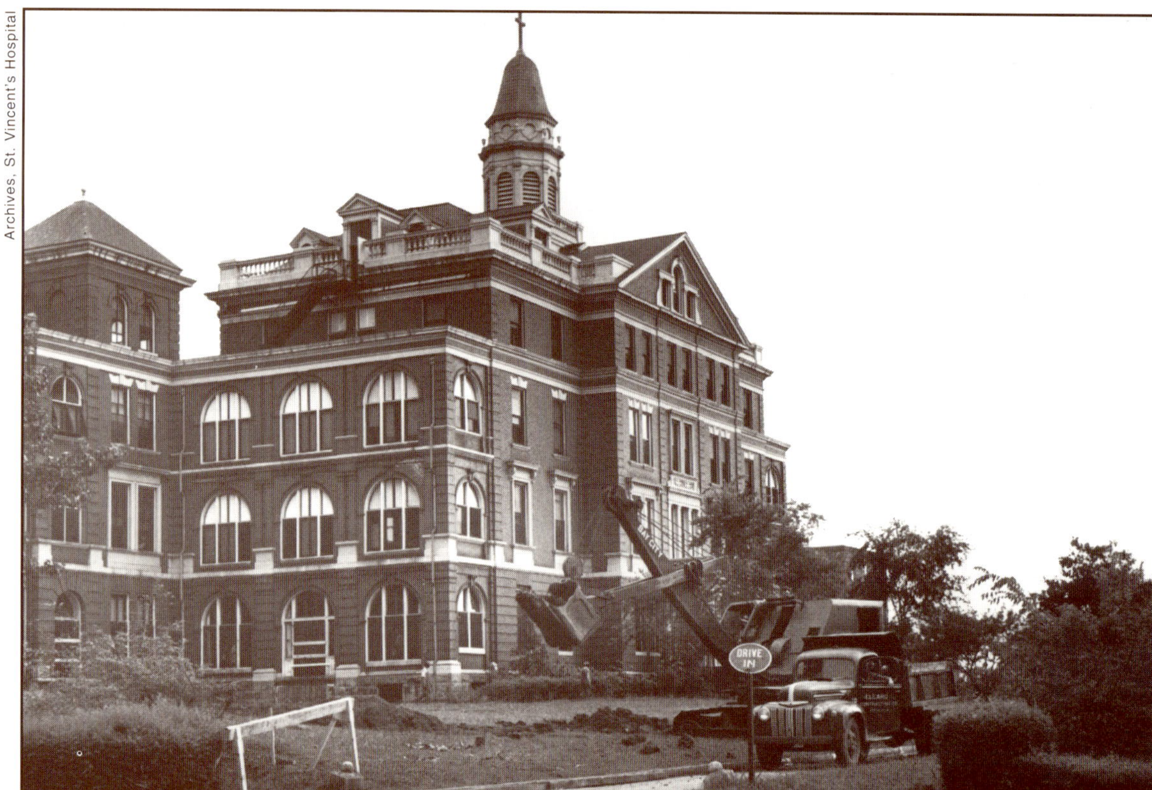

Work begins on the new East Wing, 1949.

After World War II ended, there was certainly a lot to celebrate. In 1946 Birmingham turned 75. And two years later, its oldest hospital marked its 50th anniversary.

Birmingham became a flurry of change and activity during the years following World War II.

The nation's demand for consumer goods, which had not been met during the war, exploded in the late 1940s, and the Birmingham economy rode the boom. Five years after the war ended, Birmingham steel mills were still working at capacity.

The Birmingham economy began to diversify for the first time. In the early 1950s, the Committee of 100 was formed to attract new industry to Birmingham, and within a few years its efforts helped bring 140 new businesses to the area.

In the post-war years, the Birmingham Barons set attendance records in the South. In 1948, a total of 445,926 attended games at Rickwood Field. In 1949, the Birmingham Zoo was founded. Also that year, WAPI and WBRC brought television to Birmingham.

During the 1940s more than 60,000 people became citizens of Birmingham, many through the annexation of Roebuck. Birmingham became the second largest metropolitan area in the South, with a population of more than a half-million.

These were years of celebration and growth not seen in decades.

And St. Vincent's enjoyed some of both.

These years saw the hospital become 50 years old, begin a new era of ambitious growth and receive the gratitude of the city it served. As columnist John Temple Graves wrote, St. Vincent's had been committed to the city as "perhaps no other institution or name in Birmingham's long story."

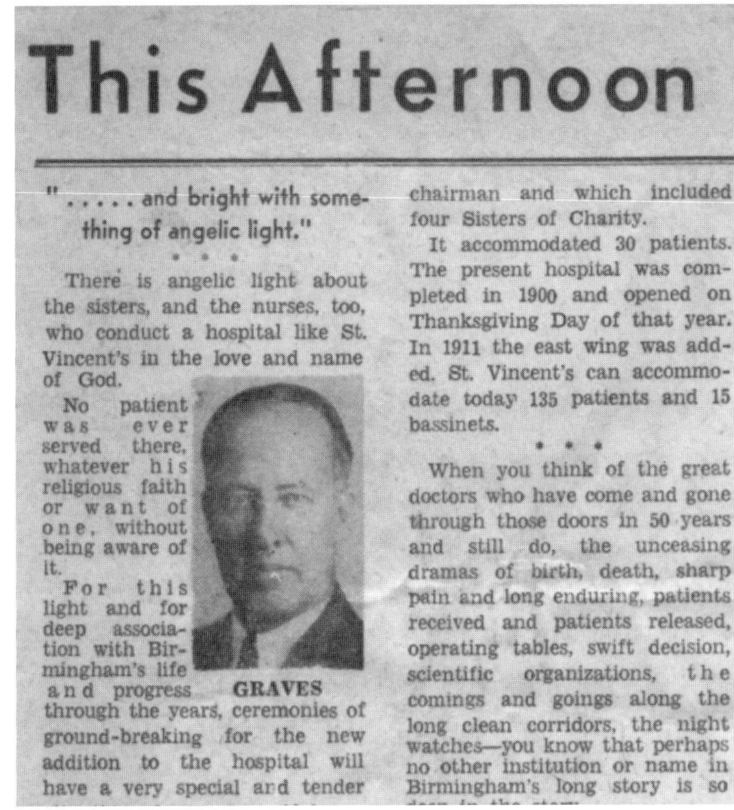

This Afternoon

". . . . . and bright with something of angelic light."

• • •

There is angelic light about the sisters, and the nurses, too, who conduct a hospital like St. Vincent's in the love and name of God.

No patient was ever served there, whatever his religious faith or want of one, without being aware of it.

For this light and for deep association with Birmingham's life and progress through the years, ceremonies of ground-breaking for the new addition to the hospital will have a very special and tender

GRAVES

chairman and which included four Sisters of Charity.

It accommodated 30 patients. The present hospital was completed in 1900 and opened on Thanksgiving Day of that year. In 1911 the east wing was added. St. Vincent's can accommodate today 135 patients and 15 bassinets.

• • •

When you think of the great doctors who have come and gone through those doors in 50 years and still do, the unceasing dramas of birth, death, sharp pain and long enduring, patients received and patients released, operating tables, swift decision, scientific organizations, the comings and goings along the long clean corridors, the night watches—you know that perhaps no other institution or name in Birmingham's long story is so

Birmingham News columnist John Temple Graves wrote frequently about St. Vincent's in the late 1940s.

Included in his loving words were these: "A hospital is always a dramatic and fundamental place, but when it has the human touch of St. Vincent's, it is a place so meaningful that you would almost expect to see a white cloud hovering over its high cross by day and a softly supernatural glow at night through the...walls."

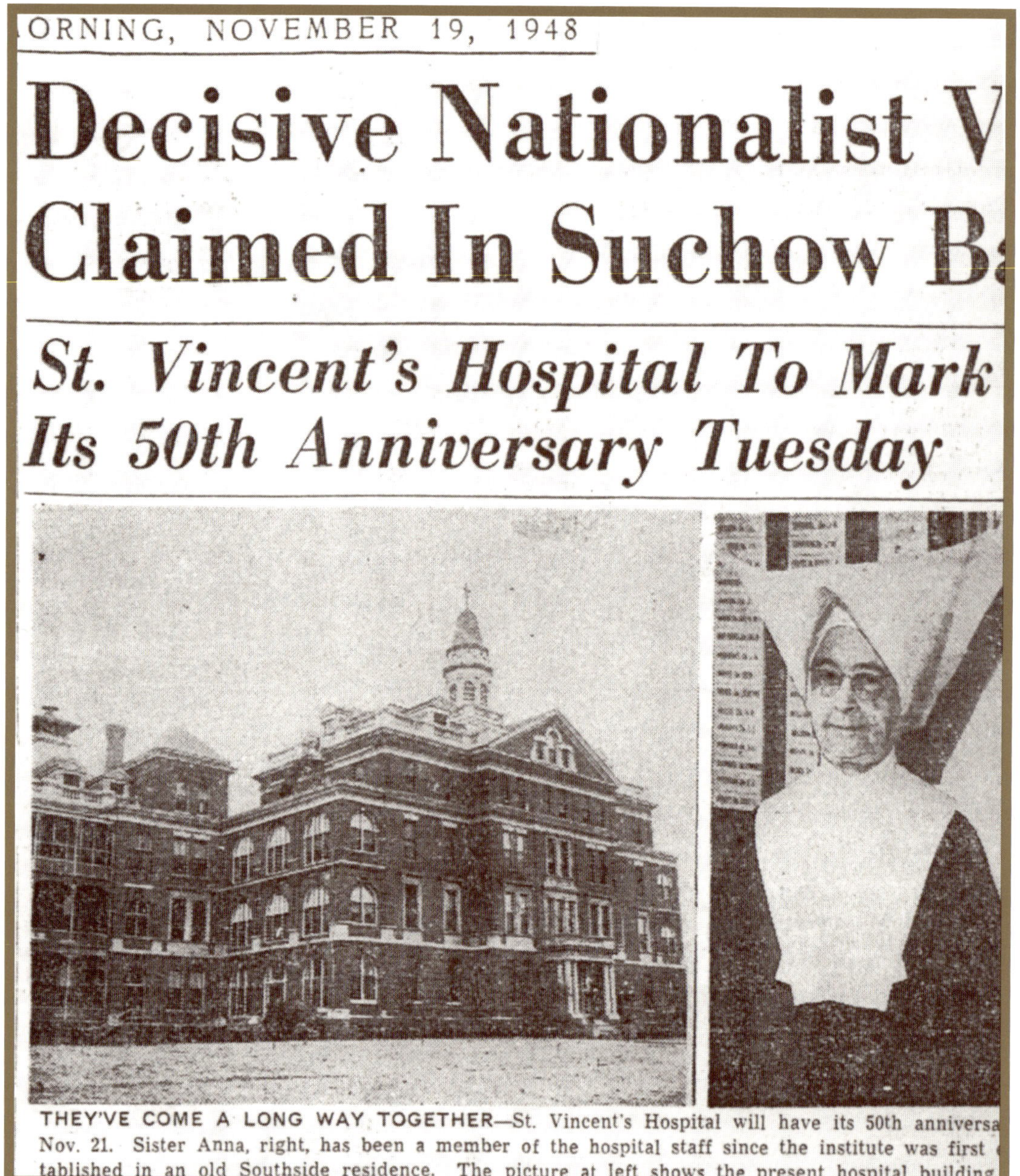

ORNING, NOVEMBER 19, 1948

Decisive Nationalist V
Claimed In Suchow B

St. Vincent's Hospital To Mark Its 50th Anniversary Tuesday

THEY'VE COME A LONG WAY TOGETHER—St. Vincent's Hospital will have its 50th annivers Nov. 21. Sister Anna, right, has been a member of the hospital staff since the institute was first tablished in an old Southside residence. The picture at left shows the present hospital building.

As St. Vincent's celebrated its Golden Jubilee in 1948, Sister Anna Thumel was soon to celebrate her 49th year in Birmingham. The last of the Sisters who had been a nurse in the DeBardeleben mansion, Sister Anna was also the second registered nurse in the State of Alabama.

A Golden (and Understated) Anniversary

Although the hospital was lauded in both morning and evening newspapers in November of 1948, Sister Mary Alice McCarthy, who had become Sister Servant of St. Vincent's in August of 1945, said the 50th anniversary would be celebrated without ceremony. The Sisters and nurses had a private chapel service on the Tuesday before Thanksgiving. The holiday had traditionally been the day the hospital's anniversary was observed.

Gold, however, was the motif for the "little private celebration" the hospital staff and patients enjoyed that Thanksgiving Day. "Tray favors with golden bells" were planned, as were gold touches in the salads and desserts. The menu for the day was printed on gold paper.

As the hospital was praised by the local press, so was Sister Anna Thumel, the last of the Sisters who had worked in the original hospital, the DeBardeleben home. Sister Anna, who had come to St. Vincent's in February of 1900, was quoted by newspapers about stories of the early days, of a hospital established "on a shoestring." "Surely the Lord was with us, or we could not have succeeded against all the odds," she said.

"In the Love and Name of God"

As it turned 50 years old, St. Vincent's had 125 beds and 16 bassinets but was sorely in need of expansion. Sister Mary Alice was intent on building a new wing of 100 rooms to accommodate 140 beds, including an expanded maternity ward that could care for 50 babies. Newspapers reported that the hospital intended to break ground in January 1949 on this new wing, which was expected to cost $750,000. The hospital began a drive to raise the $300,000 needed to begin construction.

The plans for the wing quickly changed. Soon it became evident the expansion would cost about $1 million. The new wing, as envisioned by architect Charles H. McCauley, would be "a six-story structure of red brick trimmed in stone." The number of new rooms planned for the new wing was trimmed to 80, although it was newsworthy that they would be "modern and complete with toilets." "The building will be serviced by automatic elevators," one newspaper reported.

The expansion was approved for funding under the Hill-Burton Act, which would cover one-third of the total cost. Completion was optimistically predicted for the summer of 1949.

In the News

The post-World War II days were a time of economic prosperity, brisk growth and fear of Communism. The pages of *The Birmingham News* and *Age-Herald* (weekday price: 5¢) were brimming with stories of the rise of the suburbs, stay-at-home moms and fear in the age of the atom bomb.

A Census Bureau report on December 7, 1947, listed metropolitan Birmingham as the second largest city in the South. With a metro population of 502,000, Birmingham finished behind New Orleans but ahead of Atlanta, Dallas, Memphis and San Antonio.

Construction in the unincorporated portions of Jefferson County experienced a boom in 1949, with 1,907 building permits being issued. The average cost of the 1,564 homes built in rural Jefferson County that year was slightly less than $3,400.

As the city endured an extended heat wave in June 1953, about 100 husbands in a north Birmingham neighborhood went on "strike," demanding "they shouldn't be forced to mow the lawn, spank the children or paint the porch after they came home from a hard day's work." One wife turned a hose on Jim Caldwell, ringleader of the uprising.

The April 27, 1956, *News* noted the growth of the suburbs, as two neighborhoods voted to become part of Vestavia Hills, bringing its population to about 3,000. In the four previous years, Homewood had registered a 39.8 percent population increase to 17,982.

As Americans continued to worry about "the Bomb," in October 1961 Bette Lee, the director of women's activities for WAPI radio and WAPI-TV, did a six-part series called "Life in a Fallout Shelter." She and her mother spent five days and nights in an $800 "family shelter," recommended for six people (although it was only 8 feet by 8 feet). "The question is survival," she wrote, "but we're a nation used to certain luxuries and space happens to be one of them." Stating the obvious, Lee also observed that "The problems of garbage and human waste disposal must be worked out." Her experience also led her to wonder "assuming we survive…how will we feed our families if this becomes a world without supermarkets? There seems only one answer. Urge our city to stockpile food and water."

The Birmingham Chamber of Commerce's *Birmingham* magazine hit downtown newsstands for the first time on November 15, 1961.

Of the construction, columnist Graves wrote, "There is an angelic light about the Sisters, and the nurses, too, who conduct a hospital like St. Vincent's in the love and name of God...For this light and for deep association with Birmingham's life and progress through the years...the new addition to the hospital will have a very special and tender attention from our Alabama people."

For reasons unclear, groundbreaking didn't take place, however, until that summer. This event was almost as significant as the groundbreaking of the original East Wing in 1910. Bishop T. J. Toolen officiated, and two city councilmen participated in the ceremony. Dr. Joseph A. Cunningham represented the medical staff.

Also shoveling one of the first spades of dirt was St. Vincent's beloved Dr. Cunningham Wilson, now 88 years old. The groundbreaking was one of Dr. Wilson's last public appearances, and the hospital's first chief of surgery, the city's "oldest doctor," would not live to see the new wing completed.

Upon Dr. Wilson's death later that year, columnist Graves said of Dr. Wilson, "His life was full, useful, distinguished, complete. The hands that served so many are folded...with entitlement to eternal rest..." In 1951, the hospital's library was dedicated and named for Dr. Wilson. The portrait of him that hangs there was painted by his grandson, William Symington Wilson.

The construction of the new wing also caused a problem that the hospital would eventually face again. Father O'Reilly's grave would have to be moved to accommodate the new wing. Father O'Reilly's grave would later be moved twice more to make room for hospital additions. He now rests in Elmwood Cemetery.

The new wing was five stories tall, and in addition to the 80 private rooms, it housed new obstetrical and pediatric services and a new "X-ray and radiographs department."

The East Wing opened in July 1950, and today it is the oldest part of St. Vincent's.

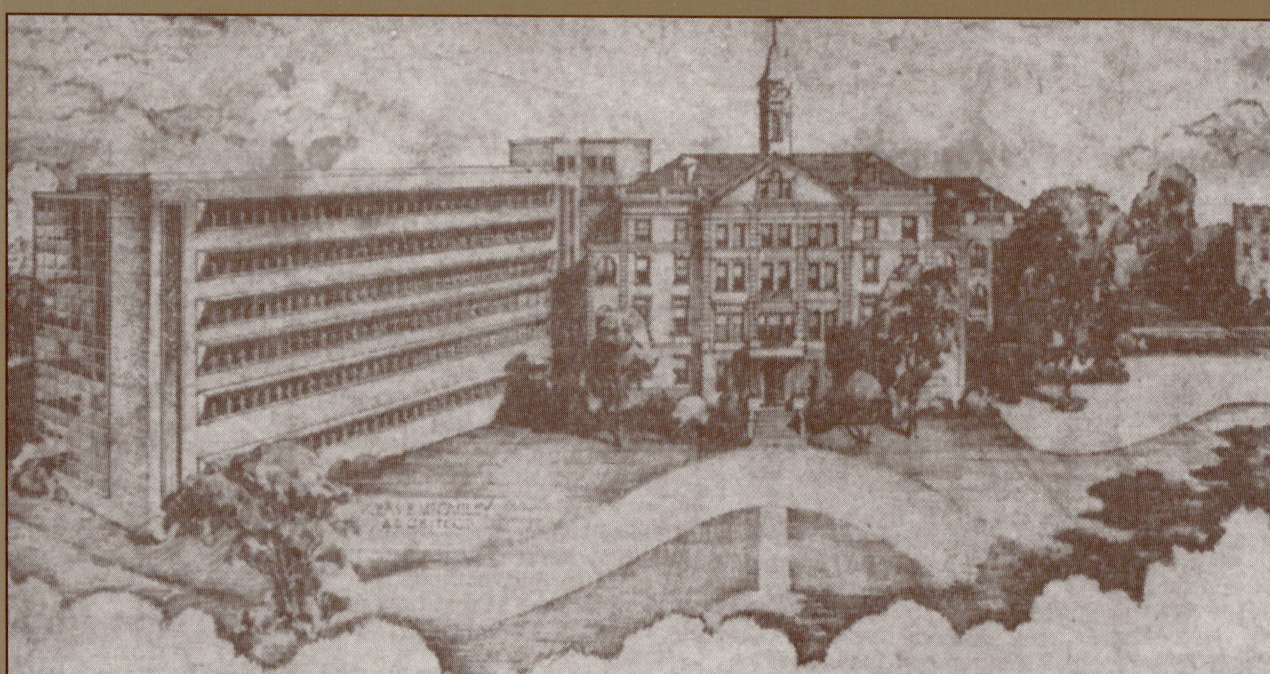

As this first architectural rendering shows, the new East Wing was originally planned as a six-story addition.

Archives, St. Vincent's Hospital

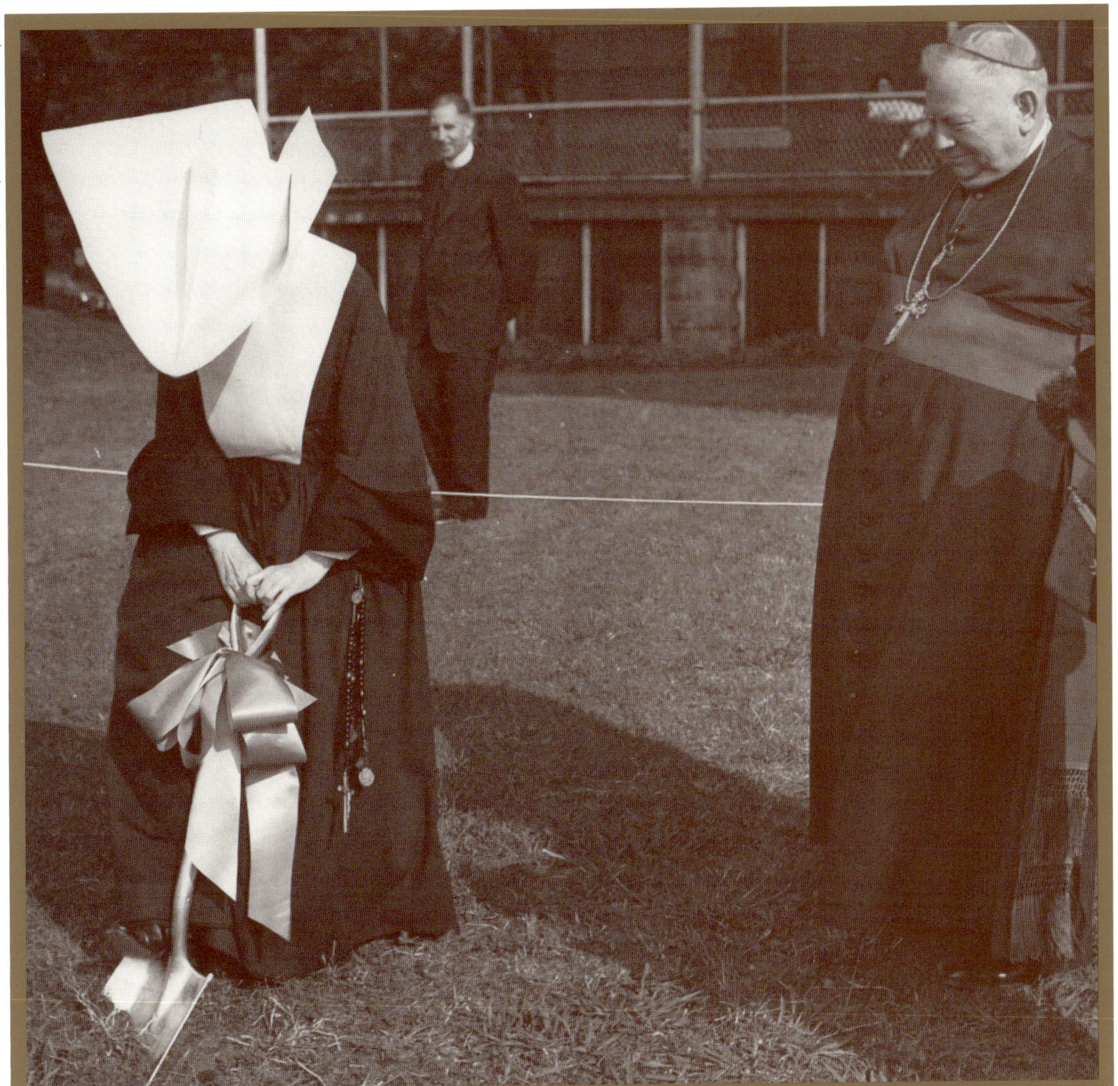

Archives, St. Vincent's Hospital

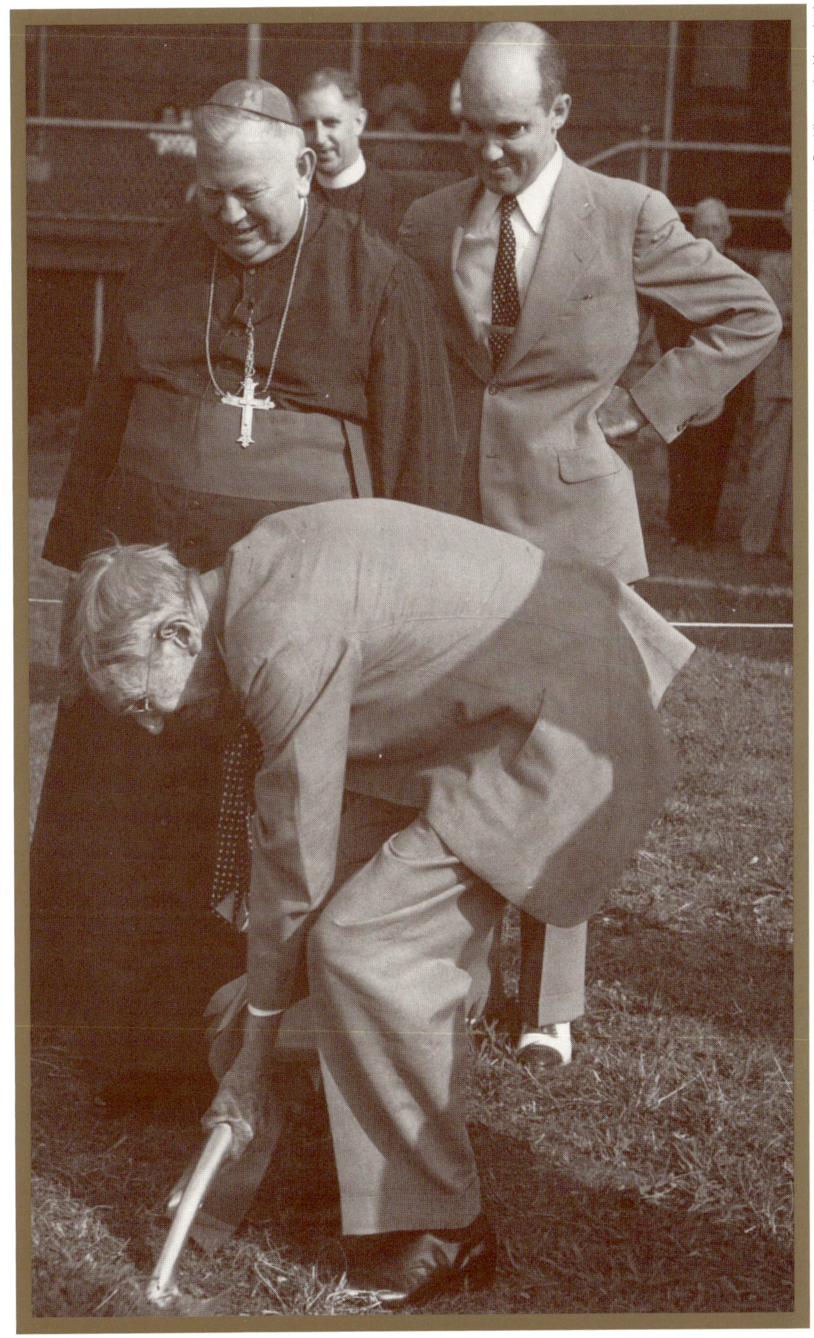

(Above) Sister Mary Alice breaks ground for the new East Wing as Bishop T. J. Toolen looks on. (At Right) Dr. Cunningham Wilson, St. Vincent's first surgeon, also takes part in the ceremony with Dr. Joseph A. Cunningham, head of the medical staff. Dr. Wilson would not live to see the new wing completed. He died later that year, after 64 years of medical service.

Archives, St. Vincent's Hospital

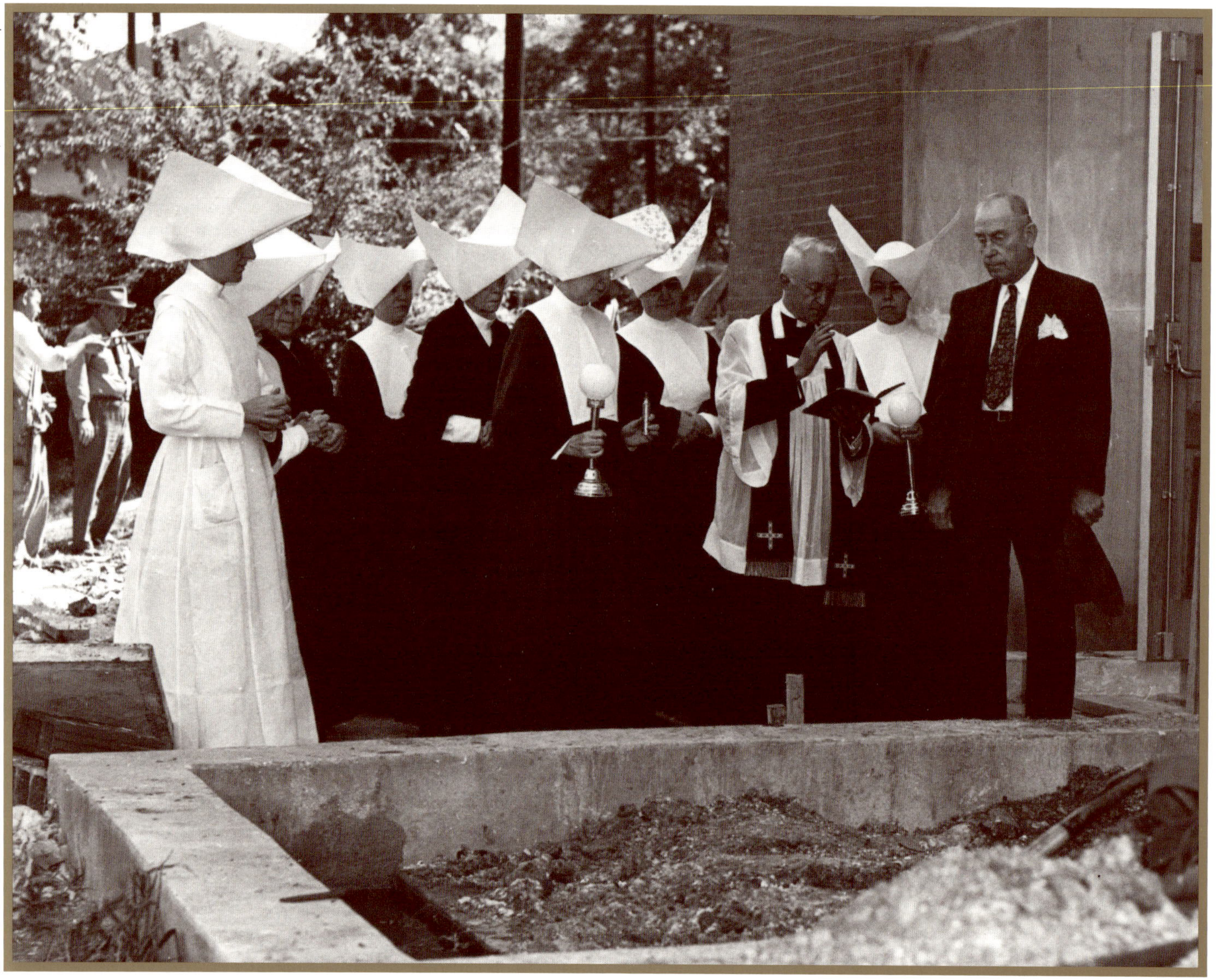

Relocating the grave of Father O'Reilly to the end of the new East Wing

The Industry of Health

Health care, today the dominant industry in Birmingham, made its first large steps during the 1950s. One factor in the growth of the medical industry in Birmingham was the Hill-Burton Act, which had provided federal funds for not-for-profit hospitals and medical centers. In the first three years, the act helped fund more than $9 million of construction in the state, much of which was in Birmingham. More than $300,000 of federal money had gone toward the new East Wing at St. Vincent's.

The University of Alabama's Medical College had moved to Birmingham in the late 1940s, and with aid from Hill-Burton, the complex quickly expanded to include a dental school, the Public Health Building, the Veteran's Hospital and the Crippled Children's Clinic.

The University's medical center soon joined the Birmingham Regional Hospital Council (BRHC), which had formed in 1944 as the Birmingham Hospital Council.

Archives, St. Vincent's Hospital

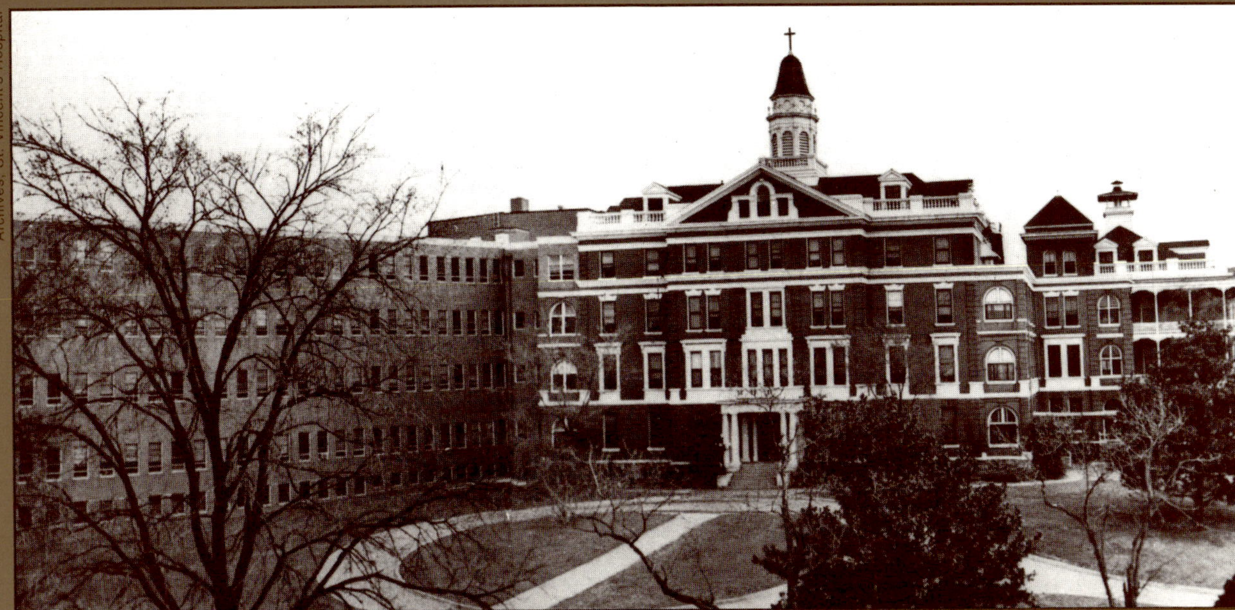

St. Vincent's, with the recently completed East Wing, December 1950

Archives, St. Vincent's Hospital

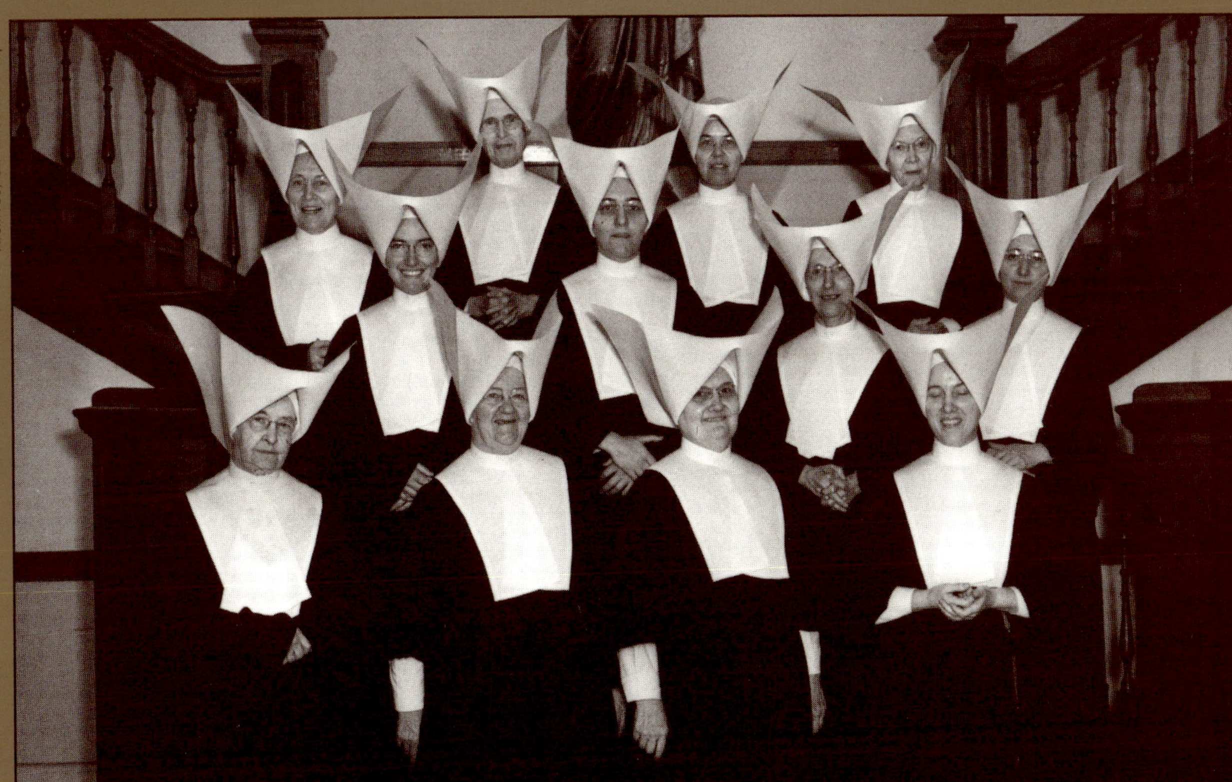

The Daughters of Charity at St. Vincent's, 1950 (left to right): (Top row) Sister Valeria, Sister Monica, Sister Baptista, Sister Bernard; (Middle row) Sister Christine, Sister Mathilda, Sister Vincent, Sister Inez; (Bottom row) Sister Anna, Sister Louise, Sister Mary Thomas, Sister Catherine

SIXTEEN THE BIRMINGHAM NEWS

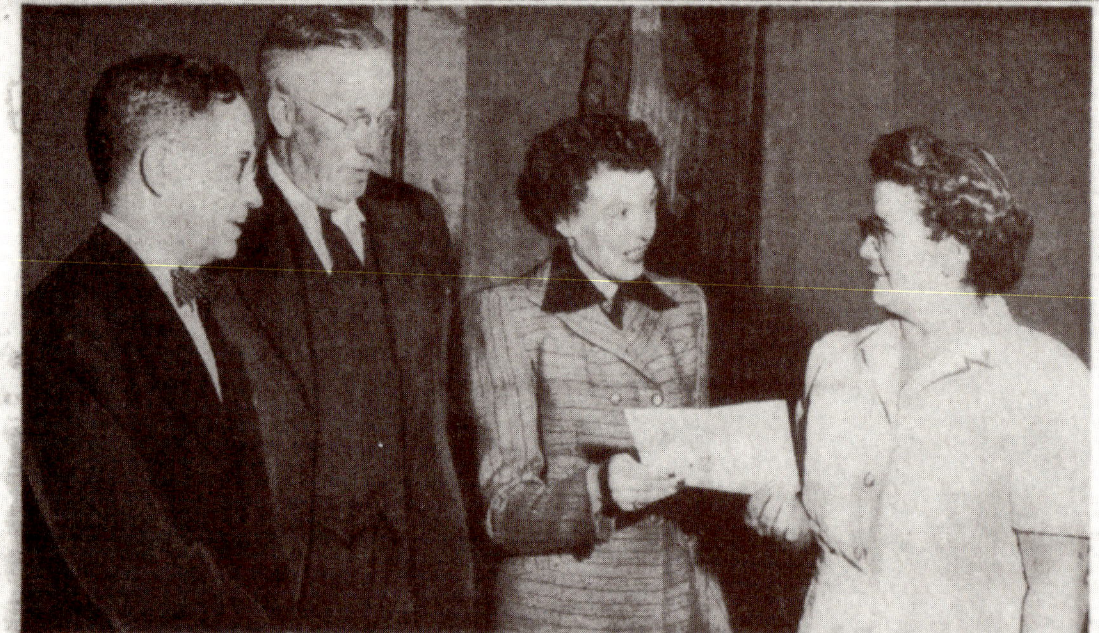

HOSPITAL STAFF CITED—Mrs. Vivian Higgins, right, a member of the kitchen staff at St. Vincent's Hospital, accepts her certificate for completing the Health Department's Food Handling Course from Mrs. Pauline McFarland, course instructor. Forty-one members of the hospital's kitchen and dietician staffs received similar certificates. The course, available to all public eating places, offers instruction in scientific handling of food. Looking on are Dr. C. J. Going, left, assistant superintendent of city schools, and V. J. Douglas, director of vocational education in the school system.

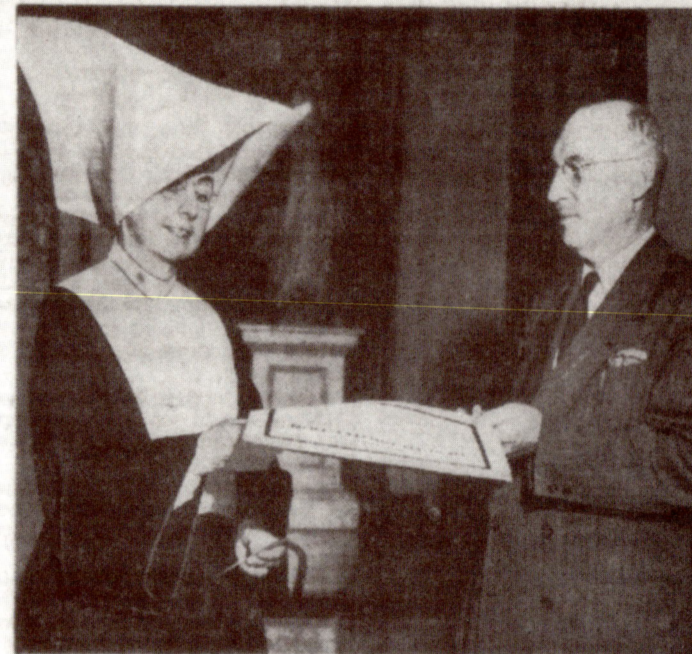

ST. VINCENT'S HONORED—Sister Mary Alice, superintendent of St. Vincent's Hospital, receives a certificate from Dr. George A. Denison, public health officer, signifying that all kitchen and dietician employes had completed the Health Department's Food Handling Course. St. Vincent's was the first hospital in the city and county whose staff completed the course.

St. Vincent's 41-member kitchen and dietitian staff was the first in Jefferson County to complete the Health Department's Food Handling Course, which offered scientific instruction concerning the handling of food.
At left, staff member Vivian Higgins accepts her certificate from Pauline McFarland, the course instructor.
At right are Sister Mary Alice and Public Health Officer Dr. George A. Denison.

St. Vincent's, under the leadership of Sister Servant Marianna Flynn, was among its original 10 member hospitals. Sister Mary Alice McCarthy, who succeeded her as administrator in 1945, became a prominent member of the Council, serving as its secretary in 1950. Sister Lydia Hoffman, who returned to St. Vincent's to replace Sister Catherine Wintz as administrator in 1956, was also a BRHC officer and a guiding force in the organization as it incorporated in 1959. The Council is now a region of the Alabama Hospital Association.

By this time St. Vincent's had already established a blood bank, according to Mrs. Frances Wideman, a lab technologist from the late 1940s into the 1960s. "We had a very active blood bank," she said, "and these were the days before the Red Cross" blood supply system.

"Sister Lydia believed in having the best and strongest medical staff possible," according to Dr. Edwin G. Waldrop, longtime St. Vincent's obstetrician/gynecologist.

Archives, St. Vincent's Hospital

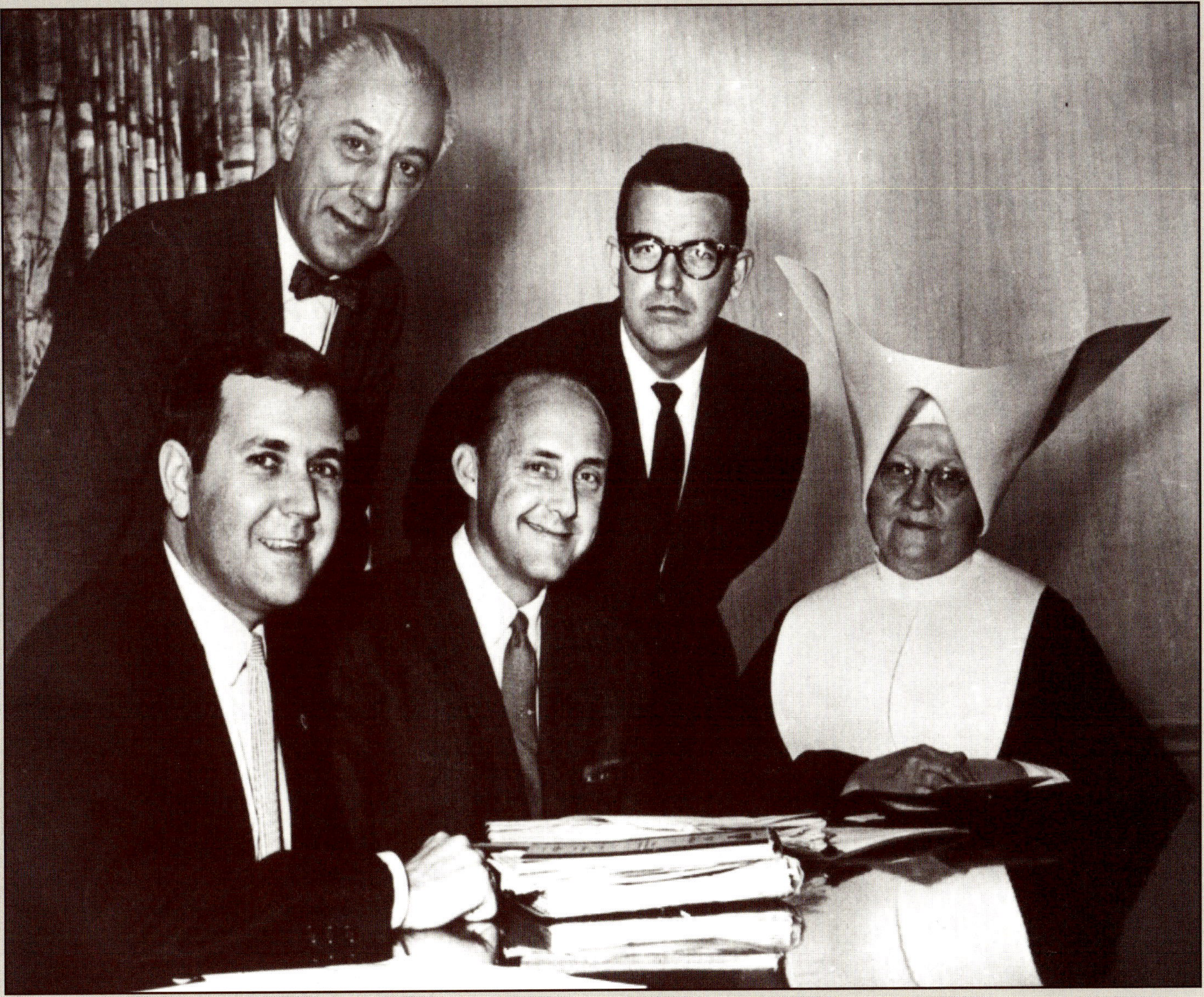

The Birmingham Regional Hospital Council, 1959 (left to right): Roy Vance of Crippled Children's Clinic and Hospital, John Howell of Carraway Methodist Hospital, Millard Johnson of Highland Avenue Baptist Hospital, Bill Thrash of South Highlands Infirmary and Sister Lydia.

Courtesy of Dr. and Mrs. Edwin G. Waldrop

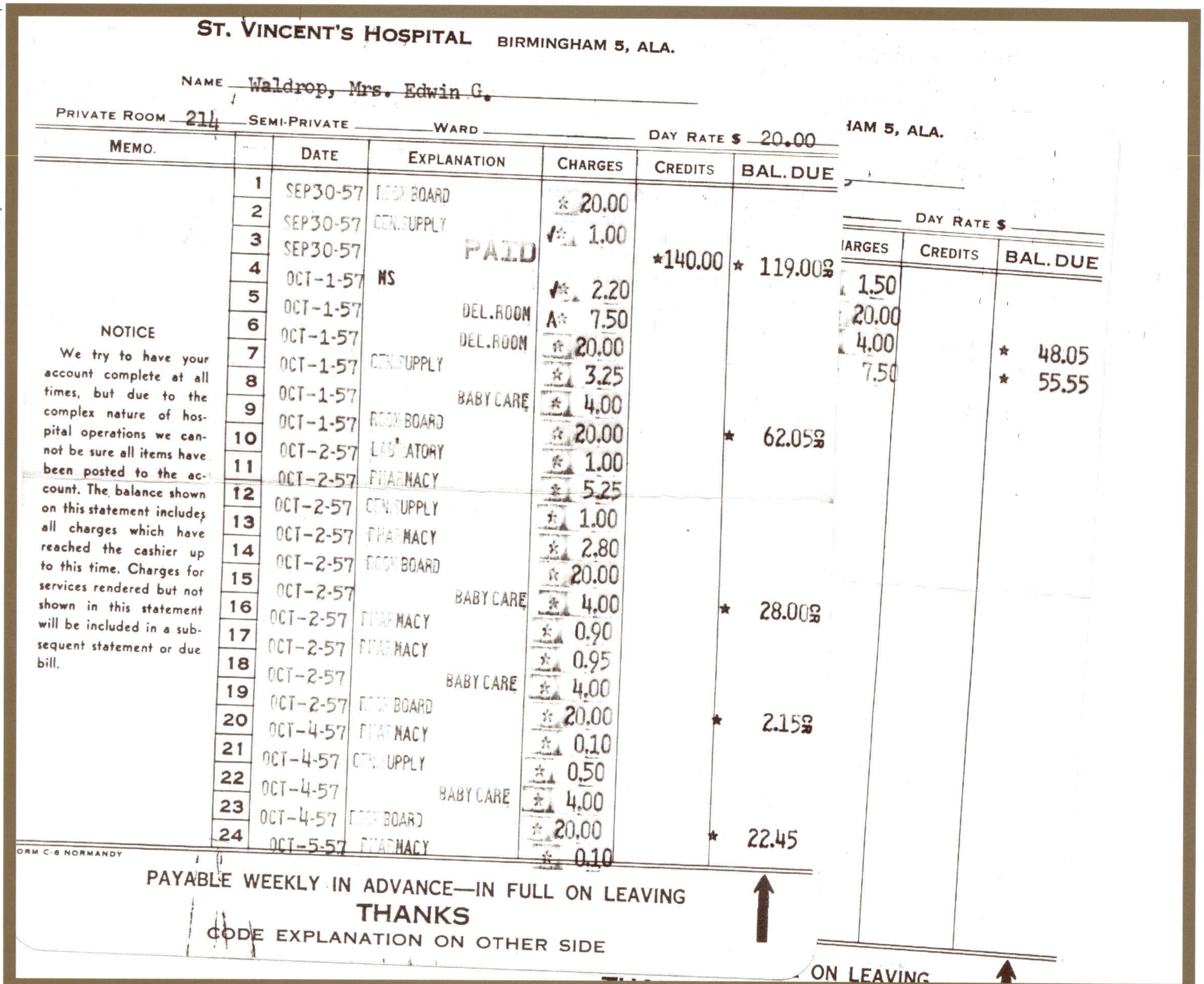

ST. VINCENT'S HOSPITAL BIRMINGHAM 5, ALA.

NAME Waldrop, Mrs. Edwin G.

PRIVATE ROOM 214 SEMI-PRIVATE ____ WARD ____ DAY RATE $ 20.00

MEMO.		DATE	EXPLANATION	CHARGES	CREDITS	BAL. DUE
	1	SEP30-57	ROOM BOARD	★ 20.00		
	2	SEP30-57	CEN.SUPPLY	✓★ 1.00		
	3	SEP30-57	PAID		★140.00	★ 119.00CR
	4	OCT-1-57	MS	✓★ 2.20		
	5	OCT-1-57	DEL.ROOM	A★ 7.50		
	6	OCT-1-57	DEL.ROOM	★ 20.00		
	7	OCT-1-57	CEN.SUPPLY	★ 3.25		
	8	OCT-1-57	BABY CARE	★ 4.00		
	9	OCT-1-57	ROOM BOARD	★ 20.00		★ 62.05CR
	10	OCT-2-57	LAVATORY	★ 1.00		
	11	OCT-2-57	PHARMACY	★ 5.25		
	12	OCT-2-57	CEN.SUPPLY	★ 1.00		
	13	OCT-2-57	PHARMACY	★ 2.80		
	14	OCT-2-57	ROOM BOARD	★ 20.00		
	15	OCT-2-57	BABY CARE	★ 4.00		★ 28.00CR
	16	OCT-2-57	PHARMACY	★ 0.90		
	17	OCT-2-57	PHARMACY	★ 0.95		
	18	OCT-2-57	BABY CARE	★ 4.00		
	19	OCT-2-57	ROOM BOARD	★ 20.00		★ 2.15CR
	20	OCT-4-57	PHARMACY	★ 0.10		
	21	OCT-4-57	CEN.SUPPLY	★ 0.50		
	22	OCT-4-57	BABY CARE	★ 4.00		
	23	OCT-4-57	ROOM BOARD	★ 20.00		★ 22.45
	24	OCT-5-57	PHARMACY	★ 0.10		

NOTICE

We try to have your account complete at all times, but due to the complex nature of hospital operations we cannot be sure all items have been posted to the account. The balance shown on this statement includes all charges which have reached the cashier up to this time. Charges for services rendered but not shown in this statement will be included in a subsequent statement or due bill.

FORM C-6 NORMANDY

PAYABLE WEEKLY IN ADVANCE—IN FULL ON LEAVING

THANKS

CODE EXPLANATION ON OTHER SIDE

HAM 5, ALA.

CHARGES	CREDITS	BAL. DUE
1.50		
20.00		
4.00		★ 48.05
7.50		★ 55.55

ON LEAVING

When Dr. Edwin G. Waldrop's wife gave birth to their first child at St. Vincent's in 1957, the delivery and one-week stay for mother and son cost less than $200.

And this medical staff made consistent contributions to the health care community in Birmingham, among them many by Dr. Waldrop and his staff.

Obstetrics at St. Vincent's had been a priority for years, particularly because most medical insurance at the time paid little or nothing toward the expense of delivering babies. Because it continued to provide services to those in need, St. Vincent's began to deliver a surprisingly large share of Birmingham's babies.

And St. Vincent's obstetrics department was one of the finest, according to Dr. Waldrop, who became chief of the department in the late 1950s.

Obstetricians at St. Vincent's pioneered a number of fetal monitoring techniques in Birmingham, including the first use of Doppler technology to monitor the fetal heartbeat during delivery, the strongest indicator of whether the fetus is in distress. Also, physicians at St. Vincent's were the first in Birmingham to use pH testing of the fetal scalp to make sure there was adequate oxygen flow to the child during delivery.

Courtesy of Dr. William V. Weldon

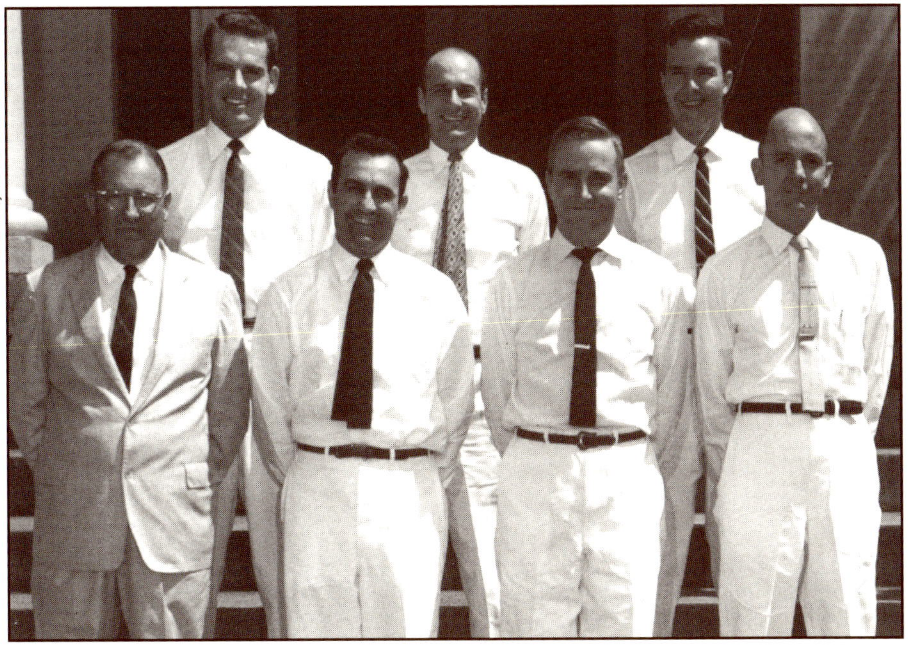

For almost 20 years beginning in 1947, St. Vincent's offered an internship program under the direction of Dr. E. B. Glenn. The Internship Class of 1957 (left to right): (back row) Dr. Jack Lewis, Dr. Ballard Phillips, Dr. William V. Weldon; (front row) Dr. Glenn, Dr. Harold Wilson, Dr. Richard Armbrester and Dr. Luther Cooper.

The First "Emergency Room on Wheels"

The baby had been large, and the new mother was in danger of a hemorrhage. Dr. Edwin Waldrop stayed with her for two hours following the birth, until her condition had stabilized.

Unexpectedly, the mother did begin to bleed in the wee hours of that night in 1955, and her blood pressure dropped "so low they couldn't measure it," according to Dr. Waldrop. As the staff repeatedly revived her, they had to send someone to central supply on numerous occasions for the medicines needed.

The mother's life was saved, and the crisis of that night produced something that has saved many lives since: the "crash cart."

"There wasn't one in Birmingham," Dr. Waldrop said of the portable, self-contained resuscitative unit that is now standard at every hospital. So he began working with the central supply nurse to make a list of items the cart should stock. "She got the carpentry shop to make the cart, essentially an emergency room on wheels," Dr. Waldrop said.

The result was a great advance for health care in Birmingham and maybe the first device of its kind in the world.

In response to the local shortage of medical technologists, Dr. Joseph A. Cunningham formed the School of Medical Technology in 1951.

"At that time we had difficulty finding people trained to do the kind of lab work we needed," Dr. Cunningham said. "It was a national problem."

The school, one of the first of its kind in the country, was small, usually with only three or four students per class, but it produced highly trained and badly needed graduates. "It was an apprenticeship of sorts," said Mrs. Frances D. Wideman, one of the hospital's lab technologists when the program began. "It was really hands on."

The program was influential across the country. "We were instrumental in setting up the medical technology curriculum nationally," Dr. Cunningham said. Students in the program won national awards and had papers published in journals, Mrs. Wideman said.

After the one-year program, graduates went on to take the national board exams. "We never had anyone fail," Mrs. Wideman said.

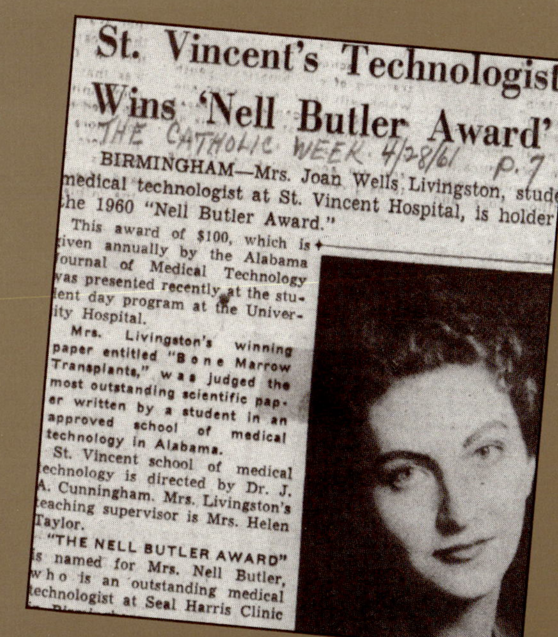

St. Vincent's Technologist Wins 'Nell Butler Award'

THE CATHOLIC WEEK 4/28/61 P. 7

BIRMINGHAM—Mrs. Joan Wells Livingston, stud[ent] medical technologist at St. Vincent Hospital, is holder [of] the 1960 "Nell Butler Award."

This award of $100, which is given annually by the Alabama Journal of Medical Technology was presented recently at the student day program at the University Hospital.

Mrs. Livingston's winning paper entitled "Bone Marrow Transplants," was judged the most outstanding scientific paper written by a student in an approved school of medical technology in Alabama.

St. Vincent school of medical technology is directed by Dr. J. A. Cunningham. Mrs. Livingston's teaching supervisor is Mrs. Helen Taylor.

"THE NELL BUTLER AWARD" is named for Mrs. Nell Butler, who is an outstanding medical technologist at Seal Harris Clinic

A Theatrical Anniversary

July 30, 1959, had marked Sister Lydia's 25th anniversary as a member of the Daughters of Charity. The Solemn High Mass celebrating the event was noted by a newspaper story the next week.

Almost half of Sister Lydia's 25 years had been at Birmingham's St. Vincent's, and her second term had been one of great achievement.

Since she had returned in 1956, the hospital had received full accreditation by the Joint Commission of Hospital Accreditation. The School of Nursing also got full national accreditation during these years, and the School of Medical Technology's accreditation was expanded.

During 1959 St. Vincent's saw 9,949 patients. An additional 5,194 were treated at the Outpatient Clinic.

Physically, the hospital changed as well, with the conversion of an unused hallway into a well-equipped eight-bed recovery room and a renovation of the hospital chapel.

In 1960 Sister Lydia oversaw the $150,000 renovation of the 60-year-old West Wing, which included two "ultra-modern nursing stations." The renovation created 14 new private rooms and four semi-private rooms, "each with its own toilet facilities" and introduced centralized heating and cooling with individual room controls.

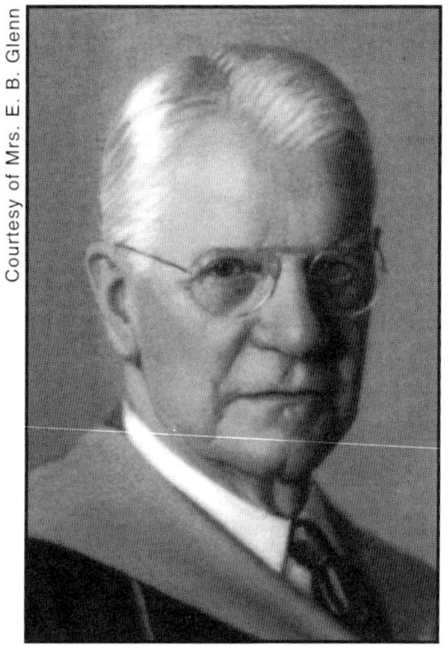

Courtesy of Mrs. E. B. Glenn

Dr. Mason Jr.

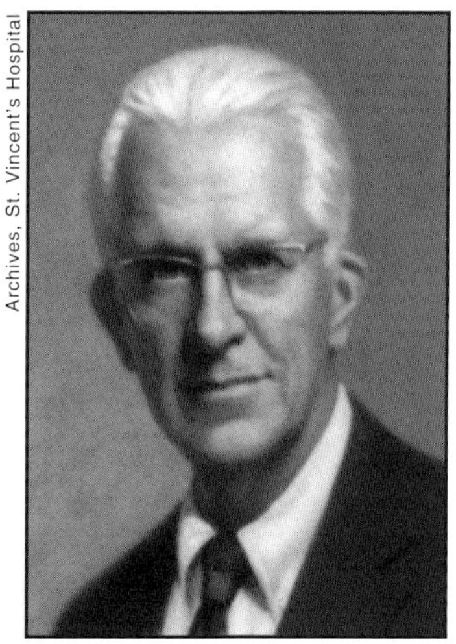

Archives, St. Vincent's Hospital

Dr. Mason III

The Drs. Mason

Dr. James Monroe Mason Jr. finished medical school in 1899 and moved to Birmingham, becoming one of the early members of St. Vincent's surgical staff. One of the pioneers in the advancement of surgery in Birmingham, Dr. Mason made two tours of the most well-known clinics in Europe during the early years of the hospital. Before his retirement in 1941, Dr. Mason had become the foremost vascular surgeon in the State of Alabama.

Dr. Mason served in many leadership roles in his field, including president of the Jefferson County Medical Society, the Medical Association of the State of Alabama, the Birmingham Surgical Society and the Southern Surgical Association. In 1936 he was vice president of the American Surgical Association.

Playing a key role in bringing a four-year medical school to Birmingham, Dr. Mason later became the first head of the Department of Surgery at the new school.

Dr. Mason served in the Army medical corps during World War I, the only time he practiced medicine outside the city of Birmingham. He published 56 articles in medical journals, the last appearing as he approached his 80th birthday.

James Monroe Mason III finished his surgical residency at Johns Hopkins in 1942, then left to serve his country in Europe during World War II. During the invasion of Italy, the younger Dr. Mason received the Bronze Medal and seven battle stars as chief surgeon for a field hospital's mobile surgical team. His pioneering development of field surgical procedures during battle earned him the Legion of Honor.

Following his discharge, Dr. Mason returned to Birmingham to join his father's surgical practice, and in 1945 he joined the staff of St. Vincent's. Dr. Mason was president of the hospital's medical staff in 1951 and became chief of surgery following the death of his father. Dr. Mason III was a tireless supporter of St. Vincent's until his untimely death in 1975.

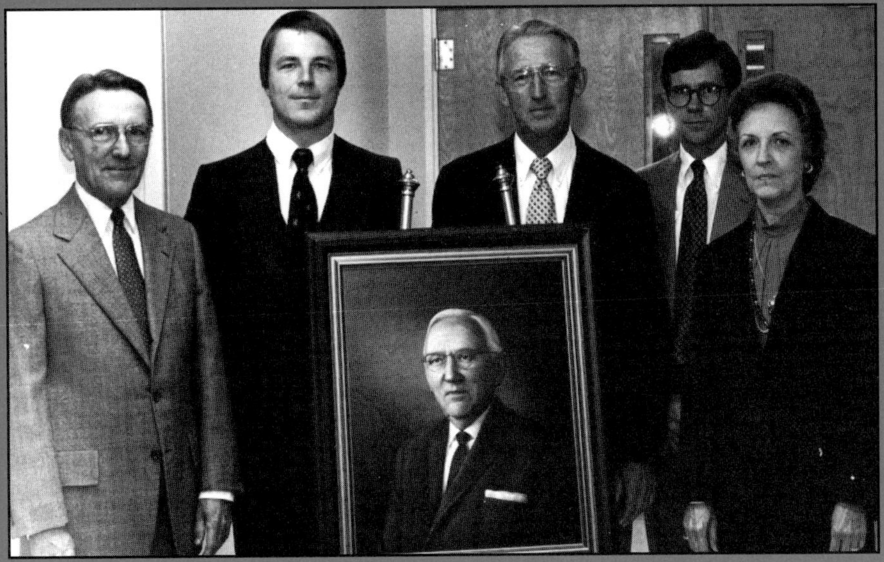

Radiology Department founder Dr. James A. Meadows was honored with a portrait, unveiled in a ceremony on November 9, 1982. Standing left to right: Dr. Edward R. Meadows, artist Danny Moore, Dr. James A. Meadows Jr., Dr. John Paul Mussleman and Dr. Meadows' daughter, Mrs. Guerry M. Denson.

Radiology – A Family Business

The Drs. Meadows and the Drs. Kesmodel

The Sisters' Diaries recorded on July 8, 1903, that an "X-ray tube was ordered today." With this purchase, only seven years after an X-ray unit was first used in a hospital environment, St. Vincent's became a leader in X-ray and imaging services.

In 1915 St. Vincent's became the first hospital in Alabama to have an X-ray Department, and Dr. James A. Meadows, a St. Vincent's intern who had recently completed his residency in radiology at the Mayo Clinic, became Alabama's first radiologist.

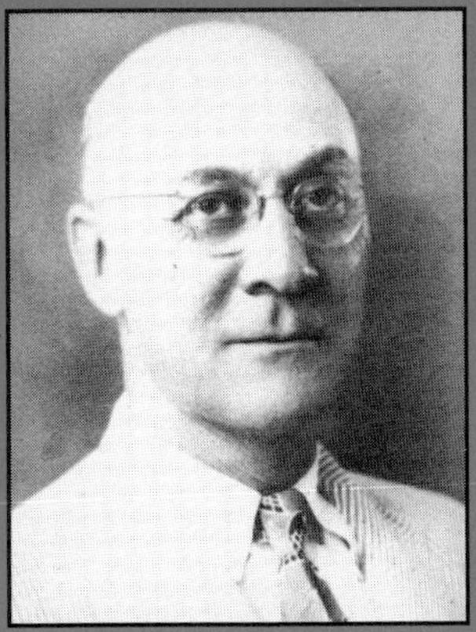

Dr. Kesmodel Sr.

During his 44-year career, Dr. Meadows was also chief of radiology at South Highlands Infirmary, Highland Avenue Baptist Hospital and Children's Hospital. Dr. Meadows instituted the first X-ray therapy and cobalt-60 units in Alabama.

Both of his sons, Dr. James A. Meadows Jr. and Dr. Edward R. Meadows, followed their father into the field of radiology and worked at St. Vincent's.

Major Karl F. Kesmodel Sr. gave up his original desire to become a surgeon because the Army needed radiologists. Like Dr. Meadows, Dr. Kesmodel had interned at St. Vincent's, and after his military career ended, he returned to join Dr. Meadows in 1925.

Dr. Kesmodel Sr. also served at South Highlands, Highland Avenue Baptist and Children's hospitals, as well as at the Hillman Hospital, where he organized the first Tumor Clinic and Registry in Alabama.

Dr. Karl F. Kesmodel Jr. also followed his father into radiology, beginning his practice in the late 1950s with the three Drs. Meadows.

During the 30 years the younger Dr. Kesmodel and Drs. Meadows served St. Vincent's, they worked to keep the hospital at the forefront of rapidly changing technology.

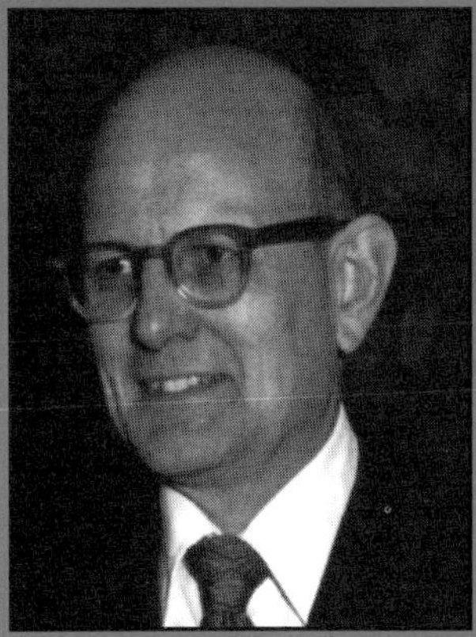

Dr. Kesmodel Jr.

Archives, St. Vincent's Hospital

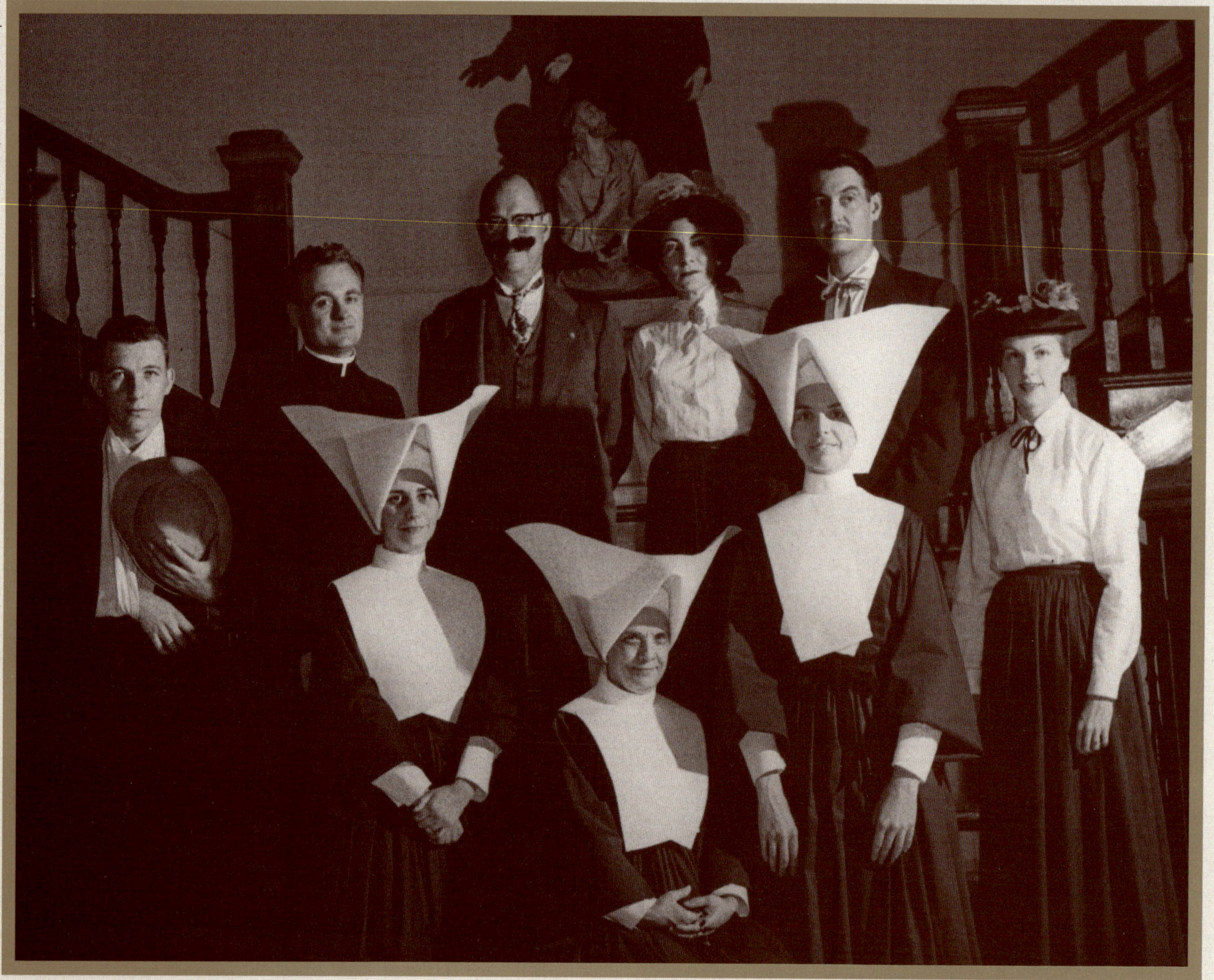

The cast of "The House That Charity Built," a four-act drama celebrating the 60th anniversary in 1960 of the opening of the original hospital (left to right): (back row) Harlan Waldrop as a Miner, J. Larry Sims as Father O'Reilly, Frank Posnich as the Mayor, Madeline Mitchell as Mrs. Wilson and J. T. Alldredge as Dr. Fitzsimmons; (front row) Marjorie King as Sister Anna, Julia Studinka as Sister Chrysostom, Joanne Meadows as Sister Margaret and Gail Lohner as Student Nurse

Archives, St. Vincent's Hospital

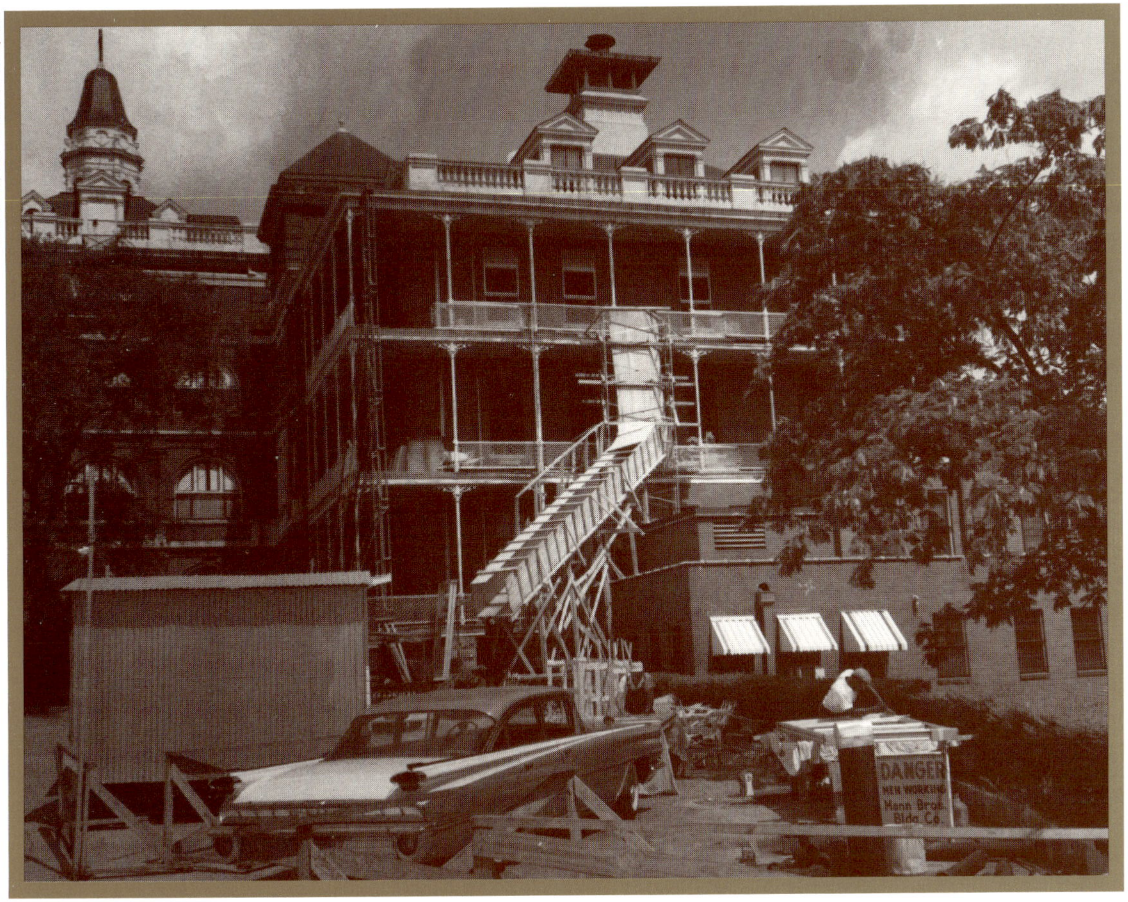

The original West Wing received a $150,000 renovation in 1960.

The hospital's capacity was now 200.

One month before the renovated wing opened, the hospital celebrated the 60th anniversary of the building. In honor of the event, personnel director and avid hospital historian, J. Larry Sims wrote a four-act play "The House That Charity Built." With Sims as Father O'Reilly, the play told the story of the hospital's founding and climaxed with the 1900 opening of the building. The play ran for six performances.

When Sister Lydia departed on September 4, 1961 – five years to the day after beginning her second tour of service in Birmingham – to become administrator at St. Anne's Home in St. Louis, she had taken important steps toward preparation of the hospital for a future that would be rapidly changing.

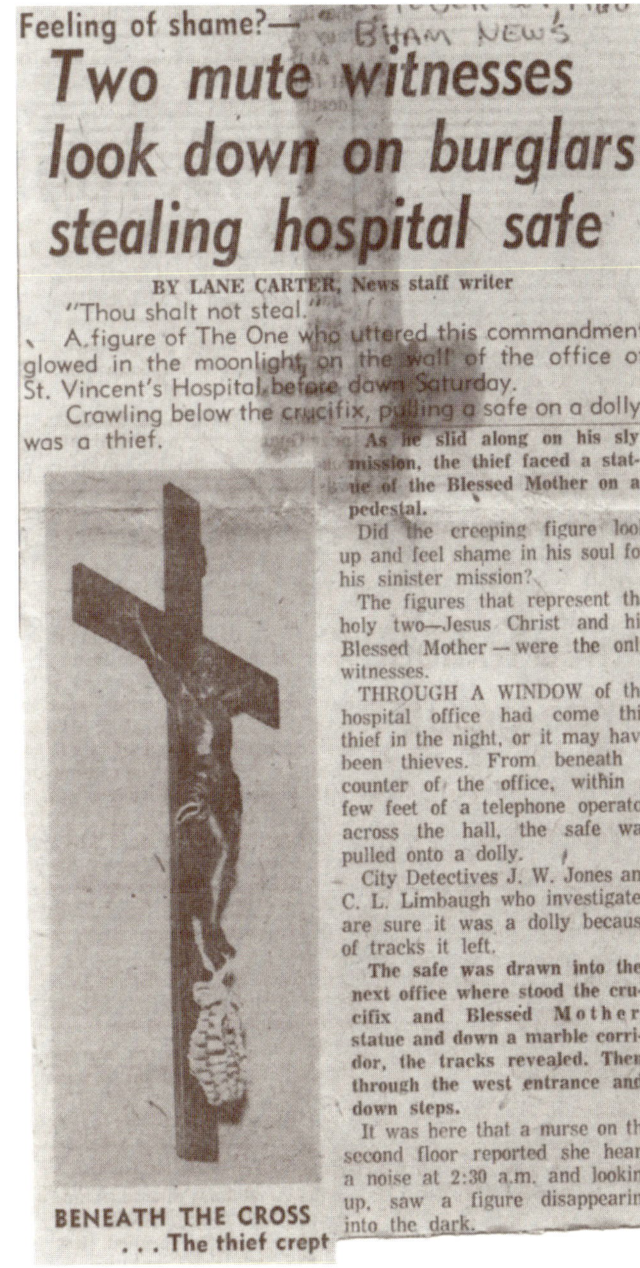

Feeling of shame?—

Two mute witnesses look down on burglars stealing hospital safe

BY LANE CARTER, News staff writer

"Thou shalt not steal."

A figure of The One who uttered this commandment glowed in the moonlight on the wall of the office of St. Vincent's Hospital before dawn Saturday.

Crawling below the crucifix, pulling a safe on a dolly, was a thief.

As he slid along on his sly mission, the thief faced a statue of the Blessed Mother on a pedestal.

Did the creeping figure look up and feel shame in his soul for his sinister mission?

The figures that represent the holy two—Jesus Christ and his Blessed Mother—were the only witnesses.

THROUGH A WINDOW of the hospital office had come this thief in the night, or it may have been thieves. From beneath a counter of the office, within a few feet of a telephone operator across the hall, the safe was pulled onto a dolly.

City Detectives J. W. Jones and C. L. Limbaugh who investigated are sure it was a dolly because of tracks it left.

The safe was drawn into the next office where stood the crucifix and Blessed Mother statue and down a marble corridor, the tracks revealed. Then through the west entrance and down steps.

It was here that a nurse on the second floor reported she heard a noise at 2:30 a.m. and looking up, saw a figure disappearing into the dark.

BENEATH THE CROSS . . . The thief crept

On October 29, 1960, Sister Mary David discovered the theft of the hospital safe, which had been rolled out the front door on a dolly. In his escape, as The Birmingham News wrote, "the thief faced a statue of the Blessed Mother...Did the creeping figure look up and feel shame...?"

Nursing School Student Life

During the 1950s the Nursing School grew from its smallest enrollment since its founding to a highly acclaimed program with a thriving social life for its students.

When the decade started, there were only six graduates, but by 1959 the school was regularly graduating classes of 15 or more nurses.

The Nursing School routinely included students from all parts of Alabama and many other states as well. In 1957 six different states were represented by members of the student body.

In addition to a basketball team (complete with cheerleaders), the students chose one girl to represent the class as Miss St. Vincent's, who led the dancing at the nurses' Spring Ball with the doctor the girls voted as their "favorite." And in 1957, student nurses were for the first time allowed to live off the hospital campus.

During these years, the program was affiliated with St. Bernard's College in Cullman, and students attended classes there three days a week.

The program received accreditation in 1957 from the National League of Nursing.

Courtesy of Dr. Walter C. McCoy

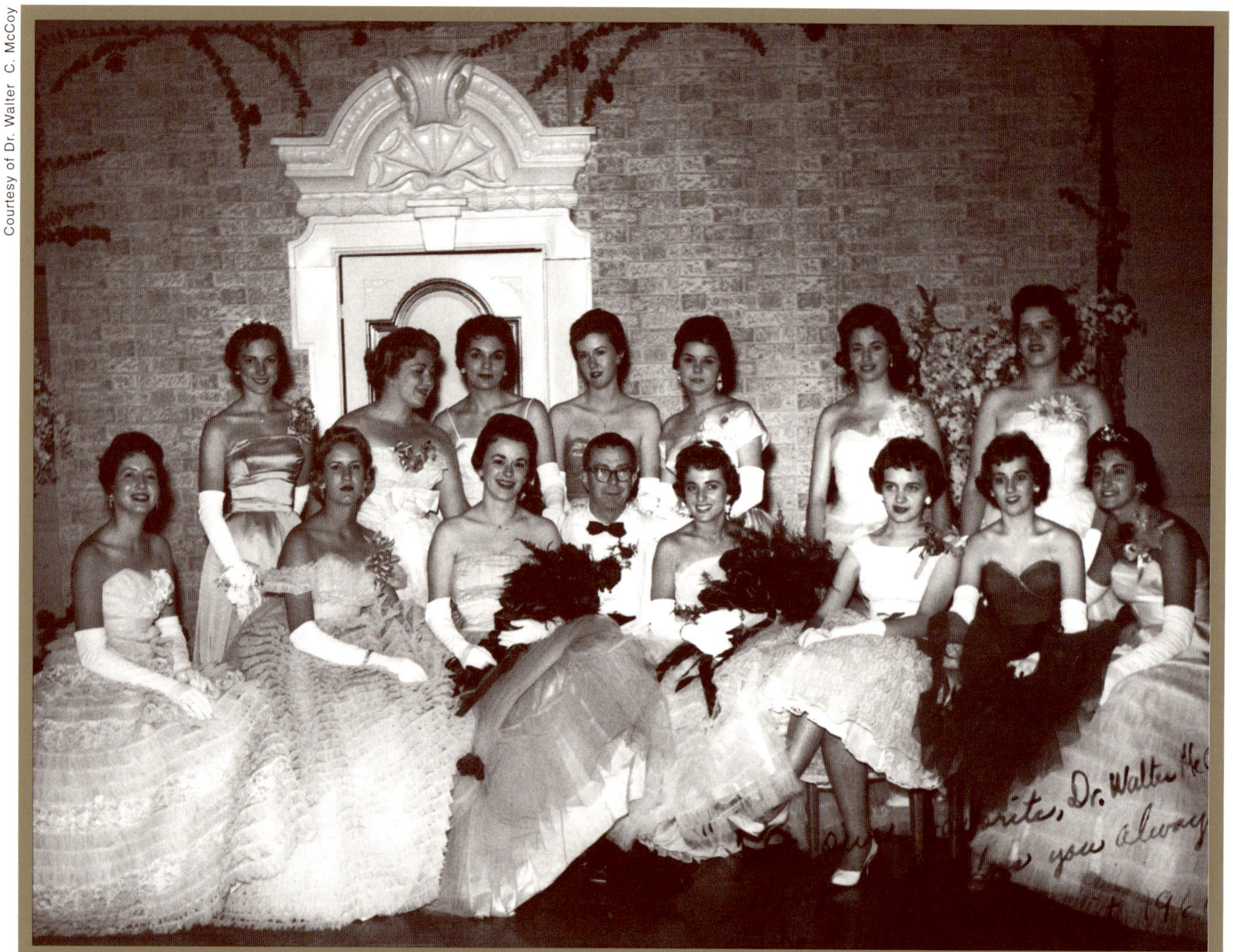

The Class of 1960 at the Spring Ball, with their "favorite," Dr. Walter McCoy

Archives, St. Vincent's Hospital

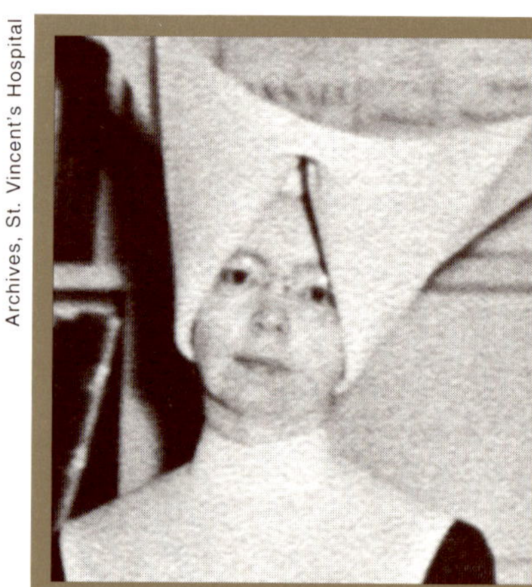

Sister Mary Agnes Tehan, School of Nursing Director

St. Vincent School of Nursing beauties in the 1959 Veterans Day parade

Photos: Archives, St. Vincent's Hospital

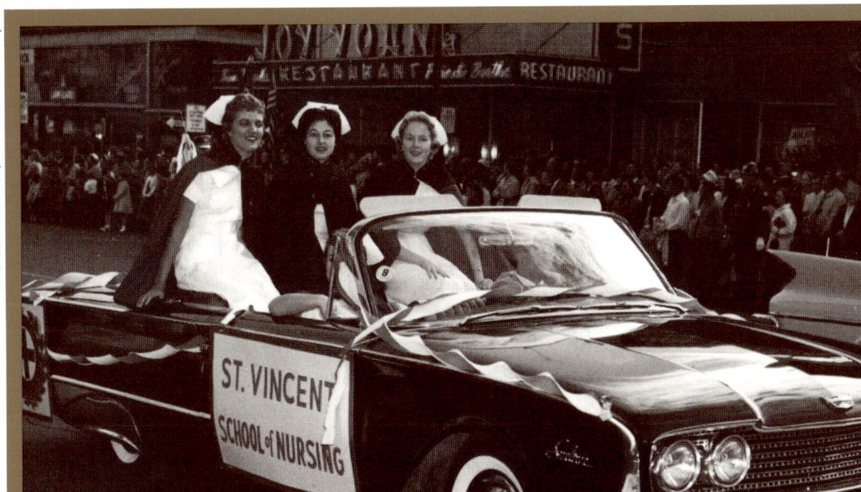

Graduation, circa 1960

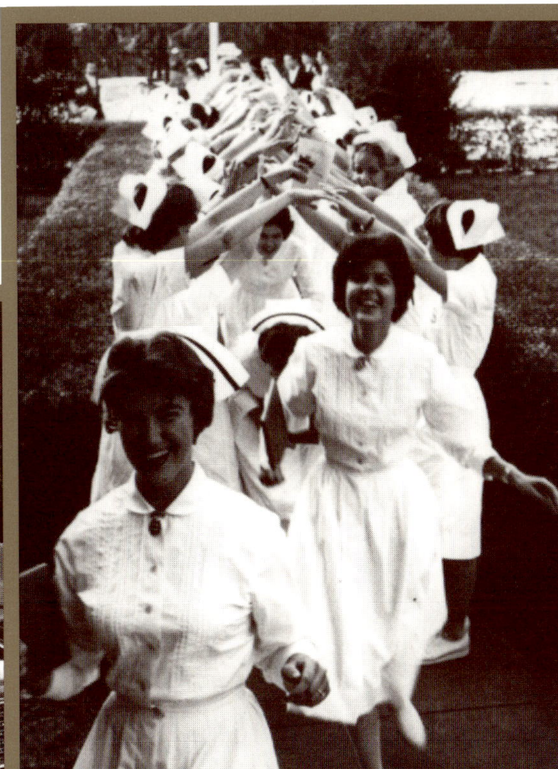

The "Cullman Bus," acquired in 1959

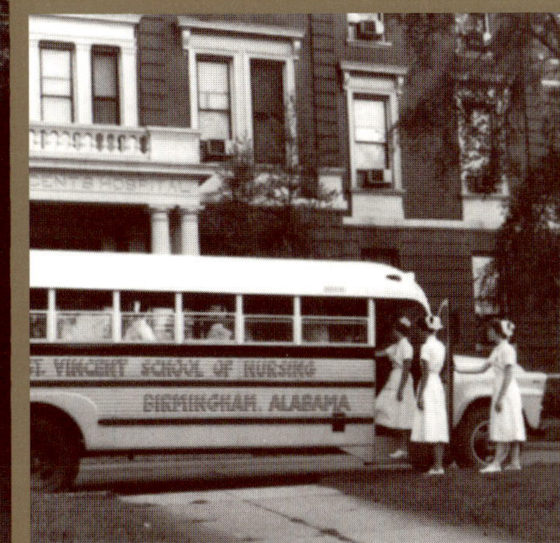

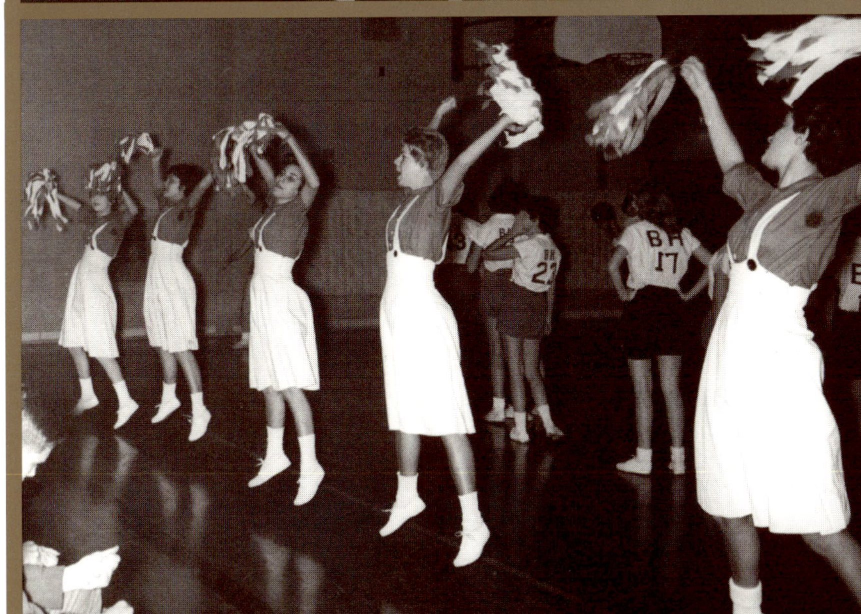

School of Nursing basketball game, 1960

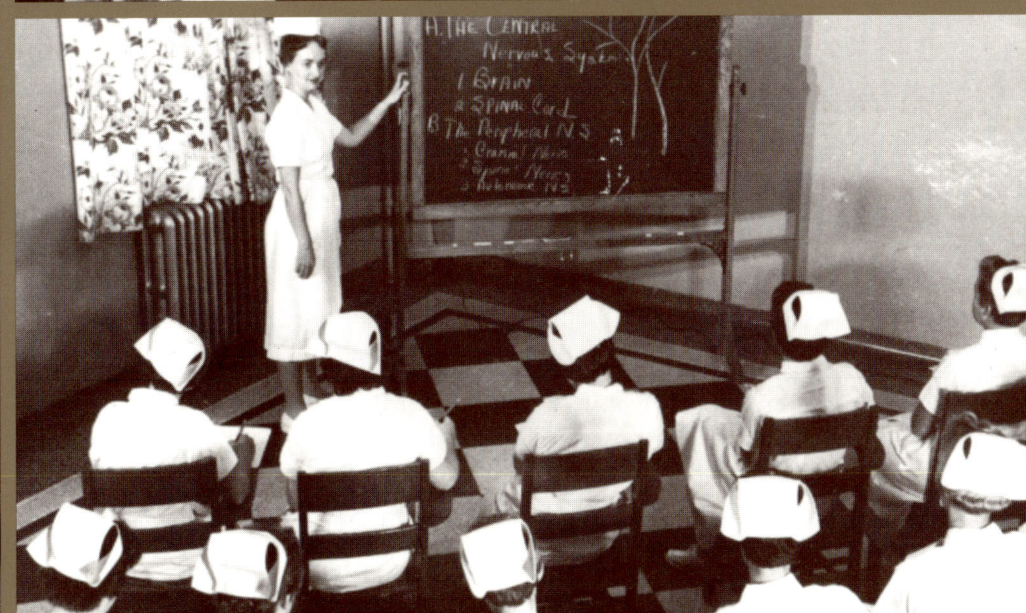

In the classroom, circa 1958

CHAPTER SIX

Winds of Change

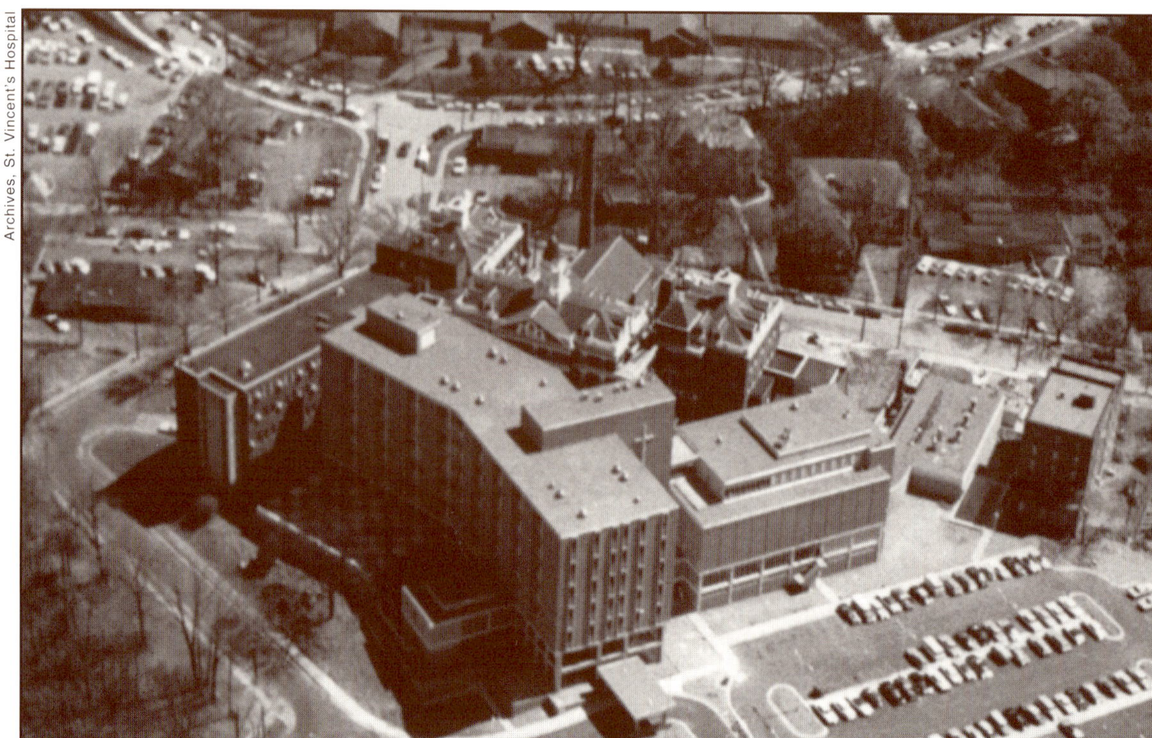

Archives, St. Vincent's Hospital

The new hospital stands near completion as the old one awaits demolition, 1972.

Change was in the air everywhere in the 1960s.

The social changes that were sweeping the country during these years were felt hard in Birmingham, as racial unrest made national headlines and the city's major industry faced a slump and increased foreign competition.

The 1960s began with Birmingham citizens voting to change its form of government from a commission structure to a mayor/council form. But when City Commissioner Eugene "Bull" Connor was defeated in the elections of 1963, he and the other commissioners refused to vacate their offices.

As a focal point in the national Civil Rights Movement, the city reeled from protests, violence and thousands of arrests.

The Times They Were a Changin'... *And So Were the Habits*

After three centuries, the Daughters of Charity underwent a significant change in 1964 as they gave up their signature cornettes.

The new habit was one piece and six inches shorter than the previous one. A blue coif covering a white headdress replaced the cornette.

The new, more practical habit made almost any activity easier for the Sisters of St. Vincent's (especially driving an automobile).

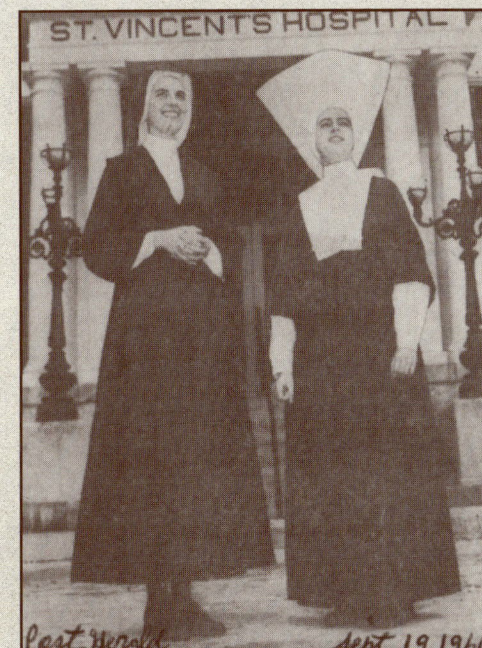

CHANGE OF HABIT—The Daughters of St. Vin cent de Paul will change to the new habit shown o the left. The old is pictured on the right. Showin the habits are Sister Vincentia, left, instructor of th School of Nursing and Sister Rita Irene, St. Thoma Home on the Hill.

After 3 Centuries—

Sisters Are Ready For Habit Change

The St. Vincent's Hospital Auxiliary

The St. Vincent's Auxiliary was formed on February 28, 1963, with 17 members and Mrs. Bonnie G. Chew as its the first president.

The group began by volunteering in the Admitting Office and with the distribution of mail to the patients. The group quickly added new departments and grew rapidly.

By the end of its first summer, the group had 27 members.

The first director of the Auxiliary, Zuma Elgin Brentnall, served the group for 30 years.

"St. Vincent's was the most wonderful place to run an auxiliary," she said. "Everyone wanted volunteers, and we were so fortunate that we had the best volunteers."

The Auxiliary also became an effective fundraising group, purchasing an electro-encephalograph machine for the hospital in only its second year.

During the next few years the Auxiliary furnished waiting rooms, bought color televisions and held fundraising events to contribute to hospital building efforts.

Since its founding, the Auxiliary has raised more than $1.5 million for the hospital, including a large contribution toward the construction of the new West Wing.

Now serving more than 30 departments at St. Vincent's, the Auxiliary has a "diverse group of 300 volunteers," including 193 volunteers with active assignments and 44 life members, according to the current manager of volunteer services.

"We have everything from college students and small business owners to retired physicians and former corporate CEOs," she said.

St. Vincent's Auxiliary Presidents

1963-65	Mrs. Bonnie G. Chew
1965	Mrs. Tom Flanigan
1965-67	Mrs. Milton Collins
1967-68	Mrs. David McCoy
1968-70	Mrs. Margaret C. Hillhouse
1970-71	Mrs. Charles Moses
1971-72	Mrs. Robert Baker
1972-73	Mrs. Hugh M. Smith
1973-74	Miss Jane Lamkin
1974-76	Mrs. J. E. Abbott
1976-78	Mrs. Coleman Kennedy
1978-80	Mrs. Hugh M. Smith
1980-82	Mrs. Patricia B. Jones
1982-84	Mrs. J. Stanley Mackin
1984-86	Mrs. Edward A. Karl
1986-88	Mrs. J. K. Weed
1988-90	Mrs. Herbert J. Loerch
1990-92	Mrs. J. E. McKinnon
1992	Mrs. J. H. Springrose
1993-94	Mrs. John R. Lewis
1994-96	Mr. John W. Higgenbotham
1996-98	Mrs. Hutch Cole

Bluebirds Cheer Spirits Of St. Vincent Patients

BY ROBERT SAOINSOT

Patient morale is running high at St. Vincent Hospital because of 110 Bluebirds flitting around the halls

A patient, Dr. David McCoy, said, "They are the finest organization of all volunteer groups. You couldn't find a better group anywhere in the U. S.

Teen Volunteers

The "Blue Birds of happiness" were St. Vincent's first teen volunteer group, beginning in the mid-1950s.

The all-female organization gave their time to help out the hospital staff and "cheer up" the patients, according to a newspaper feature story.

Under the guidance of Sister Felicita, the group's membership had grown to 200 by 1960, with almost every school in the Birmingham area represented by members.

A *Birmingham News* reporter wrote the following in 1969 about the Blue Birds after his 8-year-old daughter's stay at St. Vincent's:

"We came away with a fresh, new conviction – that today's teenagers are simply great...I think the future is in good hands."

Today the spirit of youth volunteerism thrives through the 60 young men and women of St. Vincent's Teen Volunteers organization.

Years of Progress

In health care, outside parties became dominant sources of revenue, as health insurance plans became broader and Medicare made the government responsible for many hospital costs for thousands of people. Birmingham, for many years a city with inadequate health care, became a city with no fewer than 12 hospitals, and the University Hospital medical center completed a number of large expansions. "Competition" for paying patients increased.

For all the bad publicity it received, Birmingham adapted quickly in the next few years. The city's outlook changed as it rapidly became racially integrated, elected two blacks and two women to the city council, and began to diversify its economy to include jobs in finished goods, services, research and health care. Birmingham changed its look as a building boom brought seven new high-rises that reshaped the city's skyline.

For St. Vincent's, the 1960s were times of uncertainty, but as it was for Birmingham, it was ultimately a time of great progress. This was a decade when St. Vincent's also took stock of itself, recommitted itself to its mission, and moved forward without looking back.

Archives, St. Vincent's Hospital

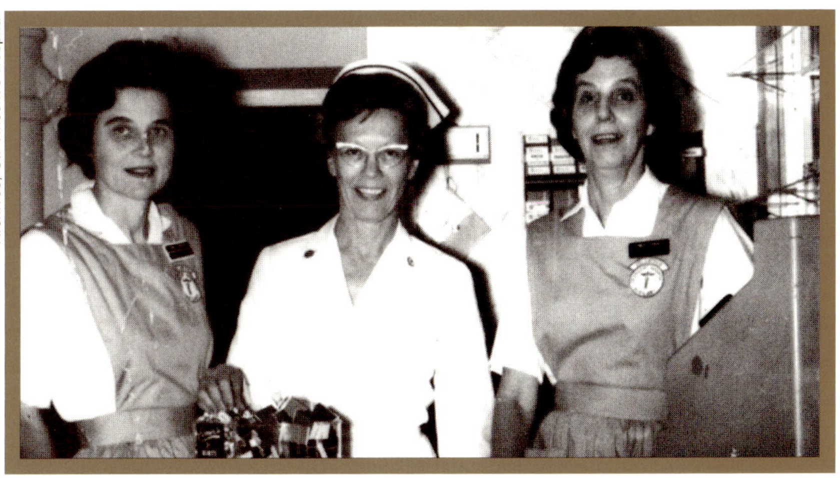

In a closet next to the staircase, St. Vincent's Auxiliary opened "Le Shoppe" in January of 1964. Above are (left to right) Mrs. Lillian Ann Moses, Zuma Elgin and Mrs. Bonnie (Mary) Chew.

In 1965 the group began sending holiday season newborns home in handmade, decorated, holiday stockings, a tradition that continues today. At near right Mrs. Glenn Blankenship holds daughter Cynthia Leigh, and at far right Mrs. Allison H. Stanton holds son Alan Leslie.

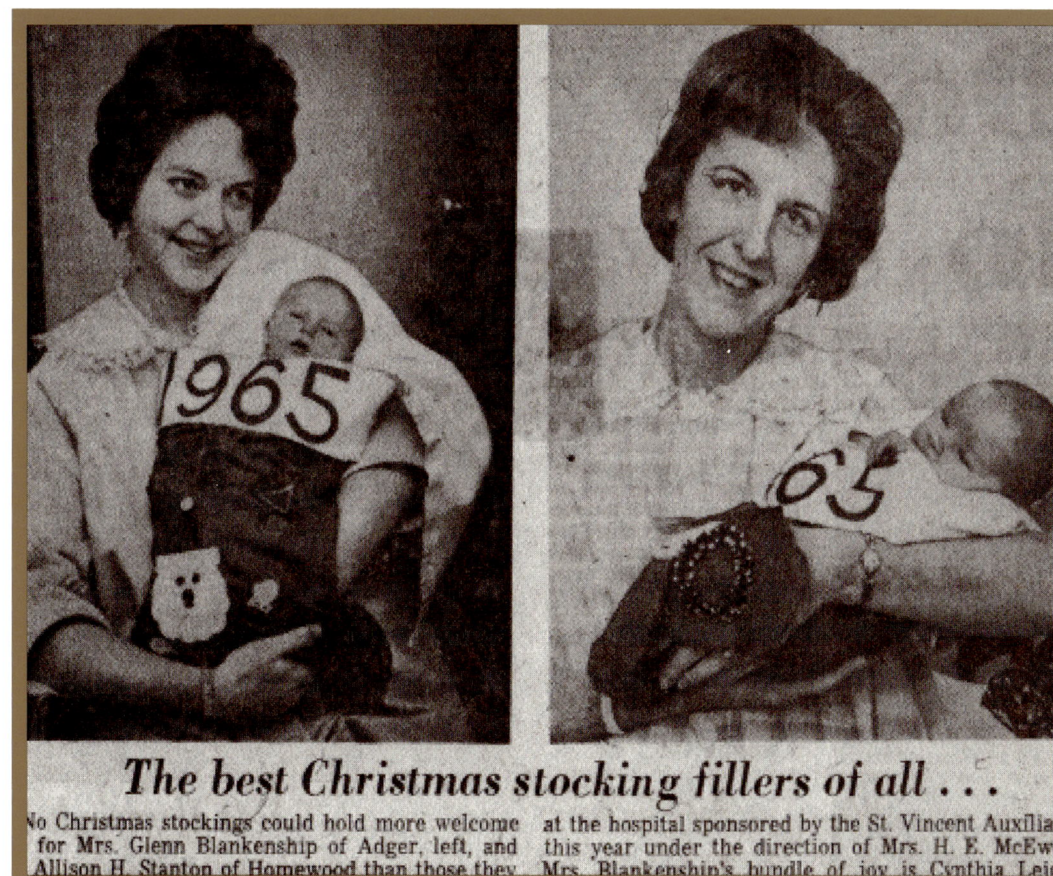

The best Christmas stocking fillers of all . . .

No Christmas stockings could hold more welcome for Mrs. Glenn Blankenship of Adger, left, and Allison H. Stanton of Homewood than those they at the hospital sponsored by the St. Vincent Auxilia this year under the direction of Mrs. H. E. McEw Mrs. Blankenship's bundle of joy is Cynthia Lei

Leaving Mount St. Vincent's?

When Sister Carlos McDonnell arrived to become administrator of St. Vincent's in 1961, she found a facility whose mission was becoming increasingly unclear and more challenging.

Rumors had floated around for the past few years that the hospital was going to be closed. In fact, when Sister Carlos arrived, she thought her mission would include shutting down St. Vincent's.

But what were the alternatives? The structure completed in 1900 was certainly now outdated. Sister Carlos told a newspaper that the hospital was "crowded all the time," and medical/surgical-bed occupancy was running close to capacity. Costs were unnecessarily high because the obsolete nursing units required larger numbers of employees than those of more modern facilities. And Sister Carlos lamented that the aging grand structure wasn't even "fire-resistant."

The once "unpopulated" area around the hospital was now a bustling and crowded neighborhood that left St. Vincent's almost no room for significant expansion. And the health care environment in Birmingham was changing so fast that definitive action would be required to make St. Vincent's future secure.

The University Hospital complex was growing rapidly, including the construction of Children's Hospital, which precipitated St. Vincent's decision to give up acute pediatrics. The Baptists were beginning

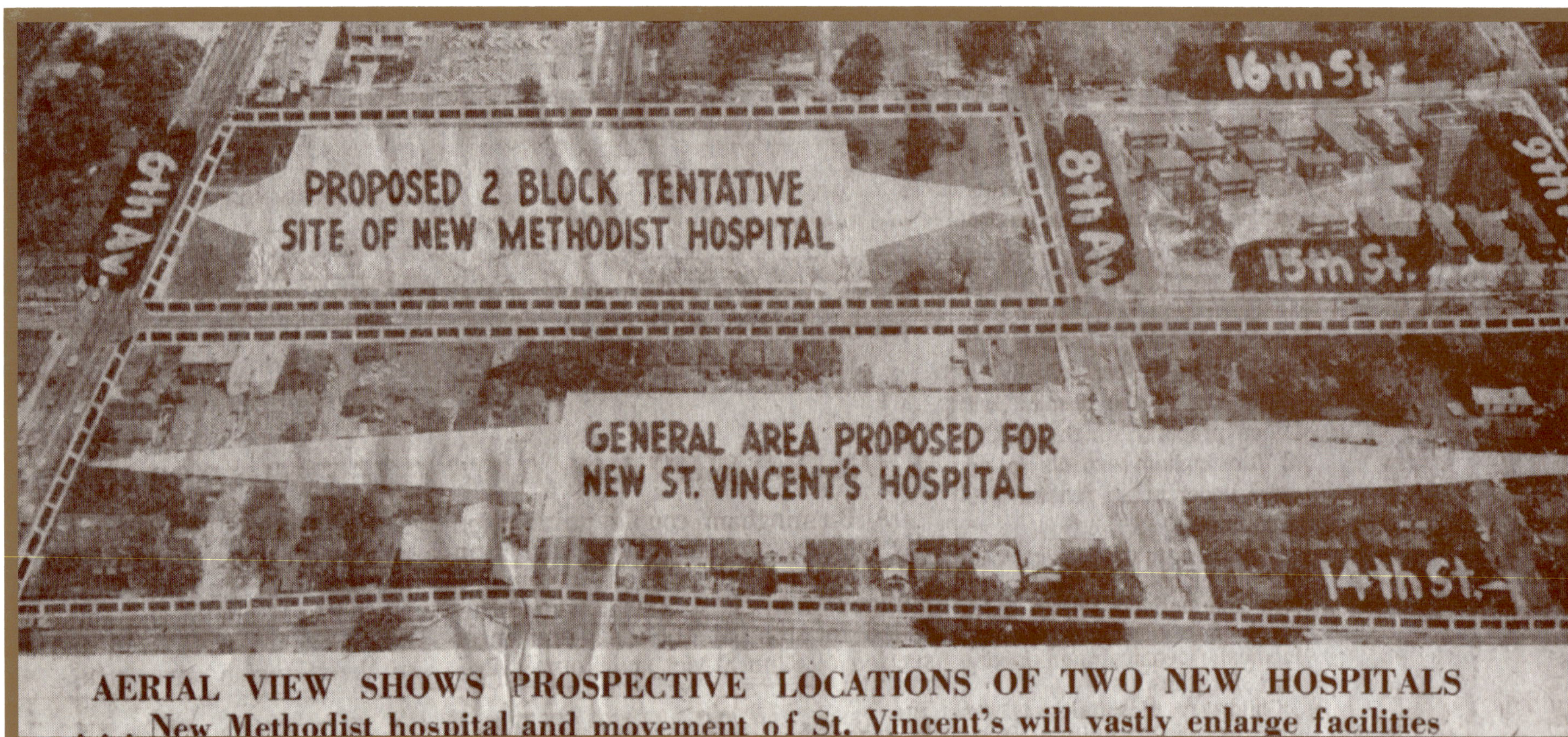

This 1965 newspaper article illustrated the site near the University Hospital Medical Center where St. Vincent's proposed the construction of an eight-story, 350-bed hospital.

efforts to expand West End Hospital and were putting together a plan for a hospital in Shades Valley. The Methodists, as well, began discussions to build a new hospital.

On top of this, bids had been let in 1962 for the proposed Red Mountain Expressway, for which the State of Alabama acquired more than two acres of St. Vincent's property, almost one-fourth of all the hospital owned. Any expansion on this site seemed impossible.

It seemed that the only solution was to move the hospital. Sister Carlos began to look at new property, including the Ramsay High School property, and the Hillcrest Country Club on Oxmoor Road near Greensprings Avenue, as well as a piece of land "over the mountain" that would later become the Mountain Brook Office Park complex. There were also informal discussions with the city about acquiring the hospital.

But none of these seemed to be the appropriate solution.

Envisioning that escalating health care costs would require greater cooperation among all hospitals, Sister Carlos took bold action.

In early 1965 Sister Carlos announced that St. Vincent's would

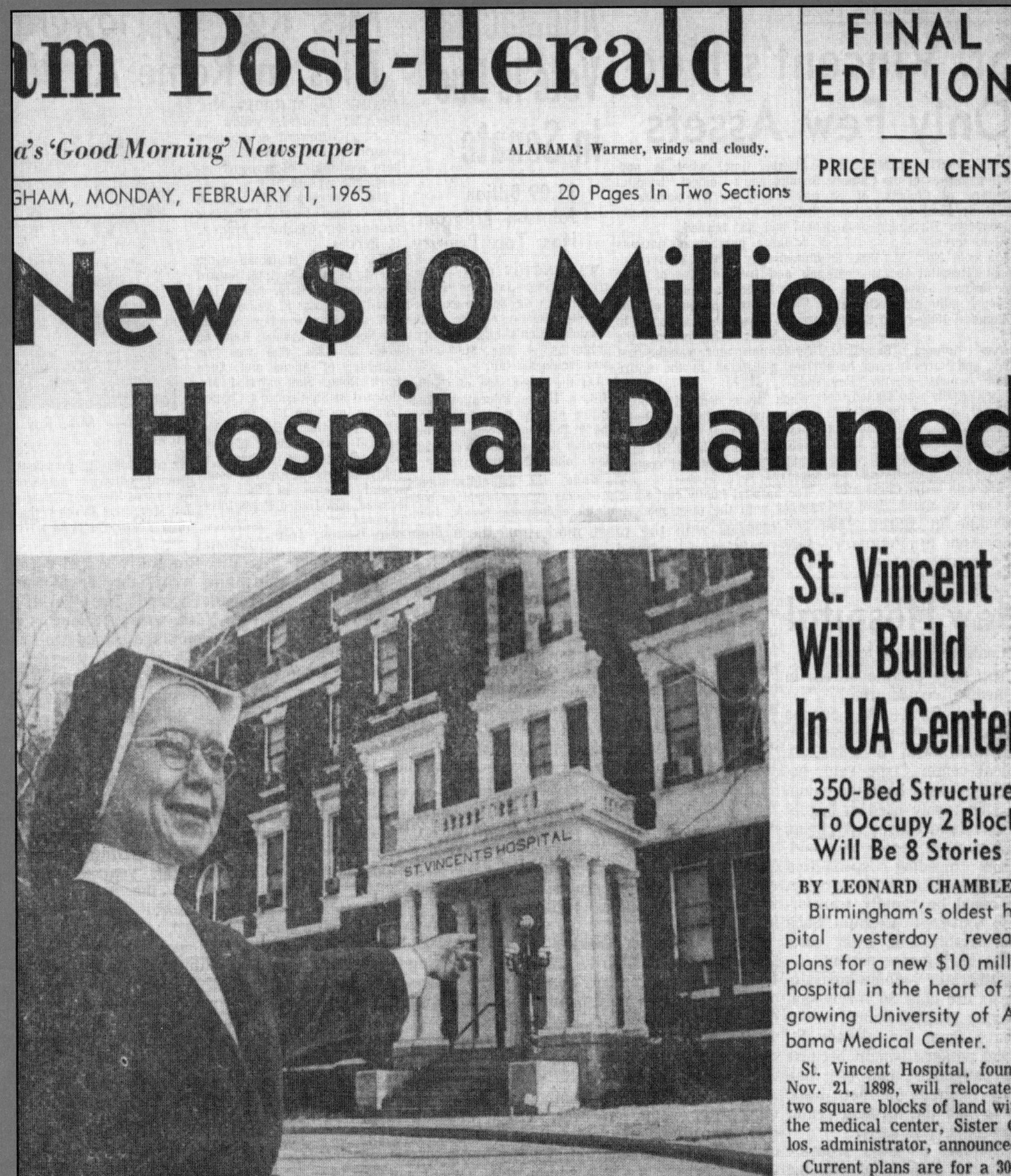

...m Post-Herald

...a's 'Good Morning' Newspaper

ALABAMA: Warmer, windy and cloudy.

FINAL EDITION

PRICE TEN CENTS

...GHAM, MONDAY, FEBRUARY 1, 1965

20 Pages In Two Sections

New $10 Million Hospital Planned

St. Vincent Will Build In UA Center

350-Bed Structure To Occupy 2 Blocks Will Be 8 Stories

BY LEONARD CHAMBLEE...

Birmingham's oldest ho... pital yesterday reveale... plans for a new $10 milli... hospital in the heart of t... growing University of Al... bama Medical Center.

St. Vincent Hospital, found... Nov. 21, 1898, will relocate ... two square blocks of land with... the medical center, Sister Ca... los, administrator, announced.

Current plans are for a 300...

The plan Sister Carlos unveiled to build a new St. Vincent's in the University of Alabama Medical Center complex was later abandoned.

In the News

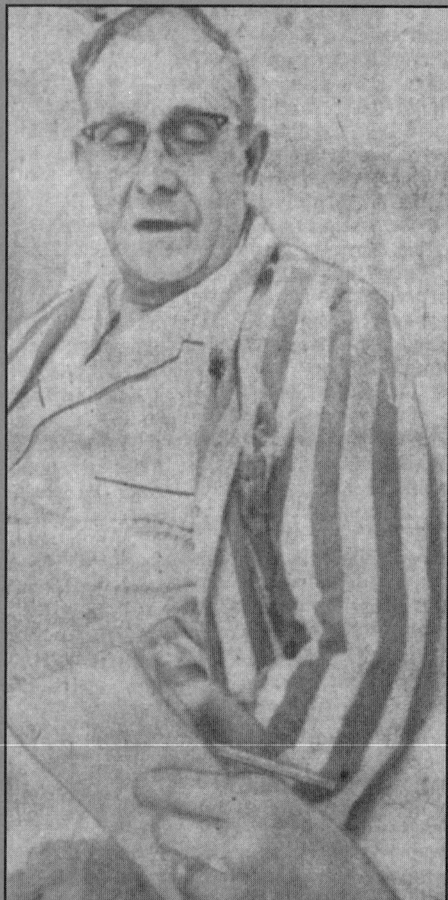

Mayor Albert Boutwell being interviewed after his appendectomy at St. Vincent's

Some things changed, some stayed the same, and some gave small glimpses into the future. From the pages of *The Birmingham News* and Birmingham *Post-Herald* of the 1960s:

On September 2, 1962, the impending construction was announced of Birmingham Cabana, a $3.25 million, 240-room "luxury motor hotel." The 11-story facility, opened as the Parliament House and located on 20th Street between Fourth and Fifth Avenues South, would be the largest motor hotel in Alabama and one of the largest in the Southeast.

Baby boomers were expected to cause overcrowding in the 35 schools of Jefferson County, reported *The Birmingham News* in the fall of 1962. Census figures reported 164,264 people between the ages of 6 and 20, an increase of almost 12,000 in four years.

Former Birmingham City Commissioner Eugene Connor defeated incumbent Jack Owen to take the Democratic nomination for Alabama Public Service Commission president on June 2, 1964.

In June 1964 the U.S. Supreme Court invalidated the state's apportionment of Alabama Senate and House of Representatives members, ordering the state to follow a formula of one state senator for every 93,335 people and one house member for every 30,818. At the time, the state's three largest counties had only one senator each, although they accounted for half of Alabama's population.

Mayor Albert Boutwell suffered an attack of appendicitis on Februrary 25, 1964, and underwent surgery at St. Vincent's the next day. Amid the flood of flowers and get-well cards, the mayor continued to do paperwork during his nine-day hospital stay.

Birmingham's new corps of 32 female traffic crossing guards began its third week of work on November 17, 1965, amid high praise from city officials. The women worked about three hours each day and earned $80 a month.

On January 2, 1967, the University of Alabama beat the University of Nebraska 34-7 in the Sugar Bowl to cap an unbeaten, untied season. "This is the greatest college football team I've ever seen or been been associated with," said Coach Paul "Bear" Bryant. The team would be named National Champions later in the week.

The *Post-Herald* reported on January 18, 1967, that traffic lights would be installed on Highway 280 at Rocky Ridge Road and Pleasant Valley Road. Guard rails were added, and lane lines were painted on this "dangerous" strip of the highway.

build a $10 million hospital on two blocks "in the heart of the growing" University of Alabama Medical Center complex. The new hospital would be eight stories with 350 beds, adjacent to a site on which the Methodists were planning to build a hospital.

Dr. Joseph F. Volker, the University of Alabama's vice president for health affairs, was "very pleased with this decision." Some St. Vincent's physicians liked the idea as well; after all, 85 percent of them held faculty positions at the medical school, and many had private offices there.

The newspapers lauded the announcement of the move, but at St. Vincent's opinions continued to be mixed.

No action had been taken on the move when Sister Carlos became president of the Birmingham Regional Hospital Council in January of 1966.

In this post, Sister Carlos assumed a high-profile in the business community. She represented the BRHC when it joined Operation New Birmingham, and she was part "of the effort to make Birmingham one of the finest" health care centers in the U.S., according to *Catholic Week*.

St. Michael's

In the days of a segregated South, the ward for blacks at St. Vincent's was called St. Michael's, named by Sister Mary Frances Loftin when she was in charge of the ward's renovation in 1957.

"No other ward had a name," said Dr. Edwin G. Waldrop, longtime obstetrician at St. Vincent's. "I think the Sisters dignified the ward by giving it the name 'St. Michael's.' And they gave the patients there the best care they could."

St. Michael's had one 10-bed ward, one six-bed ward, two semi-private rooms and one private room. St. Michael's was located on the first floor of the original building.

Betty Eaford came to work at St. Vincent's in 1960 after receiving her B.S. at Tuskegee Institute. One of the first black RNs at St. Vincent's, she became head nurse of St. Michael's the next year. "There were some very sick people there. It was a place where a nurse could learn a lot quickly."

When integration came to Birmingham's hospitals, the positive attitude of the physicians at St. Vincent's was of great value. "Integration was very easy at St. Vincent's," according to Dr. Joseph Cunningham. "The whites and blacks had always been operated on by the same doctors."

Prior to any civil rights legislation, St. Vincent's had taken a number of steps toward integration – including the admission of blacks to the School of Nursing, the hiring of blacks as nurses and in technical and supervisory positions, as well as the integration of the cafeteria and waiting areas – actions that no other Birmingham hospital had taken at this time.

"We were more of a family here, and that made it easier for St. Vincent's," Mrs. Eaford said. "And we had the Sisters, and that made a difference."

After integration, St. Michael's became First South, and in 1969 it became St. Vincent's first intensive care unit. Mrs. Eaford was its head nurse.

Mrs. Eaford, who met her husband of 34 years at St. Vincent's, has been a nursing director at St. Vincent's since 1984.

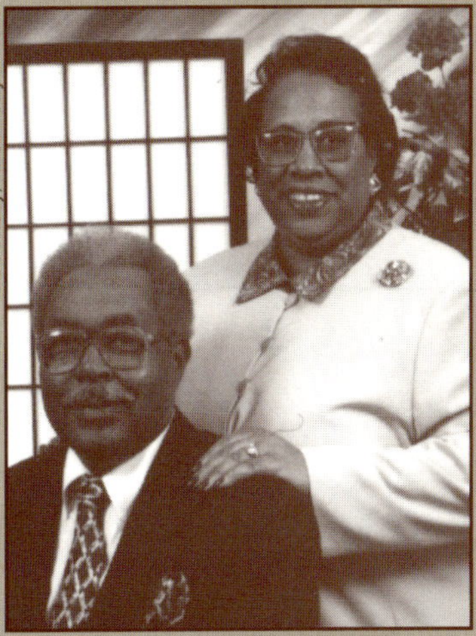

Courtesy, Mrs. Betty Eaford

Betty and Herbert Eaford

It came as a bit of a surprise that summer when Sister Carlos was required elsewhere. She announced on July 16 that she would take over as administrator at St. Vincent Hospital in Indianapolis in less than two weeks.

The BRHC presented Sister Carlos with a resolution recognizing not only her contributions to the organization but also, as South Highlands Infirmary's Bill Thrash said, " her unselfish devotion to many other organizations in the interest of hospitals and this community."

The achievements of Sister Carlos in these five short years at St. Vincent's were indeed significant. During her administration, the hospital met the strict accreditation requirements to become a Medicare provider and brought one of the first EEG machines to Birmingham. Sister Carlos had also implemented St. Vincent's first retirement plan in 1965.

And, Sister Carlos had laid a plan for the hospital's future.

In parting, Sister Carlos thanked the "fine medical staff" of St. Vincent's and said, "I love Birmingham and have been pleased with what we've been able to do in...patient care and internal organization here at St. Vincent's."

St. Vincent's Advisory Board

In 1965, Sister Carlos reactivated the St. Vincent's lay Advisory Board.

The Board, which was originally formed in the late 1950s, helped to foster a stronger relationship with the Birmingham community and to gain public support for St. Vincent's and its mission to provide health care for the Birmingham community.

During the next three decades, some of the city's most prominent and respected citizens served on St. Vincent's Advisory Board, including John S. Jemison Jr., H. Neely Henry, William R. Lathrop Jr., Frank Dominick, Joseph H. Brady Sr., C. Dowd Ritter, Carlton Baker, Harvey "Red" Terrell, Ron Kuehn, Elmer Harris, Sam M. Boykin, Louis Willie and Joseph S. Bruno, as well as prominent St. Vincent's physicians Dr. Joseph A. Cunningham and Dr. E. B. Glenn.

The Advisory Board voted to disband in 1996. The St. Vincent's Foundation had previously assumed the Board's fundraising activities, and the hospital's Board of Directors included lay leaders from the community.

Many of the Advisory Board's members continue to serve the hospital in other capacities.

Sister Mary Arrives

The "smiling, soft-spoken" Sister Mary Bourke accepted her first position as administrator when she arrived at St. Vincent's the last week of July 1966.

"We want to continue this fine quality personal care," she told a newspaper that week.

But the fate of St. Vincent's was still not determined.

One of Sister Mary's first public statements was that the move to the Medical Center required "more study," although she said the hospital was still committed to the site.

However, she told the Birmingham *Post-Herald* that no fundraising efforts were in place for a new hospital and that an architect would not be retained until early in 1967.

Eventually the decision was made that St. Vincent's would not move, and the Daughters of Charity committed to construction of a new hospital that would total about 300 rooms, an addition of more than 100.

Dr. Joseph A. Cunningham

Pathology

It was exceptionally hot, even for August, when Dr. Joseph A. Cunningham and his wife arrived at Terminal Station after a 24-hour train ride.

It was 1942, and the physician who provided pathology services to St. Vincent's and Hillman Hospitals had recently died. The war had stripped Birmingham of many physicians and staff.

"Things were pretty backed up," the New York native said. "I had enough to keep me busy for a year, there was so much work. And such interesting work, all sorts of fungus infections and things I'd not seen before up North."

In the early days, Dr. Cunningham's lab had one technician, "and the equipment was so slow, so crude."

His first lab at St. Vincent's was in the "40 or 50 feet of corridor next to the operating room." That lab is a far cry from the up-to-date facility that was dedicated to Dr. Cunningham and named after him in 1981, where tests that took three days to complete in the 1940s now can yield results in mere hours.

In 1951 Dr. Cunningham started the hospital's School of Medical Technology. During the 1950s, Dr. Cunningham served as president of the medical staff and chaired the hospital's executive committee for two years.

Dr. Cunningham served St. Vincent's as Chief of Pathology for 33 years.

The private lab that Dr. Cunningham started in 1943 was the first certified pathology group in Alabama, and half a century later, the practice still oversees the Pathology Department at St. Vincent's.

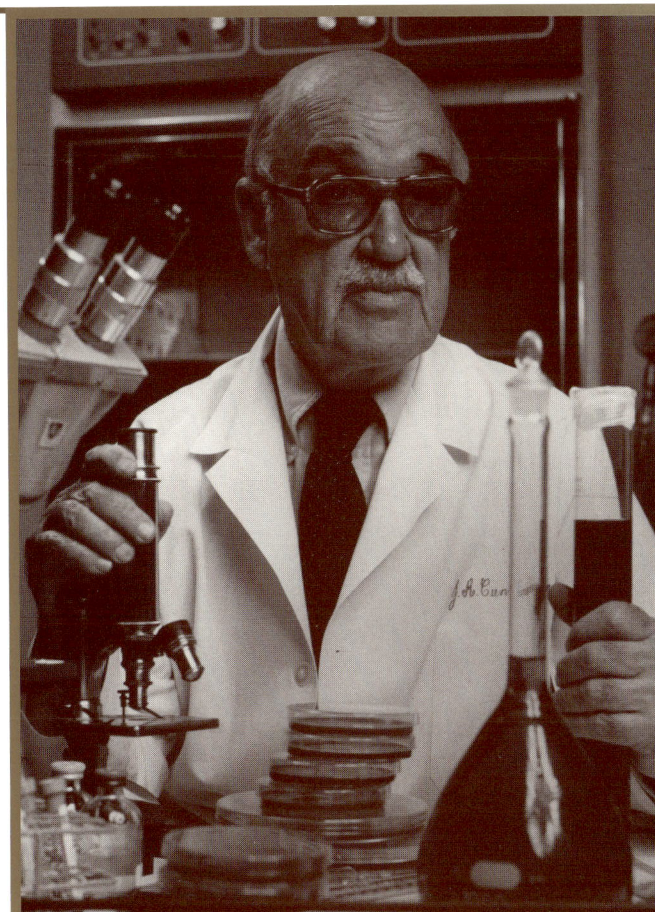

Courtesy, Dr. Joseph A. Cunningham

Dr. Joseph A. Cunningham

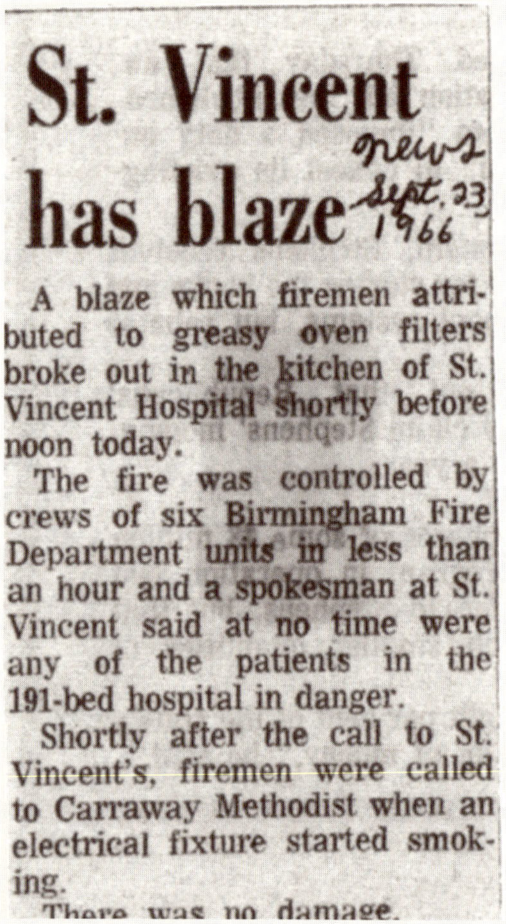

St. Vincent has blaze

news Sept. 23 1966

A blaze which firemen attributed to greasy oven filters broke out in the kitchen of St. Vincent Hospital shortly before noon today.

The fire was controlled by crews of six Birmingham Fire Department units in less than an hour and a spokesman at St. Vincent said at no time were any of the patients in the 191-bed hospital in danger.

Shortly after the call to St. Vincent's, firemen were called to Carraway Methodist when an electrical fixture started smoking.

There was no damage.

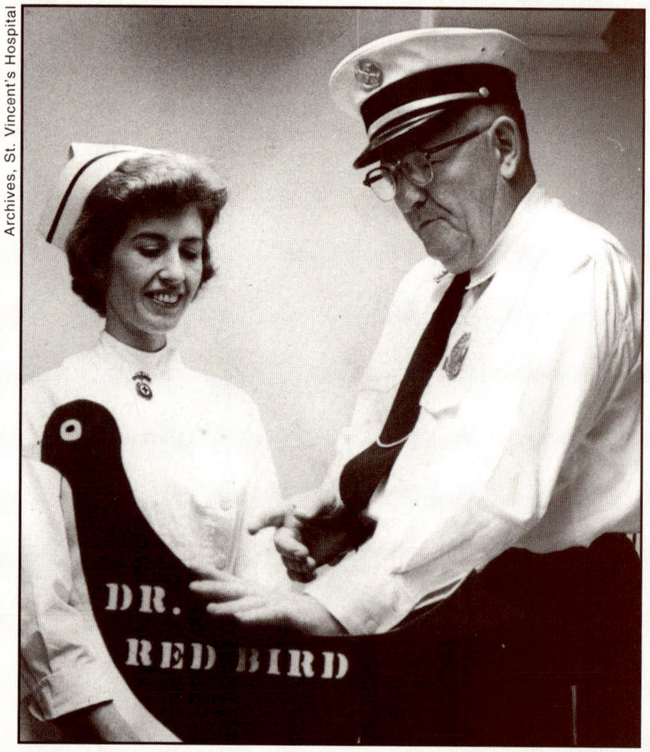

Archives, St. Vincent's Hospital

Mary Reynolds, assistant director of Nursing Services, and Birmingham Fire Department Captain Homer Allen with Dr. Red Bird, the symbol of fire during fire drills.

This blaze in 1967, blamed on greasy oven filters, illustrates a special relationship between St. Vincent's and Birmingham's firefighters.

Fire drills in the original building were critical, and the building had dozens of minor fire calls each year. To show their appreciation to the firemen, the Sisters hosted a picnic for them on the hospital grounds each year.

This relationship is still honored today with Thanksgiving and Christmas dinners that the hospital provides free each year to the personnel of the three firehouses that serve the hospital.

For several months in early 1967, St. Vincent's began purchasing land adjoining the hospital and by September had acquired more than 12 acres at a cost of more than $1 million.

Sister Mary quickly had a topographical analysis done of the new property. The hospital considered three or four different concepts for expansion, depending on the topography.

One thing was decided. The East Wing built in 1950 would remain, but the original building would be razed. Sister Mary expected the new hospital to cost more than $8 million and to be completed by early 1972.

And Sister Mary was already talking about building a physicians' professional building.

The hospital had a significant amount of cash available and was approved for several million dollars in loans, but this money would not be enough. Over the next year, the hospital waited and worked to secure enough funds to begin construction.

First, in November of 1967, St. Vincent's received a $1-million Hill-Burton grant. This brought the total building fund to $7.1 million.

But, by January 1968, it was clear that the new hospital was going to cost at least $9.1 million and that the hospital was no less than $1 million short. To raise the money, St. Vincent's began its most ambitious public fund drive to date.

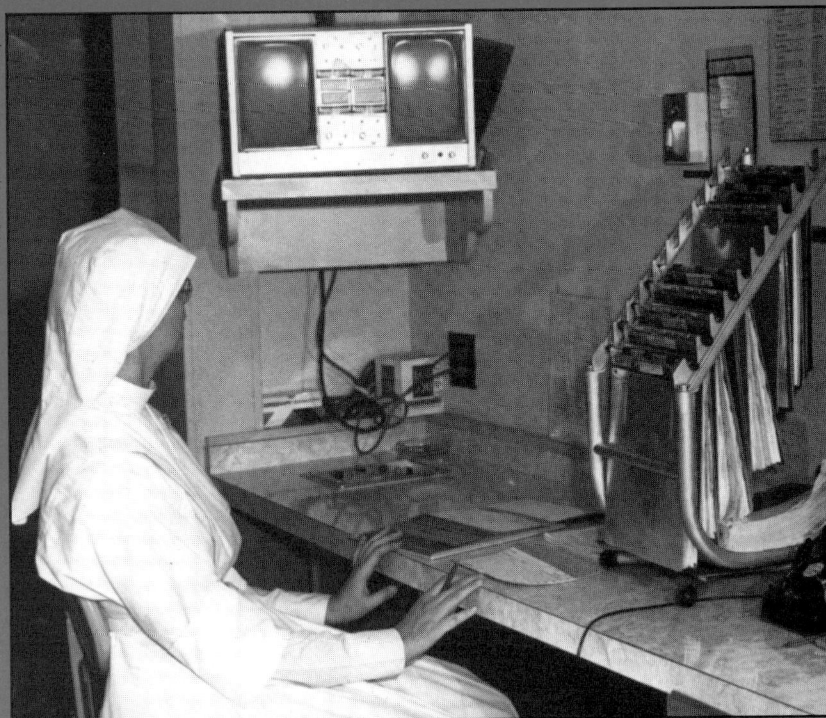

Archives, St. Vincent's Hospital

Sister Mary Elizabeth

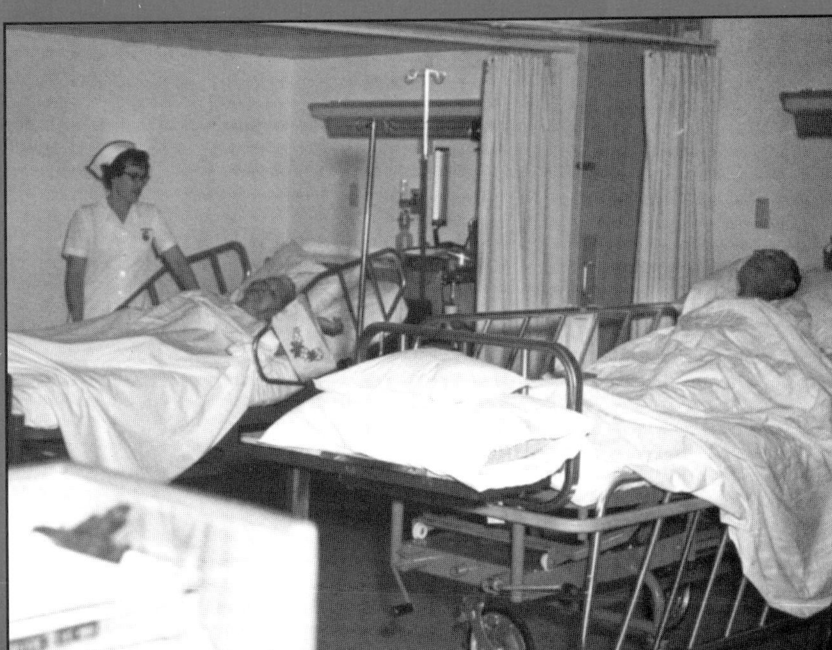

Archives, St. Vincent's Hospital

The original Critical Care Unit

Critical Care

In the late 1960s, St. Vincent's opened its first coronary care and intensive care units.

The CCU opened in 1967 under the supervision of Sister Mary Elizabeth. The five-bed unit had "the most modern in monitoring equipment." Dr. Keehn Berry was medical director of the CCU, which later moved to the East Wing and expanded to 10 beds.

When the ICU opened in First South in 1968, Betty Eaford was its first head nurse. The unit, originally four beds, moved in 1969 to Second West, with seven beds under the charge of Sister Gerald. In 1972 the unit expanded to 10 beds. Located in the West Wing since its completion in 1981, the ICU now has 14 beds.

St. Vincent opens heart patient unit

The opening of a five-bed intensive care unit to diagonose and treat persons with heart disease or suspected heart disease has been annnounced by St. Vincent Hospital.

This new five-bed coronary care unit — consisting of three private rooms and one semi-private — is operating on the third floor of the hospital. The new hospital will also emphasize private rooms, and will have no wards.

This unit is an example of the trend expected to be taken by St. Vincent in the years to come. The new hospital will place considerable emphasis on intensive care of varying types, said Sister Mary, St. Vincent administrator.

THE CORONARY unit usually has at least two registered nurses on each shift. Sometimes there are three. In addition, there are licensed practical nurses and a technician.

All have been expecially trained to use equipment and various new methods of treating and monitoring persons in the unit.

The cost of being a patient in the unit is higher than in a private room, said Sister Mary Elizabeth, who heads the unit. But she said in the long run, a stay in the unit can be cheaper.

"If a person with a severe heart ailment had an around-the-clock private duty nurse in one of the regular rooms here, he would be paying much more than he does to be in this unit, where he has access to specially trained personnel and special equipment," said Sister Mary Elizabeth.

The unit has the most modern in monitoring equipment that keeps tabs on many phases of heart activity.

IN ADDITION, there are various medicines to meet emergency situations, a defibrillator that can change a chaotic heart rhythm to a normal one and a pacemaker that can help take over when the normal heart beat is not in function.

Dr. Keelin Berry, medical director of the unit, also had a unique feature installed in the coronary care area. He suggested that windows be built in the walls separating patient rooms from either the hallway or the nurses' station.

With these windows, a nurse can pull the curtains of a patient's room and check the patient without having to disturb him by opening the door.

"These coronary care units are valuable, for now we can recognize various symptoms of trouble in the heart as soon as they show up on the monitor — rather than waiting for the sumptoms to run such a progress that they result in deadly effects before they are discovered," said Sister Mary Elizabeth.

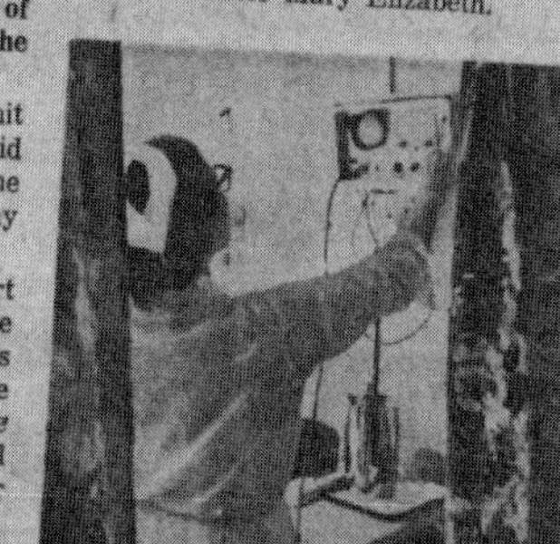

SPECIAL CARE FOR PATIENTS
. . . From Nurse Yvonne Greer

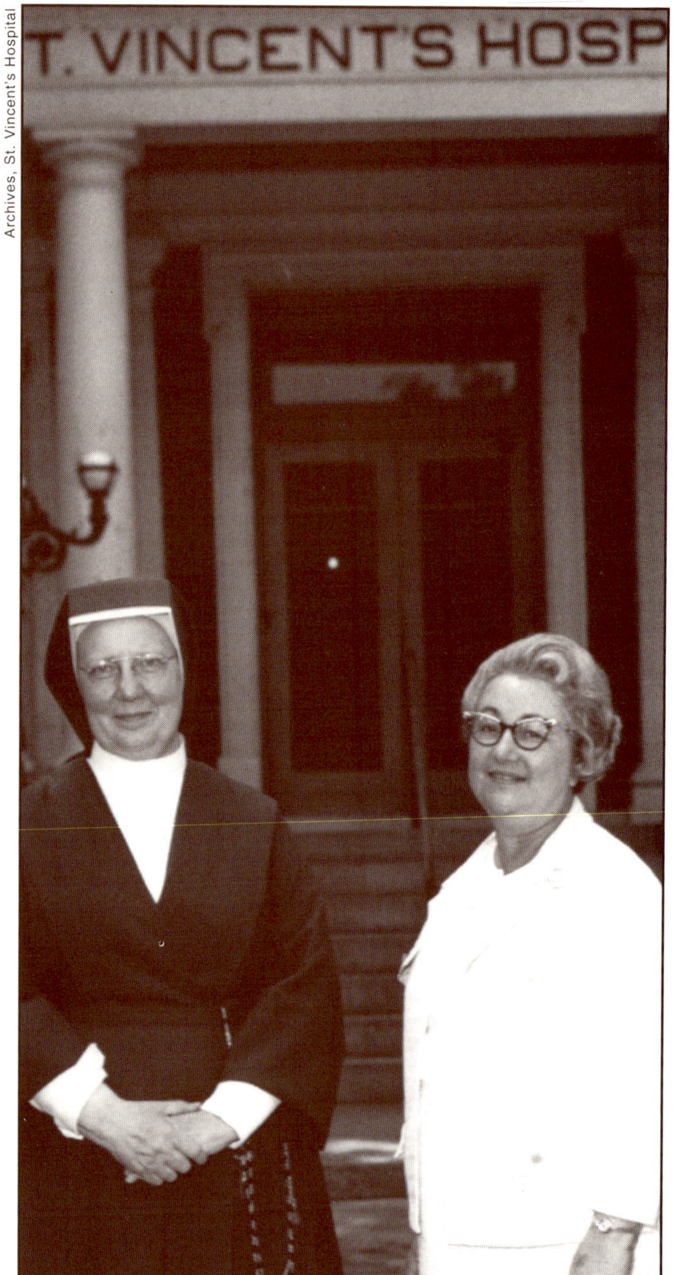

Archives, St. Vincent's Hospital

Sister Mary Bourke with Mary Catherine King, circa 1969

Mary Catherine King first arrived at St. Vincent's from Ohio in August of 1936 to become a nursing instructor. This stint lasted only a little more than a year, when her upcoming marriage required her resignation. (At the time, no married women were allowed to work at St. Vincent's.)

She moved away from Birmingham while her husband was overseas during World War II, but after the war, the Kings returned. Mary Catherine King returned to St. Vincent's in the fall of 1947.

During her years as educational director of the School of Nursing, Mrs. King saw a number of substantial improvements in the nursing curricula, as well as the first temporary and full accreditations of the nursing program.

Mrs. King became acting director of the School of Nursing in 1961 and director in 1963.

The Ohio native was named to the Alabama State Board of Nursing in 1966, serving in that capacity for 12 years. As well, Mrs. King was president of the Alabama League of Nursing and also served on the National League for Nursing accrediting team. In 1969 Mrs. King was named Jefferson County Nurse of the Year.

During Mrs. King's years as director of the program, overall enrollment in the School of Nursing soared from fewer than 100 students in the early 1960s to 221 in 1975.

Mrs. King, who retired in 1979, said her years at St. Vincent's "were the best years of my life. I wanted to make the Nursing School the best school I could."

An optimistic Sister Mary hoped that bids could be let by November and that construction would begin in January of 1969.

In support of the public appeal, the Birmingham *Post-Herald* noted that St. Vincent's and the Daughters of Charity "have served this community mightily."

And the public responded. By August, $800,000 had been raised.

With an eye toward a groundbreaking in January, Sister Mary and the large group involved with the fundraising planned a busy September.

First, Sister Catherine Mangan, with the help of Mrs. Bert Wiesel (wife of the Chief of Medicine at the time) and Mrs. Joseph M. Canary, held "The Magnificent Three," a series of fundraising fashion shows staged by local retailer Parisian.

The event, which took place at the Parliament House on Saturday, September 7, 1968, included two daytime shows and an evening show with dinner.

Each, according to the *Post-Herald*, would have "their own scintillating special effects." Pat O'Brien, "star of stage and screen," flew in from California to make appearances at all three shows.

"The Magnificent Three" raised almost $47,000 toward construction of the hospital and put the fundraising drive over the $900,000 mark.

The next week, Sister Mary hosted another fundraising event, a breakfast on the hospital lawn, followed by the opening of the metal box inside the cornerstone of the original hospital building.

The box contained a number of artifacts placed in the cornerstone in 1899, including a narrative of the hospital's founding, newspapers from the day and a collection of religious symbols, including a relic of St. Vincent de Paul.

Members of the Downtown Action Committee attended, along with the hospital's lay advisory board and the medical staff.

At the ceremony, Sister Mary put up for sale bricks from the hospital that would soon be torn down, 20,000 of them. Most of the bricks were sold for $5 each, although the ones immediately around the cornerstone went for $100. Those who purchased the bricks were given certificates commemorating the purchase.

Archives, St. Vincent's Hospital

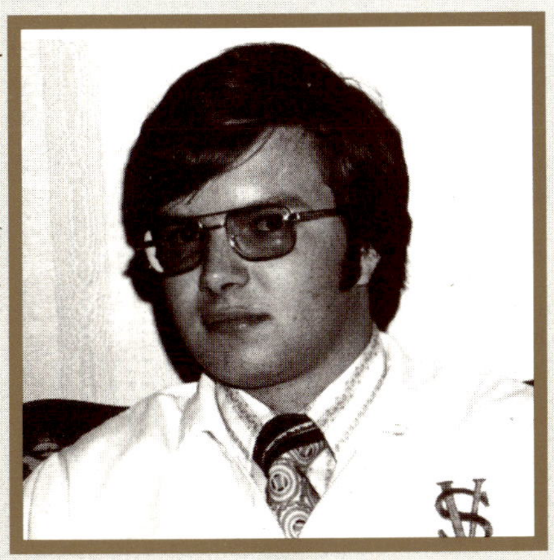

HARTSELLE'S JIMMY NIX BECAME THE FIRST MALE STUDENT AT THE ST. VINCENT SCHOOL OF NURSING IN SEPTEMBER OF 1970.

As construction on the new hospital moved ahead rapidly, St. Vincent's decided to admit male students in an effort to make sure the hospital was adequately staffed.

The former center of the Morgan County High School football team chose St. Vincent's because it "was the best school."

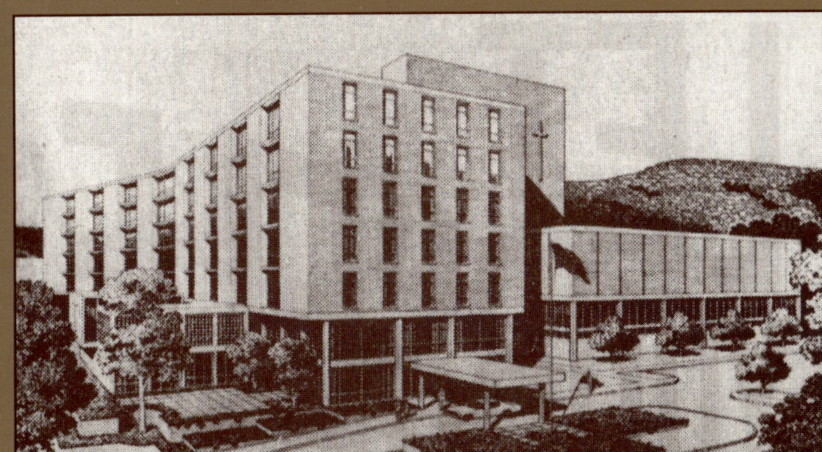

Post-Herald **Heed the Appeal** Jan. 24, 1968

For more than seven decades St. Vincent Hospital and the Daughters of Charity of St. Vincent de Paul who operate it have served this community mightily.

Once a model of a modern hospital, the red brick, galleried building in which many thousands of patients have found comfort as well as cure, no longer meets the requirements of modern medicine.

In years past St. Vincent has mod-

$8.1 million is in hand or in sight. That leaves $1 million to be raised.

Certainly there is no more appropriate place to seek that $1 million than in the community which St. Vincent has served so well.

Under leadership of William R. Lathrop a committee of laymen soon will ask Birmingham business, industry and individual citizens to provide the final essential funds to insure construction of the hospital

In its January 24, 1968, call for Birmingham's citizens to help build a new St. Vincent's, the Post-Herald said, "We can think of no recent project with a greater claim to the attention and generosity of the Birmingham area...We hope it is promptly and fully answered."

Archives, St. Vincent's Hospital

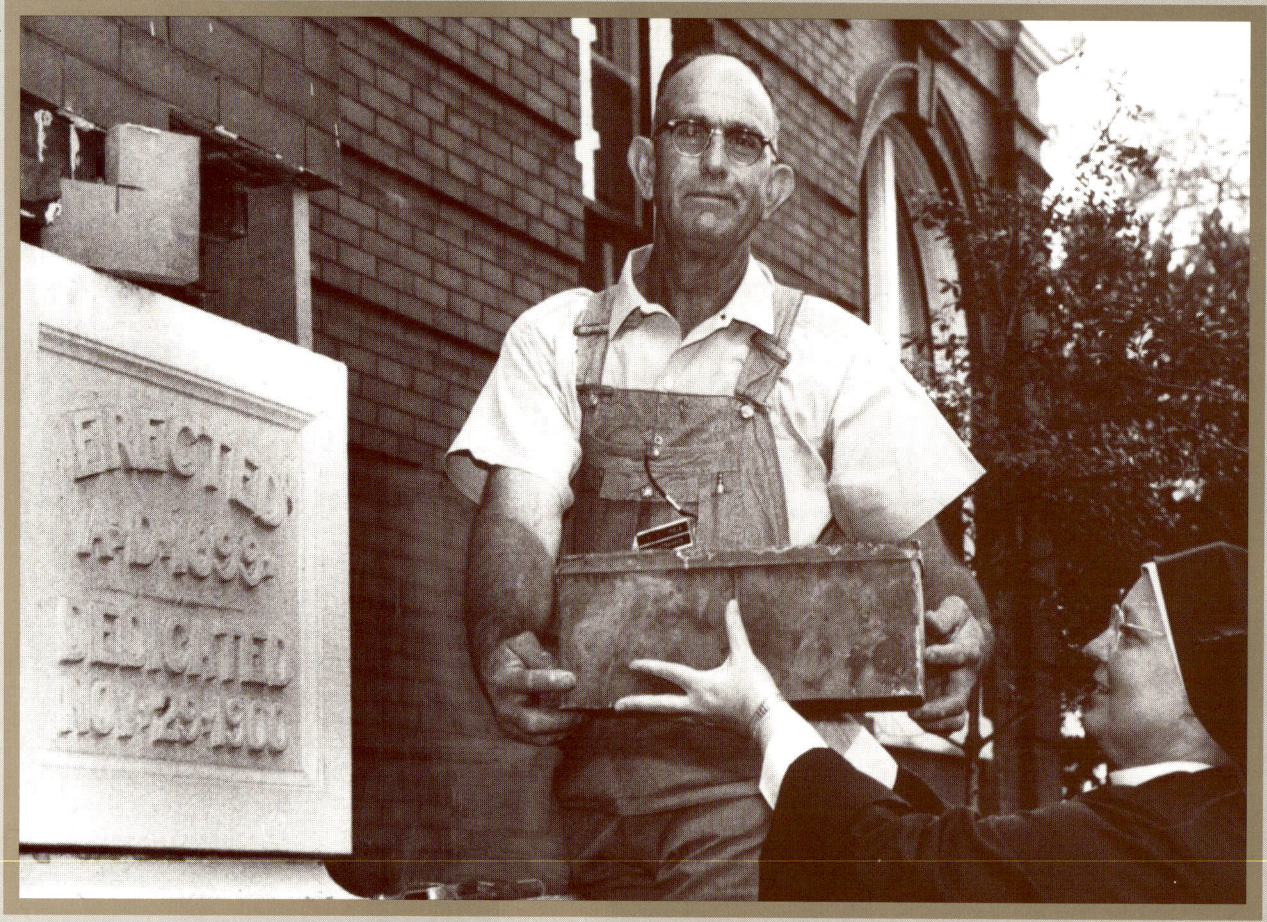

Waymond K. Ingle removes the metal box of artifacts from the original cornerstone.

The cornerstone laid in 1899 was opened in a ceremony on September 10, 1968. The bricks around the cornerstone were sold for $100 each. The cornerstone's contents included:

— The Sunday, May 28, 1899, issue of the Birmingham *Age-Herald*. The paper included a story on dinosaur bones and an article on New York as "the Western Venice" – having started "a system of building bridges" over the three rivers surrounding Manhattan "and tunnels under them." Ads in the newspaper promoted "yard goods" as cheap as 20¢ per yard, "painless" tooth extractions for 50¢ and Alabama National Bank, which was capitalized at $200,000.

— A copy of *The Birmingham News* from the day of the groundbreaking.

— An engraved plate commemorating the Rosenstihl Brothers Jewelers, the makers of the silver trowel used to lay the cornerstone.

— A 10-page document, largely decomposed, of "The History of St. Vincent's," with copper binding, signed "W. P. McCrossin, Secretary, Sisters of Charity Hospital Association."

— A green bottle containing 14 aluminum and three copper religious medals.

— A relic of St. Vincent de Paul.

Archives, St. Vincent's Hospital

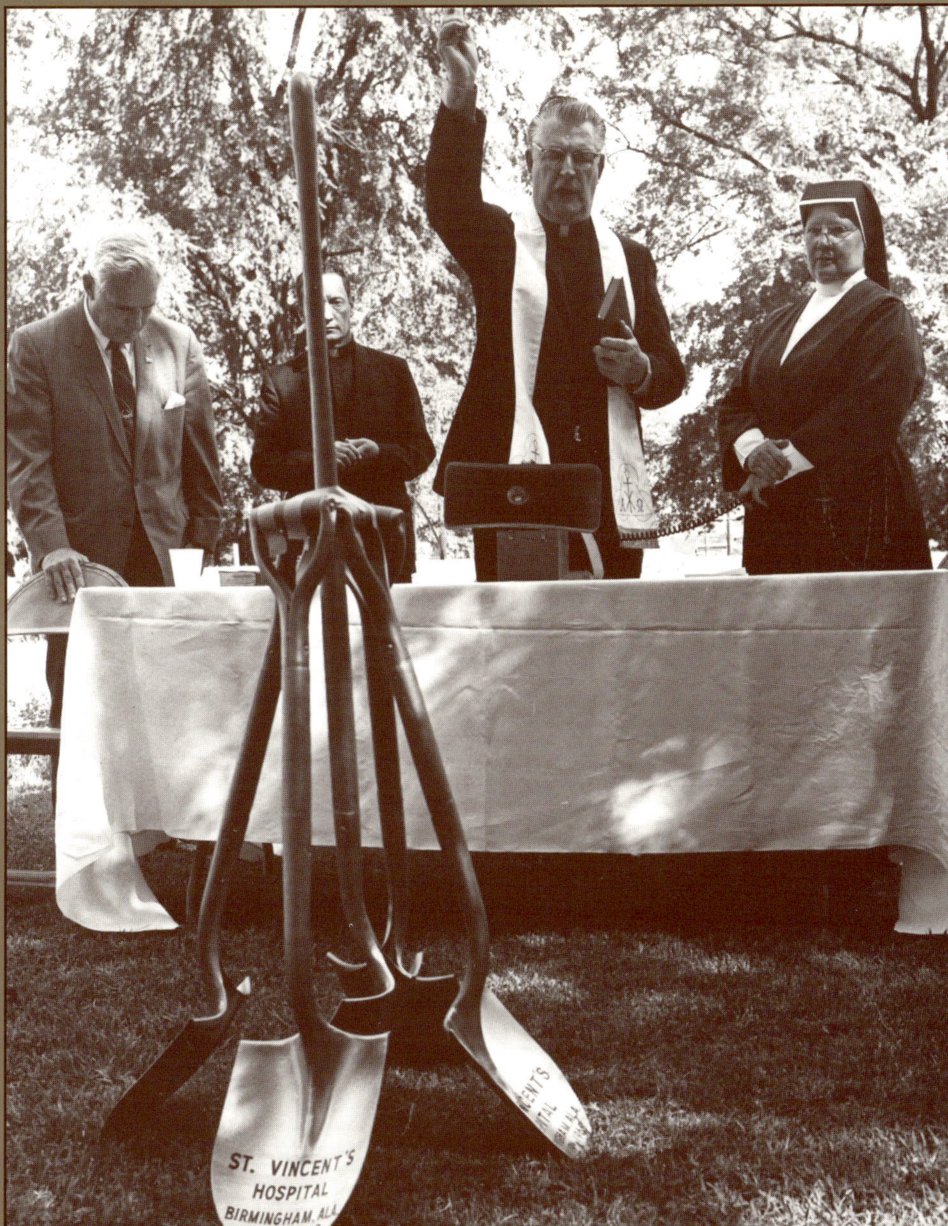

Monsignor Keyes blesses the site of the new hospital as Mayor Seibels (far left) and Sister Mary look on.

At the opening of the cornerstone, M. E. Wiggins, president of Birmingham's City Council, called the new St. Vincent's, "part of a new Birmingham."

Ground was broken for the new hospital on Saturday, July 18, 1969. On behalf of Archbishop Toolen, Monsignor George Keyes blessed the site.

The Birmingham News said the hospital marked "another chapter in its service to this community...This is an especially gratifying event because it will add still another enlarged health care center to the community's...stature as one of the region's and the nation's leading medical complexes."

"It is gratifying as well," the paper continued, "that the Sisters [sic] of Charity appealed for public support...and met with a wholehearted response from people of many religious faiths."

Chapter Seven

A New Era of Caring

Archives, St. Vincent's Hospital

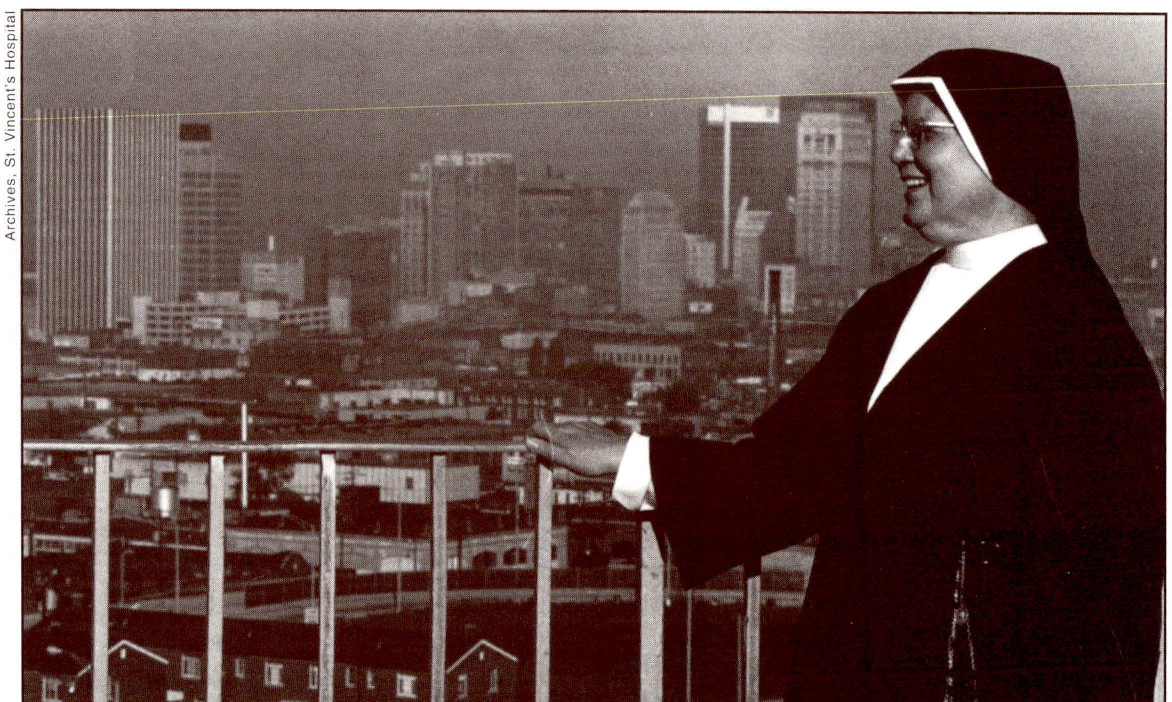

Sister Mary on the balcony of the new St. Vincent's, October 1971

The "topping out" ceremony for the new hospital was a quiet affair on May 19, 1970.

"We're saving the big event for the opening of the hospital," Sister Mary said of the "topping out," the event signaling the completion of the major steel erection of the new hospital building.

The new St. Vincent's, whose cost ultimately rose to $13 million, would have 303 rooms, including about 100 in the existing East Wing. Ninety percent of the rooms would be private.

The plans at that time called for the building to be completed in November of 1971, in time for Birmingham's 100th anniversary in December.

While construction proceeded on the new building, progress continued at St. Vincent's in many other ways as well.

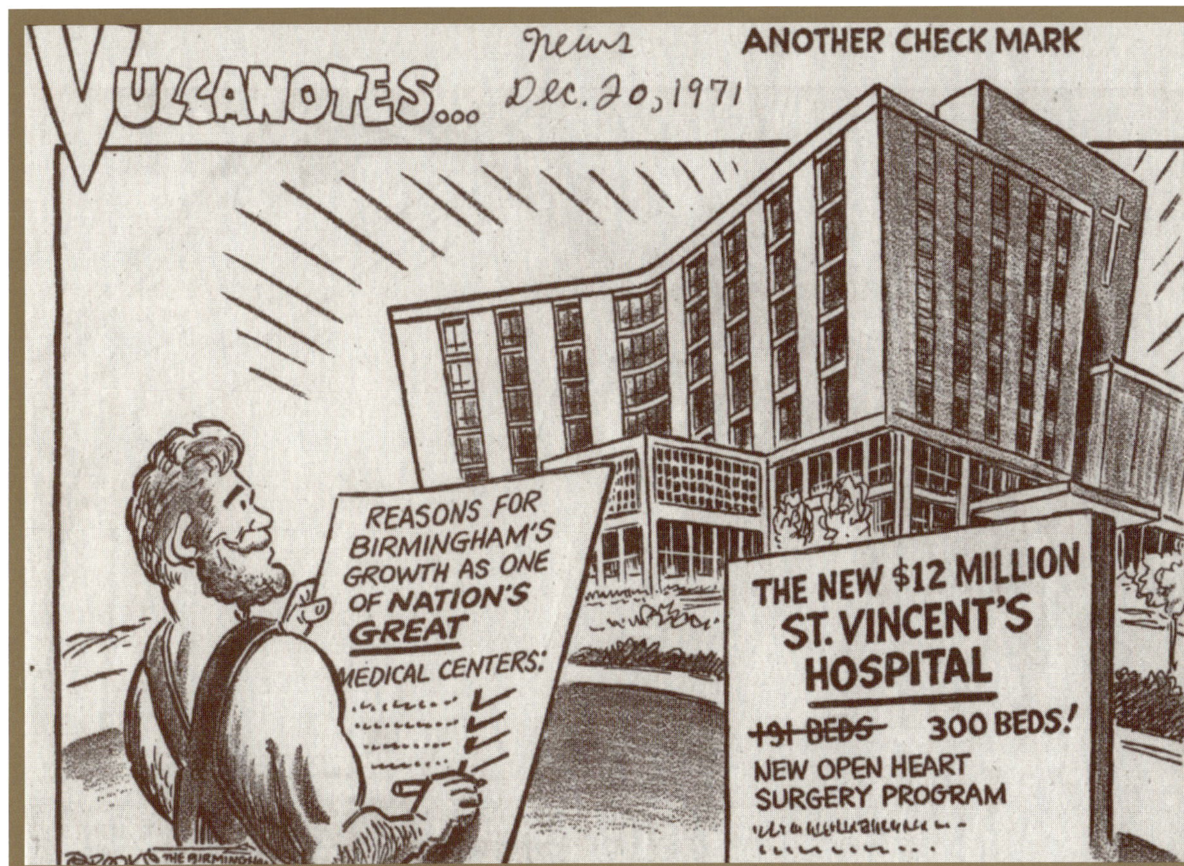
VULCANOTES...
News Dec. 20, 1971
ANOTHER CHECK MARK
REASONS FOR BIRMINGHAM'S GROWTH AS ONE OF NATION'S GREAT MEDICAL CENTERS:
THE NEW $12 MILLION ST. VINCENT'S HOSPITAL
191 BEDS 300 BEDS!
NEW OPEN HEART SURGERY PROGRAM
BROOKS

A Birmingham News *editorial cartoon by Charles Brooks from December 1971.*

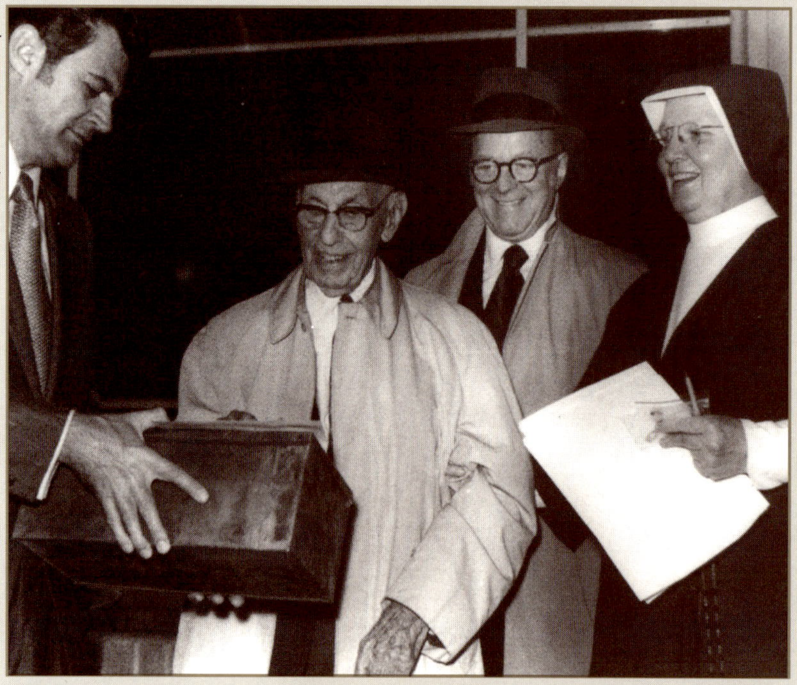

Archives, St. Vincent's Hospital

Robert Jemison Jr. saw the cornerstone laid for the first St. Vincent's, and 73 years later he watched as a new one was laid for a new hospital. From left, architect Frank Bollinger, Robert Jemison, John Jemison and Sister Mary.

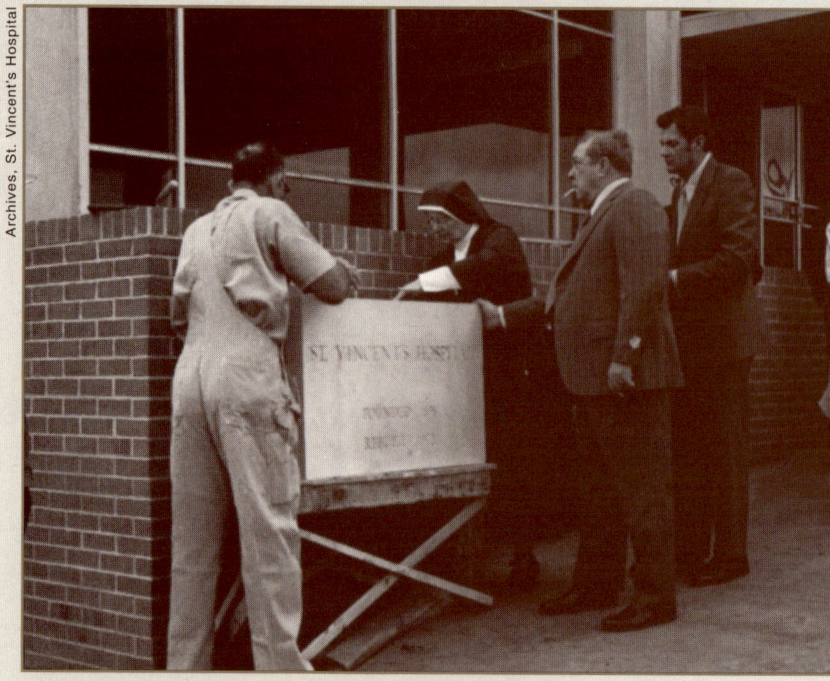

Archives, St. Vincent's Hospital

The December 21, 1971, ceremony to lay the cornerstone of the new St. Vincent's. The engraving read:
"St. Vincent's Hospital
Established 1898
Rebuilt 1972."

Advances in Care

During the early 1970s, a number of new services were offered at St. Vincent's to expand and improve care and to reduce cost.

Early in 1970 the hospital contracted for "some emergency services" with the 120-bed "Medicenter," a recuperation facility that broke ground next door to St. Vincent's in February of that year. (In recent years the Medicenter has been Hillhaven Nursing Home.)

In July 1971 Sister John Mary Robinson became administrator of the Medicenter after completing a course in management of such facilities.

In May 1970 St. Vincent's became the 10th hospital in a Daughters of Charity time-shared computer network that put itemized bills in the hands of patients as they were discharged, instead of several weeks later as was common. The system, which was expected to cut costs immediately by increasing cash flow, was projected to pay for itself in only two years, cutting costs even more at that point.

The next summer, St. Vincent's installed a gastrointestinal lab, "equipped with the latest in devices to diagnose problems of the entire digestive tract."

The facility, coordinated by local

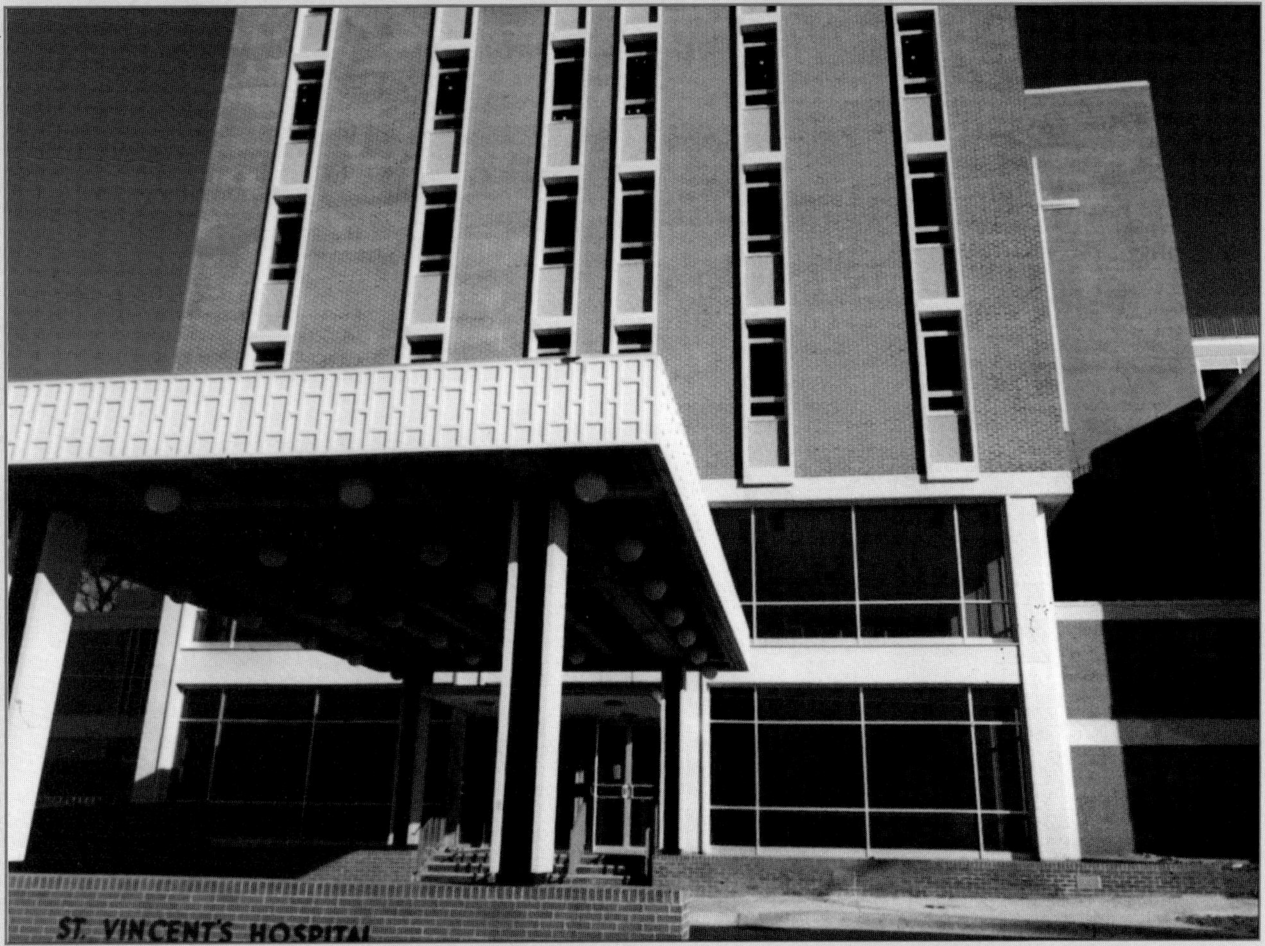

The "modern" new St. Vincent's, opened in 1972.

gastroenterologists Dr. Marshall Garrett and Dr. Gorazd Luketic, attracted patient referrals from across the city and the state.

On October 28, 1971, when Sister Lydia returned to celebrate her Golden Jubilee in Birmingham, she was thrilled to see the new building under construction, because "it was my dream when I was administrator for St. Vincent's to have a new hospital."

As the move into the new hospital drew near, the 191-bed older facility was experiencing a space problem, although newly elected medical staff president Dr. Samuel Cohn told the *News,* "Right now we're doing a good job under crowded conditions."

Among the state-of-the-art technologies in the new hospital were larger laboratory and radiology facilities, six nurseries, expanded coronary care equipment and a linear accelerator for improved treatment of cancer.

One feature of the new hospital that almost didn't happen was the balcony on the sixth floor. After a patient told Sister Mary that it made him feel better to step out onto the porch of the old hospital and look up at the stars, he asked if the new facility would have a porch. When she answered "no," the patient said, "Oh, Sister, it just must have."

Sister Mary had the plans altered to include a balcony on the floor where heart patients would be housed.

ANESTHESIA

DR. ALFRED HABEEB

The first recorded use of anesthesia at St. Vincent's was on March 9, 1901, when cocaine was used as a spinal block during an amputation. During the early years, drip ether was the most common form of anesthesia used, and it was usually administered by the Sisters or the nurses. The Diaries made mention of a few instances of physicians administering anesthetics, but it wasn't until the 1930s when Dr. Bryce Robinson of the Tennessee Coal and Iron Hospital (now Lloyd Noland) began making calls to St. Vincent's that the procedure became common there.

In 1941 a TCI intern came to assist Dr. Robinson at St. Vincent's, Dr. Alfred Habeeb. Dr. Habeeb later headed Anesthesia at St. Vincent's for more than 30 years.

"St. Vincent's had the top caliber physicians," Dr. Habeeb said. "You felt like you were working with the varsity at St. Vincent's. We had the Who's Who of Birmingham."

Sister Lydia asked the native of Lebanon to take over the department in the early 1950s.

The medical practice, where Dr. Habeeb worked originally with Dr. Robinson and college classmate Dr. Hiram Elliott, was the first in the state of Alabama to limit its focus to anesthesiology.

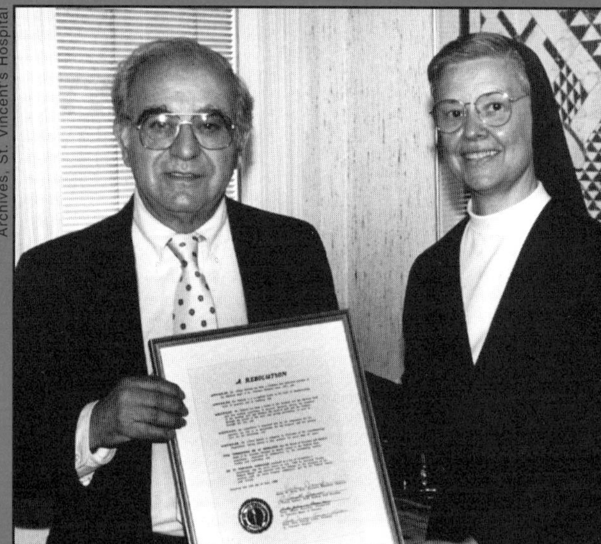

Archives, St. Vincent's Hospital

Dr. Habeeb, with Sister Juliana Beuerlein, in 1988 on the commemoration of "Freddy Habeeb Day."

"We did anesthesia for the first lung surgery and treated one of the first blue babies," Dr. Habeeb said.

Now Anesthesia Services of Birmingham, the practice has more than 30 anesthesiologists and more than 40 nurse anesthetists. Among its physicians is Dr. Elliott's son Paul, who does work at St. Vincent's and Brookwood Medical Center.

UAB named the Habeeb Chair in Anesthesiology to honor Dr. Habeeb's pioneering efforts in the field. In 1997 St. Vincent's honored Dr. Habeeb for his service to the city. Each year a St. Vincent's physician is chosen to receive the Alfred Habeeb Distinguished Physician Award for contributions to the community.

"Our hospital is a hospital planned and fashioned with the patient in mind," she said.

"REBUILT 1972"

The ceremony to lay the new cornerstone took place on December 15, 1971. The metal box that was removed from the original cornerstone was placed in the new one. Several items from the original cornerstone were included in the new one, as well as a number of newspapers and magazines from the time of the groundbreaking of the new building. Sister Mary also collected mementos from the gathered crowd to place in the cornerstone.

The new cornerstone read, "St. Vincent's Hospital...Established 1898...Rebuilt 1972."

Two special guests were in the crowd that day, longtime St. Vincent's Chief of Surgery Dr. Frank C. Wilson, whose father was one of the hospital's first doctors, and Robert Jemison Jr., now 93 years old, who had watched as the original cornerstone was laid. "I remember that cornerstone laying," he told the *News*, "and I remember Father O'Reilly. I was there when he was thrown from that horse."

As the hospital's operations slowly moved into the new facility, Sister Mary announced she would leave St. Vincent's. Her wish, however, was to see the new hospital in operation, and the dedication of the new hospital was planned before Sister Mary's departure on June 1.

Only weeks before, Sister Mary had also seen the completion of a new home for the Daughters of Charity in Birmingham. The residence, on Hanover Circle, was the gift of the Elesabeth and Barbara Ingalls Foundation and was named for the donors' grandmother, Ellen Gregg Ingalls.

The May 27 dedication of the new hospital was a small ceremony, with Sister Mary's successor, Sister Xavier Ballance, also attending the simple dedication. Cutting the ribbon on the new building was Sister Mary's last official act.

"If I ever get sick," she said that day, "I want to come back to St. Vincent's, because it has the best medical staff of any hospital I've been in."

In With the New

Sister Xavier was somewhat of a contrast to her predecessor.

"Sister Mary baked her own bread and gave it to all the doctors at Christmas," Sister Xavier said. "I went to the bakery."

So, while Sister Mary had built the new hospital, it would be Sister Xavier's responsibility to tear down the old one. She immediately realized the loyalty and attachment the people of Birmingham had for the 72-year-old building.

"There were people literally standing in the street and crying," Sister Xavier said.

The crowds also swarmed for souvenirs, taking bricks and brass fixtures.

Archives, St. Vincent's Hospital

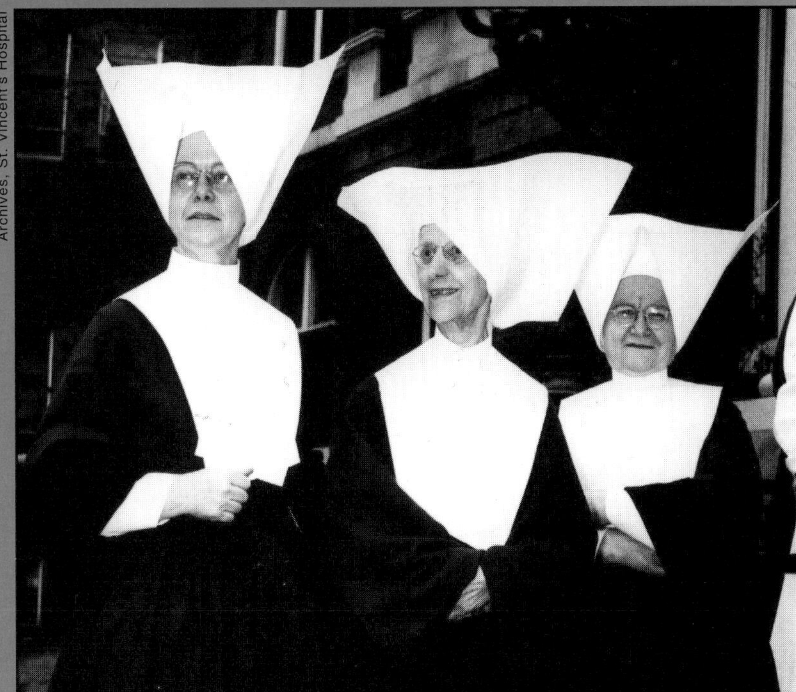

Sister Vincent (center) in 1963, with Sister Carlos (left) and Sister Anna Louise.

On March 6, 1972, St. Vincent's and Birmingham lost one of its most dedicated workers.

Sister Vincent Kurtzeman, who died at the age of 87, had been in charge of the pharmacy at the hospital from 1921 until 1962. Sister Vincent was a charter member of the American Society of Pharmacists and at the time of her death was the oldest registered pharmacist in Alabama.

After her retirement, Sister Vincent – well remembered for her ever-present smile – devoted all of her time to operating "the room for the poor," collecting and distributing food and clothing, finding jobs for the unemployed and helping the disadvantaged with their rent and utilities.

NURSING IN STYLE

A look at the uniforms of St. Vincent's nurses through the years

Photos: Archives, St. Vincent's Hospital

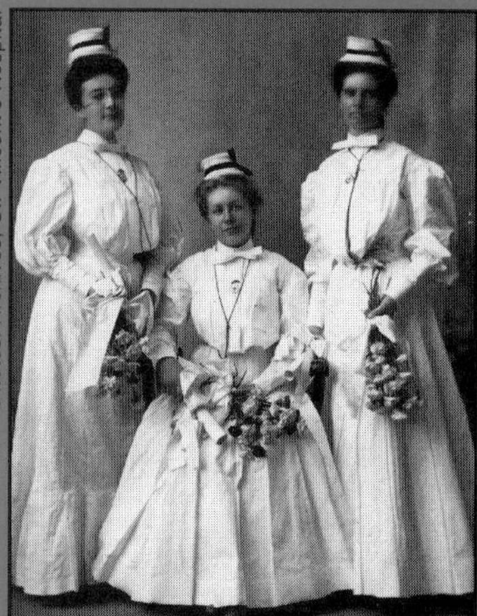

1905

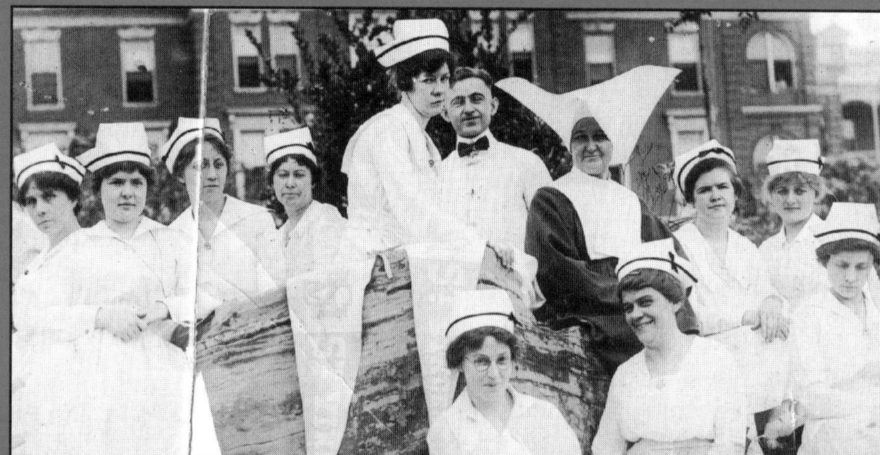

1918

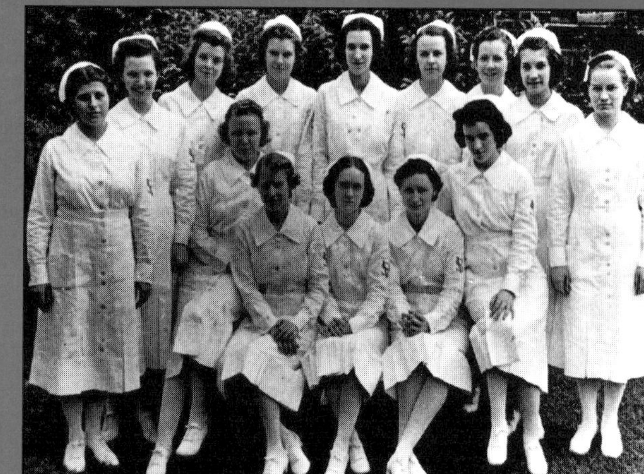

Late 1930s

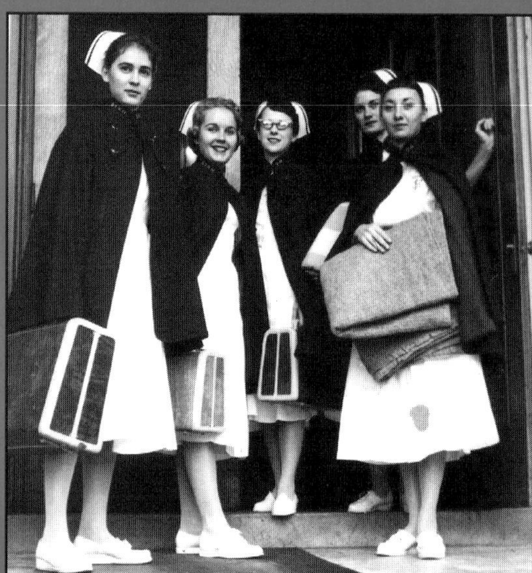

Late 1940s

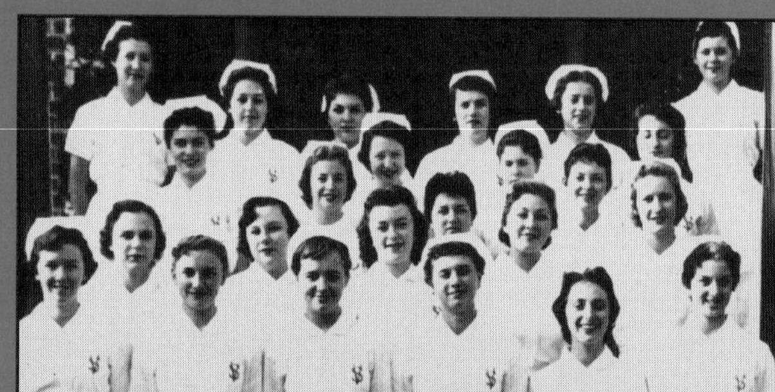

Late 1950s

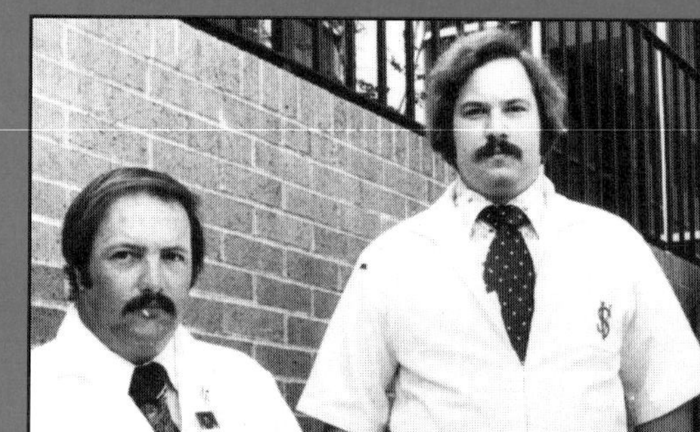

Late 1970s

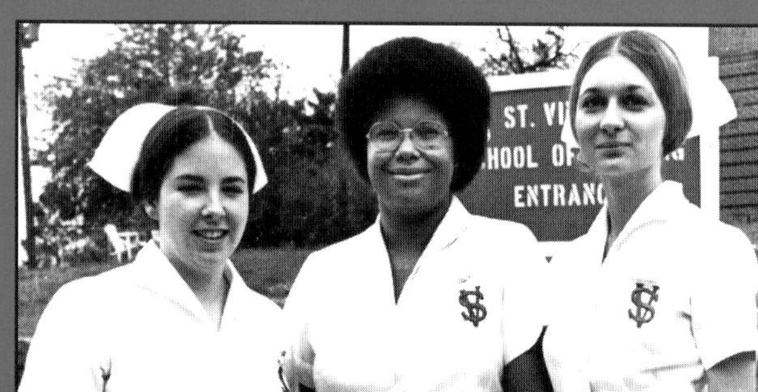

Early 1970s

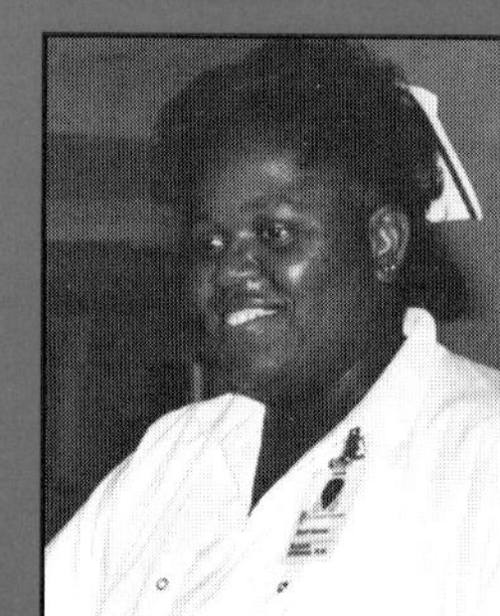

1990s

Archives, St. Vincent's Hospital

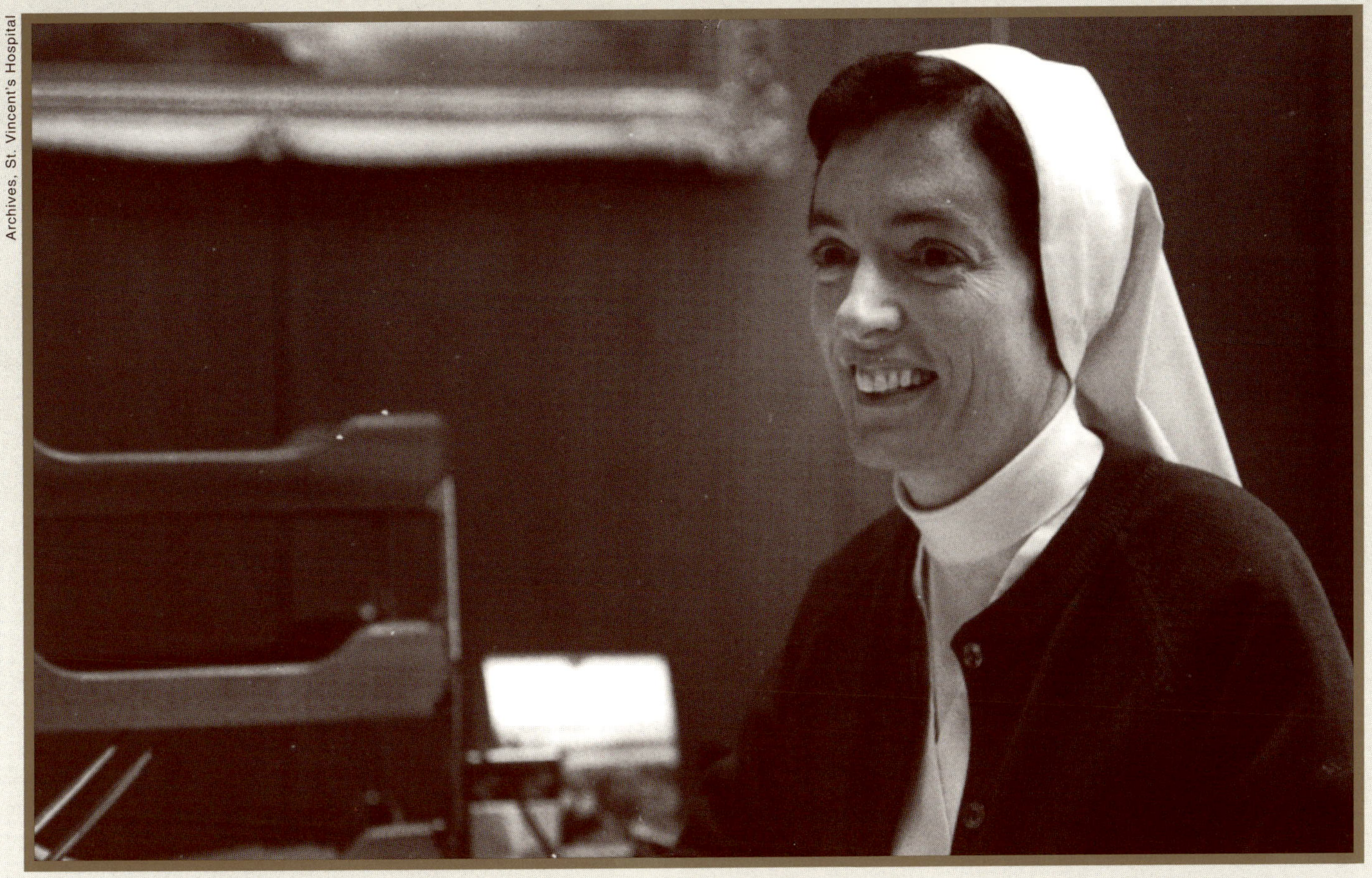

Sister Xavier Ballance

"We Opened the Unit"

The new hospital was not completely in operation on June 29, 1972, when seven Sisters from St. Vincent's were injured in a car accident only blocks from the hospital.

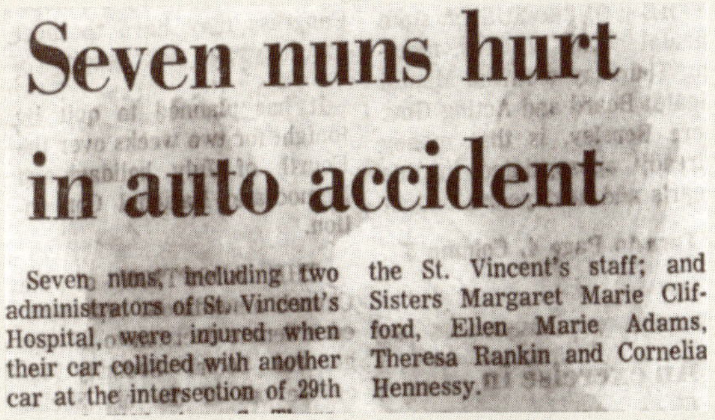

Seven nuns hurt in auto accident

Seven nuns, including two administrators of St. Vincent's Hospital, were injured when their car collided with another car at the intersection of 29th [illegible] the St. Vincent's staff; and Sisters Margaret Marie Clifford, Ellen Marie Adams, Theresa Rankin and Cornelia Hennessy.

The injured were Sisters John Mary Robinson, Gerald Mulvanny, Margaret Marie Clifford, Ellen Marie Adams, Theresa Rankin and Cornelia Hennessy – as well as the new administrator, Sister Xavier Ballance.

"The emergency room wasn't open yet," Sister Xavier remembers, "and they took us in through the morgue."

"We opened the unit there on the 6th floor that night," she says, speaking of the new location of the ICU.

Sister Xavier spent more than three months as a patient of St. Vincent's, setting up an office in her room when she was well enough to work. All the Sisters recovered from their injuries.

Sister Xavier had spent more than three of her first six months at St. Vincent's as a patient following a car accident that injured her and six other Sisters.

Overall, however, Sister Xavier called her three-year tenure at St. Vincent's "a very stable period," especially considering the volatile decade the hospital had just gone through. She even had time to paint, and her artwork hung for a month in the St. Vincent's Art Gallery.

In October, just as the old St. Vincent's was coming down, Sister Xavier announced the next phase in St. Vincent's long-range building plan: a professional office building containing 50 doctors' offices and a 280-car parking deck. A feasibility study was under way to determine the details of the project, which was expected to cost $2.5 million.

This office building, the first professional building for St. Vincent's, was the primary achievement in Sister Xavier's relatively short tenure, but it was not the most high-profile.

The three Gala events, programs which honored outstanding and internationally acclaimed women, took place under Sister Xavier's administration.

The first, Gala 75, was in conjunction with the hospital's 75th anniversary in 1973, and it was such a success that two more followed.

From 1973-75, St. Vincent's started a tradition of bringing to Birmingham some of the most renowned and glamorous women of the day.

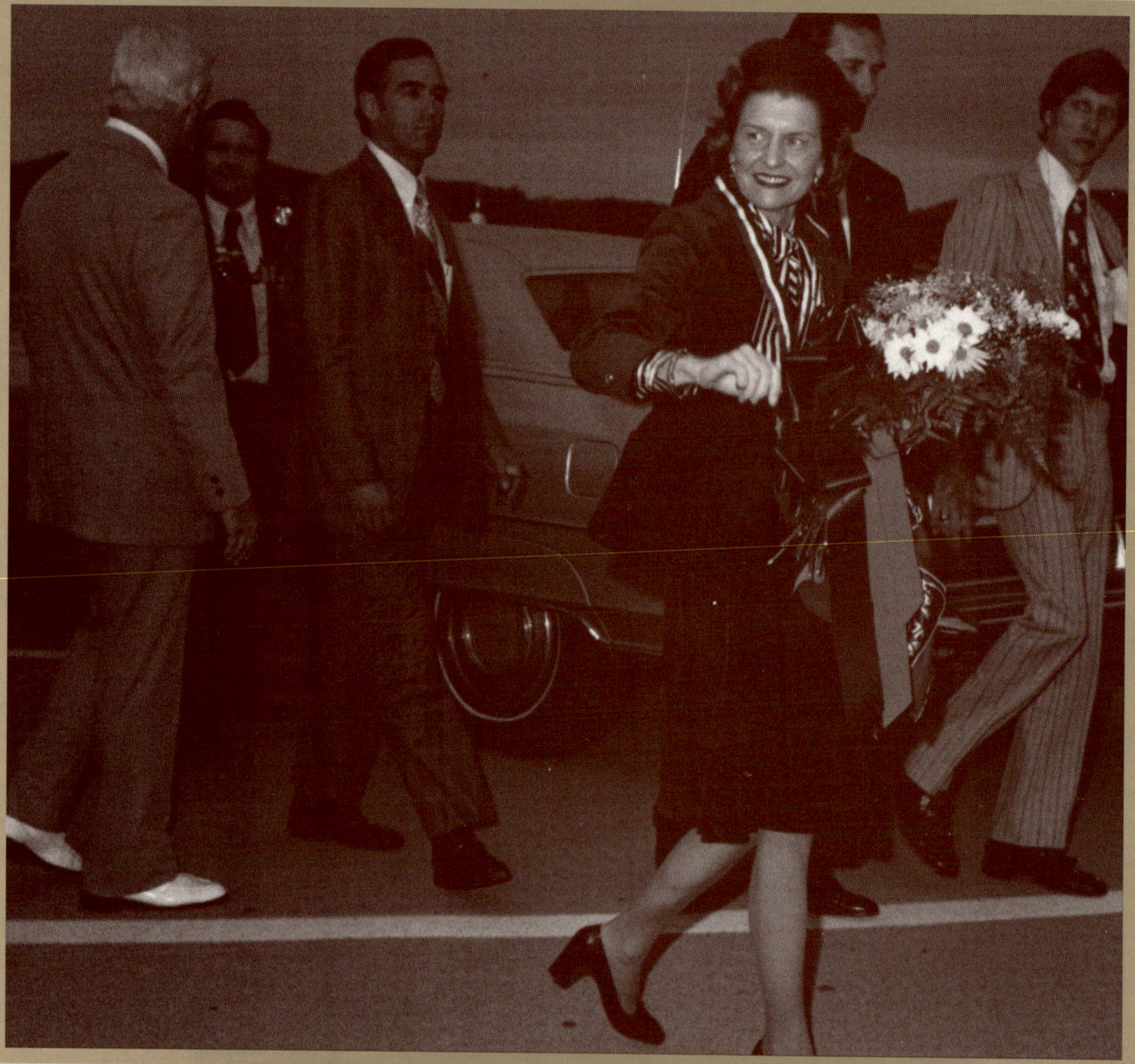

First Lady Betty Ford arrives for Gala II.

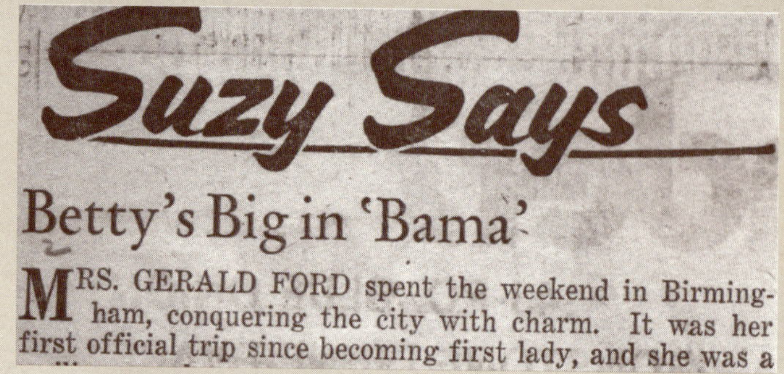

Suzy Says

Betty's Big in 'Bama'

MRS. GERALD FORD spent the weekend in Birmingham, conquering the city with charm. It was her first official trip since becoming first lady, and she was a

The Galas, which St. Vincent's sponsored for three years, brought money and awareness to the hospital, as well as famous women like Lady Bird Johnson, Nancy Reagan, Helen Hayes, Kitty Carlisle Hart, Cicely Tyson – and First Lady Betty Ford.

Cornelia Wallace, wife of then-Governor George C. Wallace was the state hostess for each Gala.

George Delfavero, a store planner at Parisian, originated the idea as a fundraising event, "Gala 75," to coincide with the hospital's 75th anniversary. The weekend of honoring women of international acclaim was so successful it spawned two encores, Gala II and Gala III.

With its high-profile celebrities, Gala became a public relations coup for St. Vincent's, garnering nationwide publicity, including mentions from national gossip columnist Suzy, a Gala II honoree.

Sister Catherine Mangan, who organized the Galas, found the potential honorees to be gracious without exception. "I wrote to each of them first, then talked to them. They were all wonderful about attending. Everyone we contacted accepted unless there was a scheduling conflict that couldn't be resolved," Sister Catherine said.

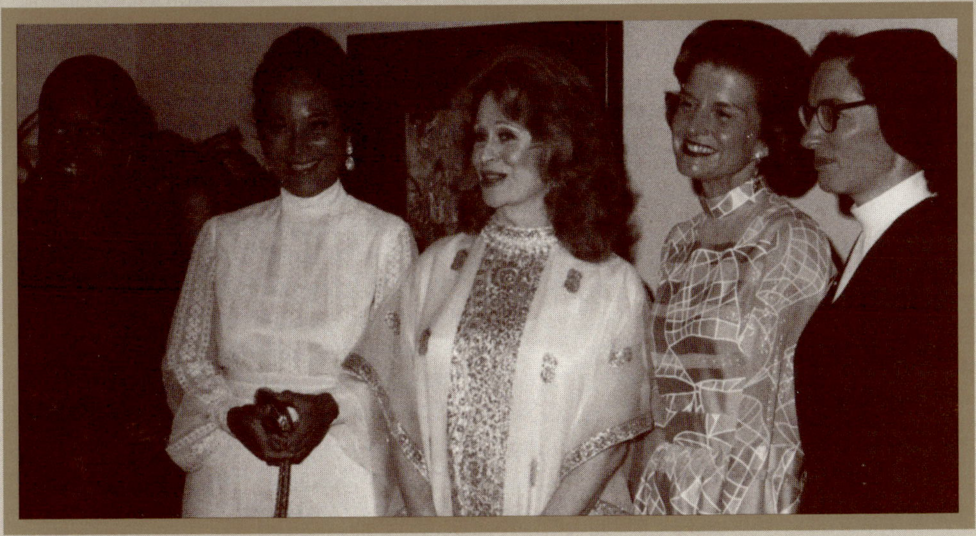

Gala II Honorees (from left) Cicely Tyson, Merle Oberon, Suzy (Aileen Elder Mehle), First Lady Betty Ford and Sister Xavier

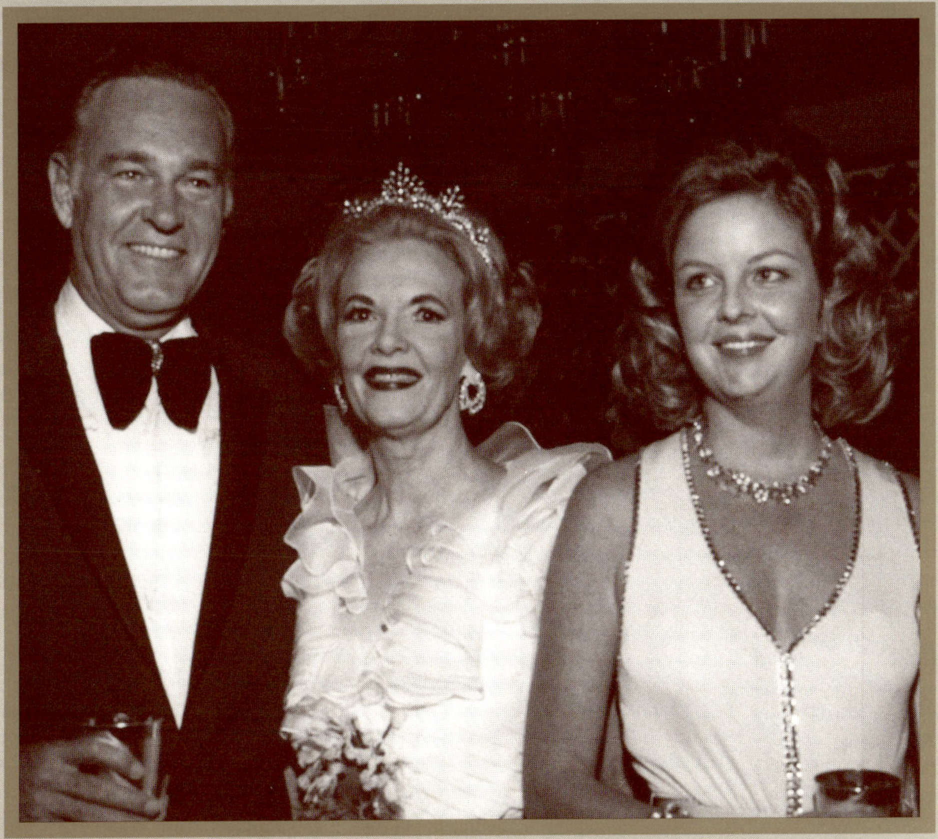

Robert and Barbara Shook with Gala 75 hostess Eleanor Kidd (center)

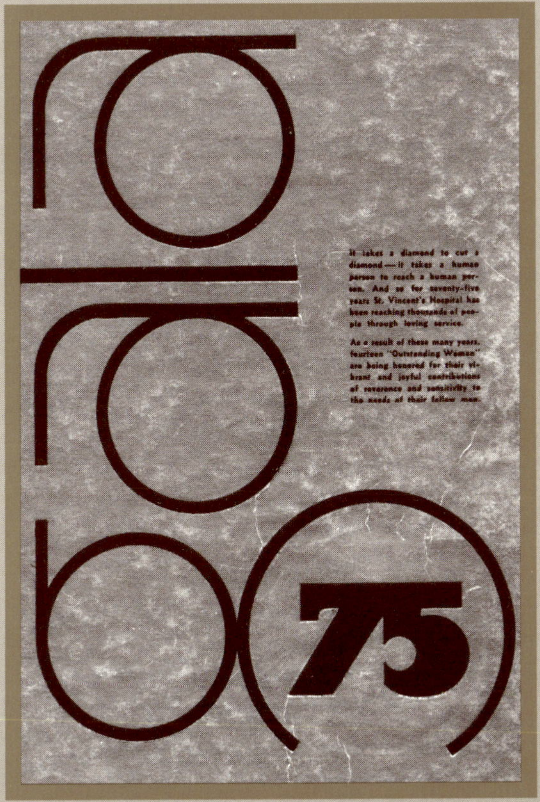

Gala 75 Program

The Galas were also excellent fundraising opportunities. The Gala 75 fundraising dinner was particularly elegant – "absolute heaven," according to one writer. Hostess and Gala 75 benefactor Eleanor Kidd greeted guests in a white Valentino gown.

Gala 75 raised almost $85,000 for equipment for the Nuclear Medicine Department, and Gala II raised more than $100,000.

Gala II also created a great deal of drama, when invitee Betty Ford became First Lady prior to the event. Her presence heightened the already strong media interest in the event, according to Larry Johnson, who worked in St. Vincent's community relations department at the time – interest that cut her visit to Birmingham short.

"President Ford called for her to come home," Johnson said, "because he was about to pardon Nixon, and he didn't want her to be on the road when that news broke."

After three annual Gala events organized by St. Vincent's, Sister Catherine was missioned elsewhere, and the hospital declined to host a Gala in 1976. The Galas, however, soon found a new home. Beginning in 1977, the Galas became biennial events under the sponsorship of Birmingham-Southern College.

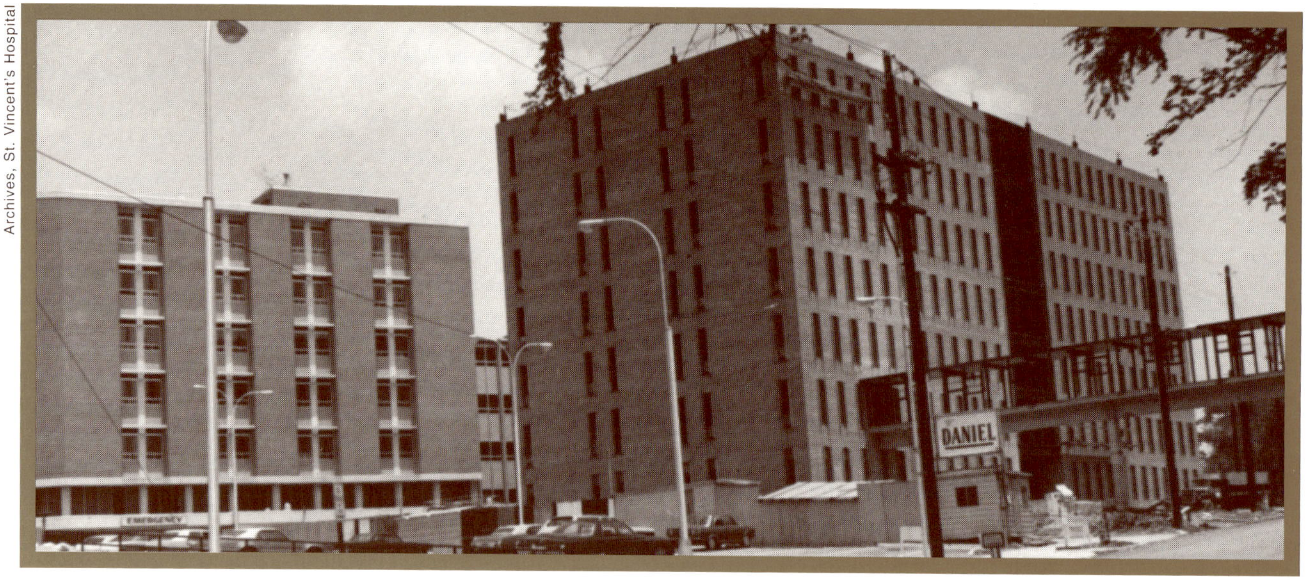

Archives, St. Vincent's Hospital

Professional Building One, under construction in 1975

Sister Xavier quickly became active in local organizations. In 1975, she was chairman of the Birmingham Regional Hospital Council, a member of the Human Use Committee for UAB and a board member of Birmingham Cable Television. She resigned these positions in October 1975, when she was called to take over the 402-bed Providence Hospital in Southfield, Michigan.

In November, Sister Xavier was succeeded by a familiar face arriving from Indianapolis.

Hello, Again

Sister Carlos returned to St. Vincent's in December of 1975. While it had been only 10 years since her departure, there had been more changes than simply a new hospital. The way health care was delivered was changing as well.

Outpatient surgery was becoming increasingly more frequent, and St. Vincent's was involved in this cost-saving approach by the mid-1970s. Minor orthopedic, gynecological, and ear, nose, and throat operations were among the first to be embraced as outpatient surgeries. From June to September 1976, there were 260 outpatient surgeries at St. Vincent's. Director of Nursing Sister Theresa Marie felt at the time the hospital could handle possibly four times the number of procedures being performed initially. Patients slowly became more comfortable with the approach.

Another new attitude that arrived in the 1970s was "family-centered" childbirth, which included a much larger role for the father on the delivery team.

St. Vincent's had been a "birthplace of Birmingham" for many years. In the late 1970s, a newspaper article claimed almost 20 percent of all births in Jefferson County were at St. Vincent's, more than at any other hospital in Birmingham. It is no surprise, then, that St. Vincent's was a pioneer in childbirth innovation, introducing the Family Centered Care program.

In addition to the father's presence in the delivery room, one of the first in Birmingham to offer fathers this opportunity, the program introduced "rooming in," where mothers could have their babies brought into their rooms as often as they requested, as well as a more family-oriented visitation policy for siblings. This commitment to providing a flexible birthing experience continued at St. Vincent's. In the early 1980s the hospital opened a birthing room, designed for labor, delivery and recovery.

But there were many more changes to come.

Sister Carlos had explored many different expansion plans for the hospital in the 1960s that she didn't have the chance to execute. Three years after her return, she did.

On October 5, 1978, St. Vincent's began a four-year construction project that would eclipse the one that had started the decade.

The dirt shoveled that day began $30.7 million of renovation and expansion, including a new wing which would become as distinctive to Birmingham citizens as the original building had once been.

And physically, St. Vincent's was about to double in size.

Archives, St. Vincent's Hospital

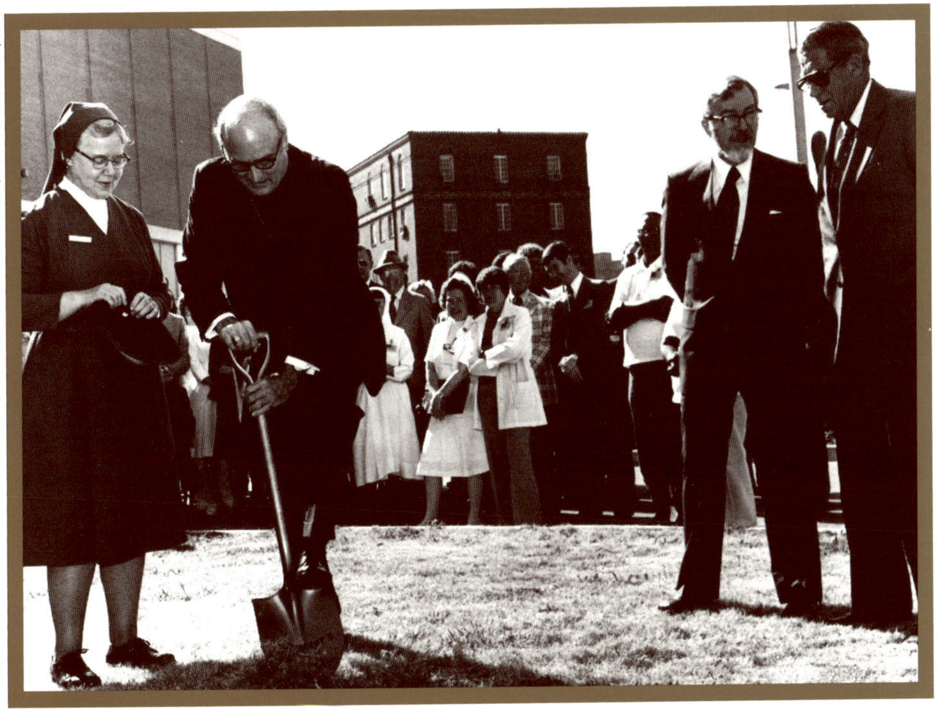

Sister Carlos watches as Bishop Joseph G. Vath breaks ground on a $30.7 expansion in 1978. Medical Staff President Walter C. McCoy (second from right) looks on with William R. Lathrop Jr., President of the St. Vincent's Advisory Board.

Photos: Archives, St. Vincent's Hospital

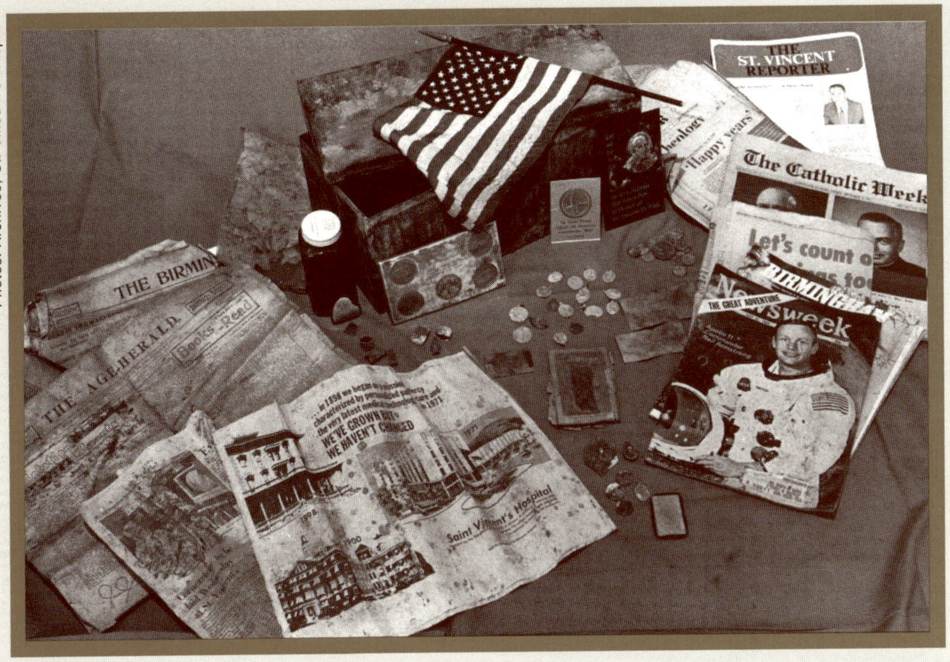

Construction of the new West Wing required that the cornerstone be opened again.

On this occasion the contents, those placed there in 1899 and in 1972, were photographed. In addition to the silk American flag used to "top" the new hospital in 1972, the copper box contained photographs of the new hospital's construction, new hospital stationery and a copy of *Newsweek* featuring Neil Armstrong walking on the moon.

Although it had been badly deteriorated for years, the original history of the founding of St. Vincent's had been placed in a sealed vinyl pouch since 1972.

All the contents were returned to the cornerstone box and resealed.

Chapter Eight

A Multitude of Blessings

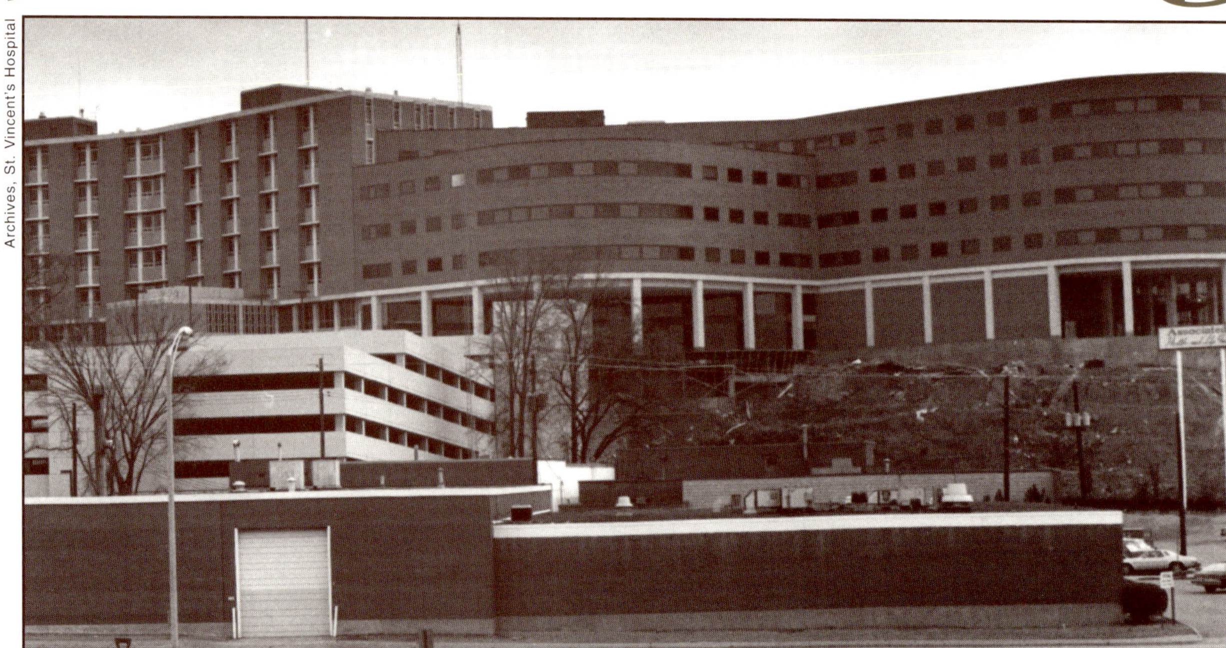

Archives, St. Vincent's Hospital

The new West Wing near completion, 1981

The construction project at St. Vincent's that marked the passing of the "disco era" took place in phases, with the new 300-car parking deck being finished first, in 1979.

The overall project moved or expanded almost every department in the hospital. And it began a time of unprecedented expansion, renovation and achievement for the hospital.

All beds were to be removed from the 1951 East Wing, and this building, now the oldest part of the hospital, was converted to administrative offices. The Nursing School also moved into the wing.

The main hospital, less than 10 years old, received minor renovations as well.

The crown jewel of the expansion project was the new West Wing. The first two floors of the wing contained a number of ancillary services, including the new pathology lab, physical therapy and nuclear medicine. A four-story patient tower rose above this two-story base. The new lobby, two floors high, featured a high glass wall with a view of the downtown skyline.

On May 22, 1981, this new wing, the Barbara Ingalls Shook Pavilion, was dedicated.

Named for the St. Vincent's benefactor who provided a large gift toward the expansion, this new, rounded wing gave the hospital 140 new patient rooms.

St. Vincent's now had 338 beds.

And the West Wing's additional 240,000 square feet basically doubled the size of the hospital. The new wing included an expanded ICU, which now had 14 beds, a CCU and neonatal ICU.

Archives, St. Vincent's Hospital

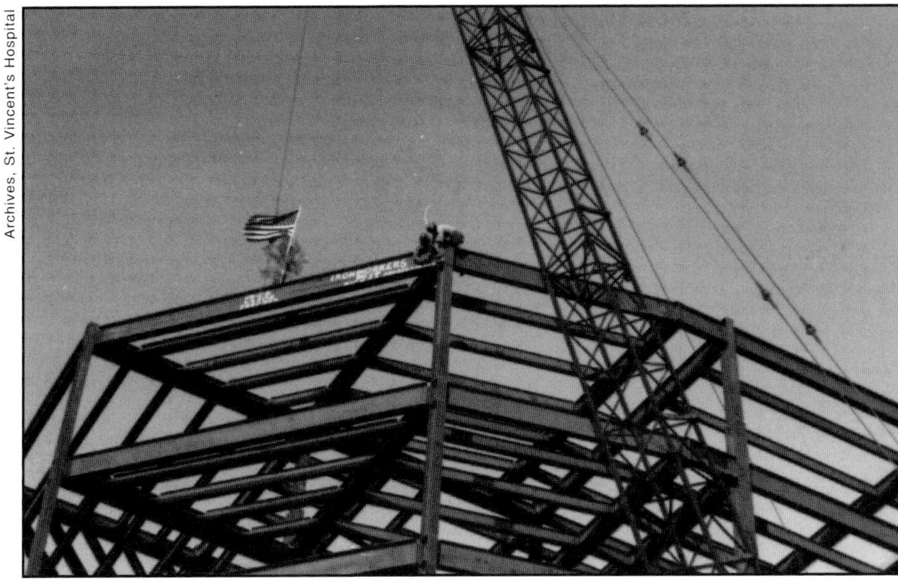

The "topping out" of the new West Wing, with the customary tree and American flag

A Decade of Continued Growth

The 1980s saw an almost continual wave of construction at the hospital. It was a decade of impressive expansion in terms of services and quality of care at St. Vincent's as well.

In 1982, the hospital began a formal Quality Assurance Plan, a reporting system to improve care, reduce cost and identify problems before they affected care.

"It was designed to provide a flow of communication," said Dr. Samuel Cohn, who was the original chair of the committee. "We needed to be able to hear what experiences the associates on the front lines were having."

Later that year, the Cardiac Catheterization Lab expanded the range of the hospital's diagnostic services for heart patients to complement the full range of acute care services that had been available in the Cardiac Care Unit since 1981. And during this time great technological leaps occurred, especially as computers began to influence almost every aspect of health care.

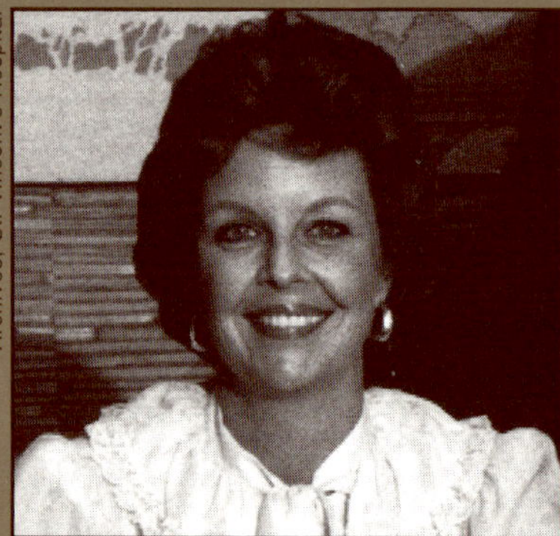
Archives, St. Vincent's Hospital

Barbara Ingalls Shook

Through the charitable foundation begun by her grandfather, Robert Ingersoll Ingalls Sr., Barbara Ingalls Shook emerged as one of St. Vincent's most generous supporters.

A cancer survivor, Mrs. Shook generously gave to the hospital where much of her rehabilitation took place. Her gift of $500,000 helped fund construction of the new West Wing, as well as renovations to the existing hospital buildings.

The wing, named the Barbara Ingalls Shook Pavilion, was completed in 1981.

This gift was the second given to St. Vincent's by the Ingalls Foundation. In 1972, Mrs. Shook and her sister Elesabeth Ingalls Boykin funded construction of the Ellen Gregg Ingalls Home, a new residence on Hanover Circle for Birmingham's Daughters of Charity. The home was named for Mrs. Shook's grandmother, who originated the effort to build the residence.

"St. Vincent's has always been very important to my family and has always taken great care of us," Mrs. Shook said. "I love the hospital, the doctors, the nuns, everyone there."

In late 1982 a new computer system revolutionized the way laboratory results were reported within the hospital, providing faster reporting and therefore faster treatment.

The next year the hospital acquired new computerized tomography equipment, which linked existing X-ray technology to a computer. This now common "CAT" scan equipment made evaluations of vital organs, blood vessels and extremities "safer, more effective and less expensive," radiologist Dr. John P. Mussleman said.

St. Vincent's, the site of many "firsts" through the years, continued this pioneering spirit through new technology.

The first cochlear implant in the State of Alabama took place at St. Vincent's in 1983. While the procedure, which was performed by Dr. Dennis G. Pappas, did not restore the patient's hearing to normal, it did allow her to hear environmental noises, such as the telephone or doorbell.

The trend toward outpatient services continued as St. Vincent's opened its Outpatient Physical Therapy Department in late 1983. Three years later the hospital acquired upgraded cancer therapy equipment in the newly renamed Oncology Center.

In 1986 St. Vincent's started magnetic resonance imaging in a temporary facility, becoming the first community hospital in Alabama to offer MRI. The next year the hospital opened its new $3.4 million MRI facility staffed by neuroradiologists and four full-time technologists.

Care for the community continued to be a priority at St. Vincent's. In 1985 St. Vincent's began Camp Bluebird, a camp for adult cancer patients, and in 1986 the hospital opened the Good Health School, a collection of lifestyle and wellness programs, including parenting, fitness and lifesaver courses. St. Vincent's also became the first hospital in the area to provide meals to shut-ins through the Meals on Wheels program.

Dedication to the community led the local Daughters of Charity in 1983 to purchase Home Health Care of North Alabama, which was financially troubled, to create Seton Home Health. Serving more than 15 counties in the beginning, Seton Home Health purchased a home health care group in the Mobile Bay area in 1986 and began service to five more counties in south Alabama, according to Sybil Burton, the organization's first executive director. Burton served until 1991, when she was succeeded by Sister Mary Ann O'Brien.

By the time Seton Home Health merged with the Baptist home health group in early 1997, the organization was providing care for more than 10,000 patients each year in 25 counties across Alabama.

Last Graduates and New Administrators

Sister Carlos didn't have the opportunity to finish her term as President of the Birmingham Regional Hospital Council in 1965, so it was only fitting that in 1984 she became head of the organization again.

During this second term as President of the BRHC, Sister Carlos emphasized the need for cooperation and consensus among area hospitals so that they could effectively address changing health care issues.

But at the end of this term, Sister Carlos announced her retirement, departing with warm words for the hospital where she had worked so hard. "The Christian climate and attitudes of the associates make it different from other hospitals. The associates of St. Vincent's truly live up to the philosophy of the Daughters of Charity."

Only months after her retirement, Sister Carlos received the Annual Brotherhood Award from the Birmingham chapter of the National Conference of Christians and Jews.

Sister Almeda Golson had been CEO of St. Margaret's in Montgomery and had spent time at St. Vincent's as assistant administrator in the late 1970s.

When she arrived to succeed Sister Carlos, the charming Sister Almeda was well prepared for the task before her.

"I have a great deal of respect for the associates, administrators and Sisters of this hospital, and I am glad to be here," she said.

Sister Almeda also had a strong vision for the hospital: to "remain faithful to our mission, to deliver quality health care in a family-centered atmosphere of Christ-like compassion," she said.

Fully aware of the rapidly changing health care environment, Sister Almeda underscored the drive that continued to distinguish St. Vincent's from other hospitals when she said, "We must find a balance in which we can accomplish this."

After 87 years and more than 1,800 graduates, the St. Vincent School of Nursing closed in 1987.

Sister Almeda lamented the declining numbers of applicants during the 1980s due to a perceived softness in the nursing job market.

One of only three remaining diploma programs in Alabama at the time, the St. Vincent School of Nursing had been facing competition from baccalaureate nursing programs.

However, a National League of Nursing study found that 83.9 percent of St. Vincent graduates described their education and clinical preparedness as adequate, a significantly higher percentage than that of baccalaureate graduates.

The last director of the school, Betty Williams, said, "It's sad, but I feel the decision was a timely one."

St. Vincent's to close nursing school after more than 80 years

By Celeste Williams
Post-Herald Reporter

The nursing school at St. Vincent's Hospital in Birmingham will close after graduating its last class in

Archives, St. Vincent's Hospital

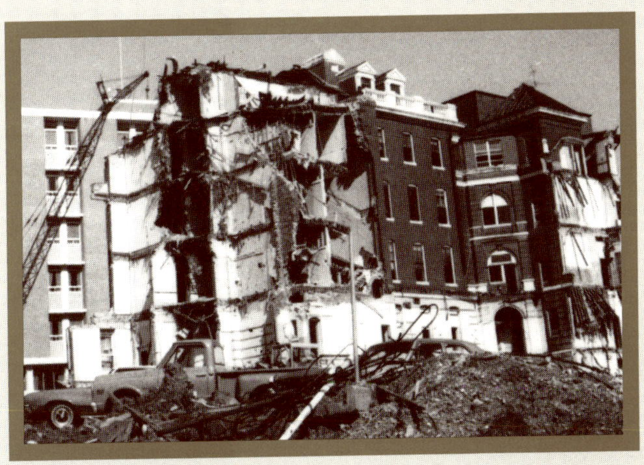

When Laboure Hall was torn down in 1982, it had not been used as a dormitory for several years. The School of Nursing classrooms and offices moved to the East Wing of the hospital because the 56-year-old Laboure Hall had become obsolete.

While St. Vincent's was growing in many different ways, there was one area that did not share the good fortune. In 1985 the declining number of applicants forced Sister Almeda into announcing that St. Vincent's would close the School of Nursing after the graduation of the Class of 1987. "Our school is second to none in quality and excellence of tradition," Sister Almeda told the *Post-Herald*. "We are simply responding to developing trends and needs."

And later in 1987, Sister Almeda was called to Montgomery to take on a governance position on the boards of all three Daughters of Charity hospitals in Alabama. Her successor, Sister Mary Frances Loftin, had a most impressive background as well, most recently having been the top executive in the regional office of the Daughters of Charity National Health System.

An Abiding Presence

One of the greatest gifts St. Vincent's offers its patients is its Sisters.

In the beginning, members of the Daughters of Charity filled every leadership position and formed the core of the nursing staff.

But as years passed, fewer Catholic women chose to give their lives in service to the Church, and as the membership of the Daughters of Charity grew smaller, so did the numbers of the order at St. Vincent's and other hospitals in the system. One by one, leadership positions once held by Sisters were turned over to lay people.

This trend became evident in 1983, when organizational changes created the position of executive vice president to handle the day-to-day operations of the hospital. Sister Carlos became president and chief executive officer.

And although today there are fewer Sisters at St. Vincent's – half as many as 25 years ago – their presence continues to make the hospital special.

Sister Gerald Mulvanny, who has been at St. Vincent's for almost 25 years, doesn't perform nursing duties anymore, but continues a vigorous work schedule managing the hospital's mail and copy center. "It is as important today as it has always been that all our employees understand there are some things we do differently from other hospitals," she said.

Sister Mary Frances also acknowledges the challenge. "In a competitive health care environment, St. Vincent's emphasizes that the focus of its work ethic is on the patient," she said.

Sister Gerald states with pride that the hospital's mission to the poor is the same as it was the day St. Vincent's was founded.

Jean S. Brandli

This prominent Pell City telecommunications executive enjoyed a close relationship with St. Vincent's.

The second-floor conference room in the new West Wing was named the Jean S. Brandli Memorial Conference Center following the gift she provided through her will in 1983.

Upon dedication of the Conference Center, Sister Carlos said, "It will serve as a center for medical and professional learning, and I know that the advancement of St. Vincent's Hospital was an area close to Mrs. Brandli's heart."

B. A. Monaghan

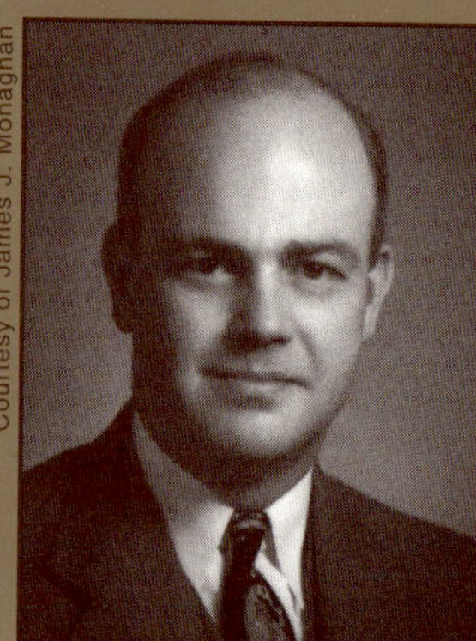

Courtesy of James J. Monaghan

B. A. Monaghan, during his tenure at Vulcan Materials

In 1987 Bernard Andrew "Barney" Monaghan bestowed one of the largest gifts ever received by St. Vincent's – more than $3.5 million – through a charitable trust established in his will.

A prominent attorney for more than 40 years, Monaghan was also a former president and CEO of Vulcan Materials.

The Birmingham native was a graduate of Harvard Law School and was a Rhodes scholar. During World War II, Monaghan earned a Bronze Star for valor during the Battle of Iwo Jima.

Before the original hospital building was razed in 1972, Monaghan had secured the crucifix from the room where his father died in 1927, which he kept until his own death.

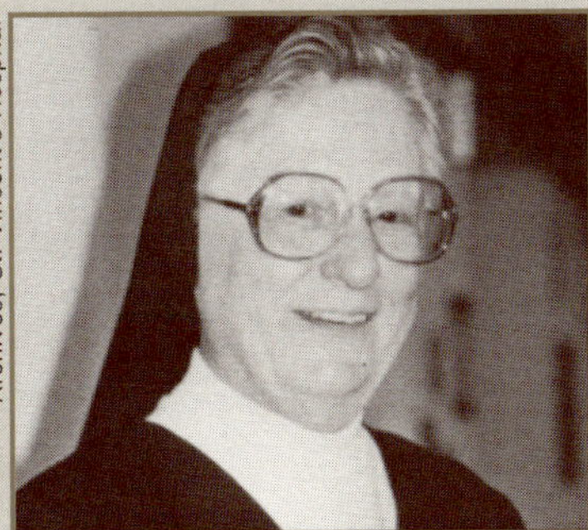

Archives, St. Vincent's Hospital

Sister Gerald

Almost 25 of Sister Gerald Mulvanny's 54 years of service as a member of the Daughters of Charity have been at St. Vincent's.

It is clear to see that Sister Gerald is still a nurse at heart and that at St. Vincent's, patient care also means caring. "Go through the hospital, and you can't tell who are the paying patients and who aren't," Sister Gerald said.

"The Sisters have always believed in treating patients as guests," said Betty Williams, former director of the nursing school. While there are fewer Sisters, that philosophy permeates the atmosphere at St. Vincent's. "It used to be that every patient saw a Sister every day," Mrs. Williams said. "Personal care is still a high priority at St. Vincent's."

Camp Bluebird

Since 1985, Camp Bluebird has been a haven for adult cancer patients as they learn to survive and to thrive.

When former St. Vincent's associate and cancer survivor Louis Josof could not find an adult camp for cancer patients, he wrote the plan for Camp Bluebird, which, with the support of Alabama's Telephone Pioneers, became the first camp of its kind in the United States. The program's success in giving patients an opportunity for recreation, crafts and peer support has since been duplicated in more than 20 locations in Alabama and other states. St. Vincent's camp, held twice each year, is funded by the St. Vincent's Foundation.

Perhaps the most symbolic of the campers' activities is the building of birdhouses, which supports the Telephone Pioneers of America's efforts to ensure the survival of the Eastern bluebird.

St. Vincent's Foundation

St. Vincent's has survived and flourished through the generosity of Birmingham's citizens. St. Vincent's Foundation was established in 1984 to foster the spirit of stewardship the community has offered St. Vincent's since its founding.

The Foundation administers gifts to the hospital and supports the activities of the hospital by encouraging philanthropic support of its ministry.

In 1997 the Foundation completed a Donor Recognition Wall in the new Bruno Conference Center to express gratitude to the friends of St. Vincent's who have helped the hospital thrive.

The Foundation has raised more than $22 million to fund hospital and community programs and projects.

William M. Moran has served as the Foundation's Executive Director since the organization's inception.

St. Vincent's Foundation Presidents

1984-86 William M. Spencer III
1987-88 C. Caldwell Marks
1989-90 Mary Jo Mackin
1991-92 Lee J. Styslinger Jr.
1993-95 Clarke H. Gillespy
1995-97 Wayne H. Gillis
1997-present Marvin R. Engel

The Pastoral Care Department helps to carry on this tradition of personal and spiritual concern to complement health care, including both Catholic and Protestant clergy.

"I see a great hunger for spirituality among so many of our patients," said Sister Regina Priller. "It's a vibrant spirit that I see in the hospital. And one wonderful thing about this part of the country," she continued, "is the willingness of people of all denominations to talk about Jesus."

In 1988 St. Vincent's began formally rewarding the spirit of the personal touch. That year well-known actor and Birmingham native Wayne Rogers established the Loula E. Rogers Award for Care Giving. The award, given to the St. Vincent's associate "most attentive to the needs of patients and their families," is named for Rogers' sister who died at St. Vincent's in 1986. The recipient receives a cash prize along with the honor.

But taking care of the Birmingham community has never stopped at the doors of St. Vincent's, and that attitude is visible in the roles of Sister Virginia Delaney, the hospital's mission coordinator, and Sister Veronica Berg, patient representative.

The hospital's community outreach includes the adoption of local schools and involvement in the surrounding neighborhoods through the leadership of the Daughters of Charity. St. Vincent's assisted the Diocese in establishing the Villa Maria retirement community, and Sister Mary Cecilia Schlebecker served as administrator for its first 10 years.

A Wealth of Generosity

The 1980s closed as they had begun, with a flurry of good fortune and construction as St. Vincent's continued to expand its facilities, again with the help of committed supporters.

Among the Greatest

Courtesy of the Burno family

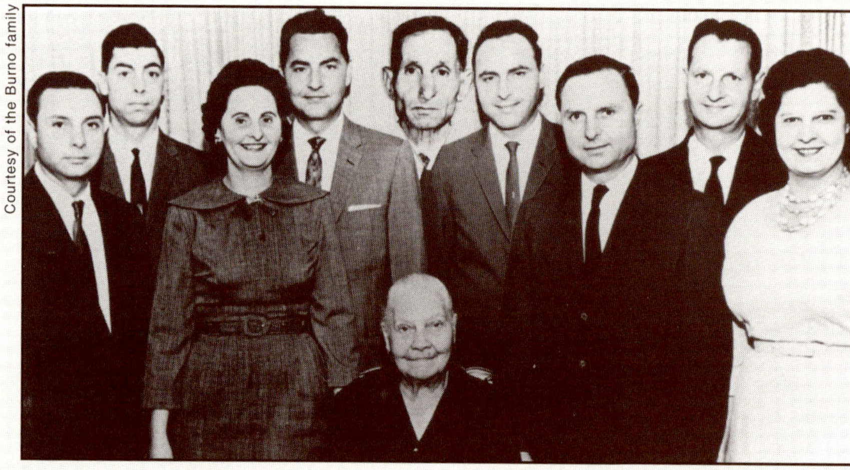

The Brunos. Standing behind Mama Theresa (seated) left to right: Lee, Ben, Theresa, Angelo, Papa Vincent, Anthony, Joe, Sam and Mary.

One of Birmingham's greatest success stories, the Bruno family has also been one of the most generous. Several facilities at St. Vincent's bear the Bruno family name. The hospital chapel was dedicated to immigrant parents Vincent and Theresa.

Bruno Memorial Heart Care Center

Dedicated to the memory of "those who made the Bruno name a legend in the Birmingham area," the Bruno Memorial Heart Care Center was dedicated on February 23, 1992. The Center combines the latest in cardiac technology with the caring of St. Vincent's Hospital, providing all heart surgery services in one location. The Center offers a comprehensive range of services for coronary patients, including cardiac rehabilitation and educational programs.

Lee J. and Nancy Bruno Rehabilitation Center

Archives, St. Vincent's Hospital

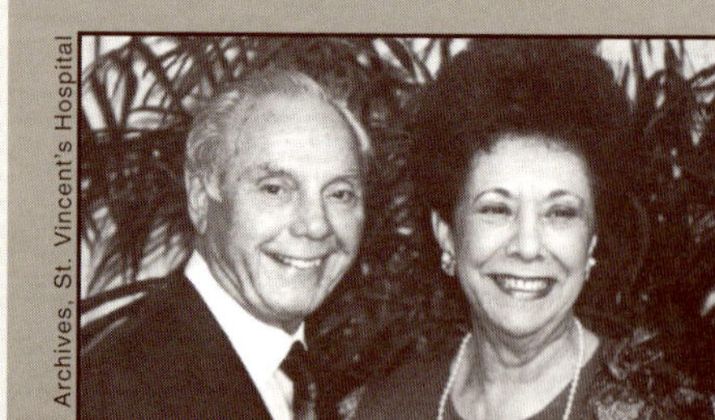

Lee J. and Nancy Bruno

f Blessings: The Bruno Family

Joseph S. and Theresa R. Bruno Cancer Center

The $1.5 million donation by the Brunos made the hospital's planned Cancer Center a reality in 1989. Longtime benefactors of the hospital, St. Vincent's started the Care Fund with a $100,000 gift from Mr. Bruno.

Archives, St. Vincent's Hospital

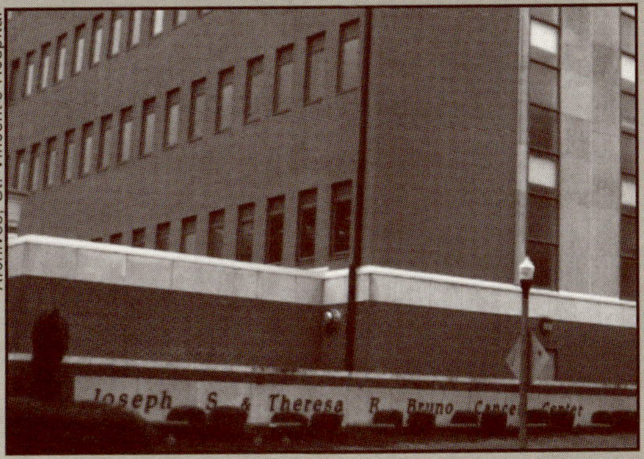

Joe and Theresa were named affiliates of the Daughters of Charity in 1990. Joe Bruno and his family also received the Heritage Award of the Daughters of Charity National Health System. Joe Bruno was the first recipient of the Cornette Award, given by the Daughters of Charity National Health System's Council of Foundations, as well as the first lay person named to the hospital's Board of Directors. St. Vincent's lost one of its dearest family members with the death of Joe Bruno in 1996.

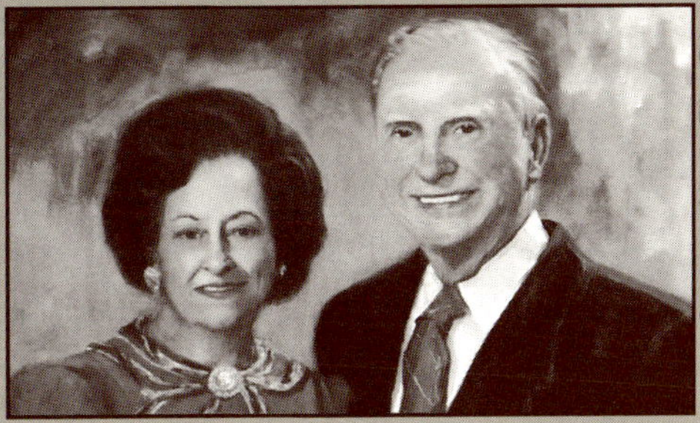

Courtesy of Linda Ellen Price

Portrait of Theresa and Joe Bruno

Archives, St. Vincent's Hospital

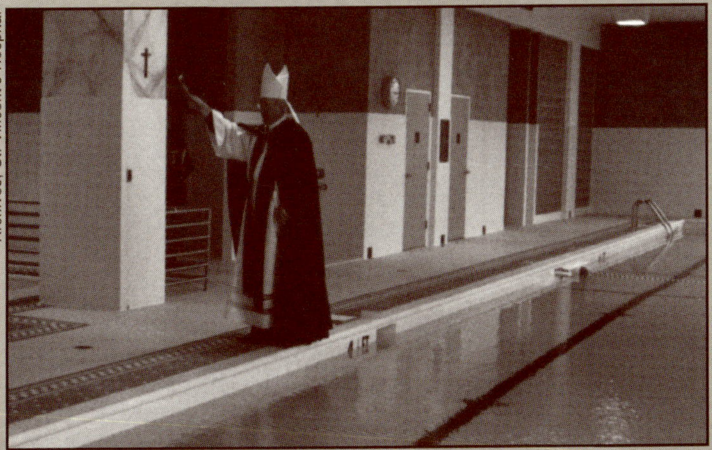

The Most Reverend Raymond Boland, bishop of the Diocese of Birmingham, blesses the Rehabilitation Center's swimming pools.

Opened in 1992 in Professional Building Three, the Center offers a full range of rehabilitation programs in one location.

The Rehabilitation Center was made possible by a $4.3 million gift by the late Lee J. Bruno and his wife Nancy, the largest gift ever given to a private hospital in Alabama.

"Now, thanks to God, I can help others who have not been as fortunate," Lee said. "Our donation to St. Vincent's is one way we can help make a difference."

Bruno Conference Center

Adjacent to the new Women's and Children's Center, the Bruno Conference Center was made possible through the generosity of sisters Mary Bruno and Theresa Bruno Russo.

Dedicated in 1997, the Conference Center – with its 300-seat auditorium, tiered lecture hall, computer lab and flexible classroom and meeting facilities – serves as an educational center for the hospital, medical staff and the community.

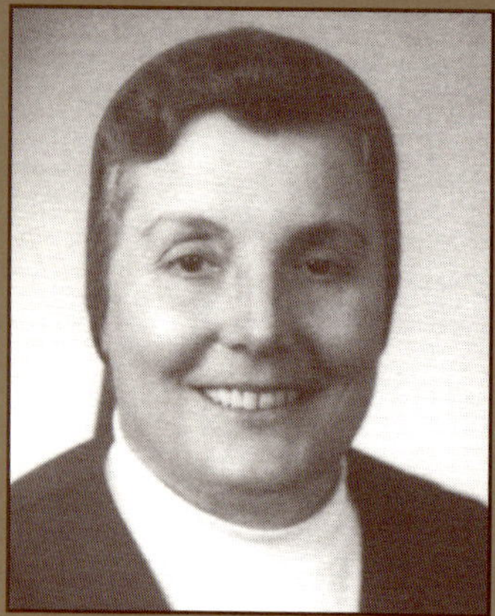

Sister Almeda

Sister Almeda Golson began her career at St. Vincent's in 1975, working part-time, and became the assistant administrator two years later. The Prattville native served as administrator of St. Vincent's from 1985 to 1987, and in 1995 returned to become chair of its Board of Directors.

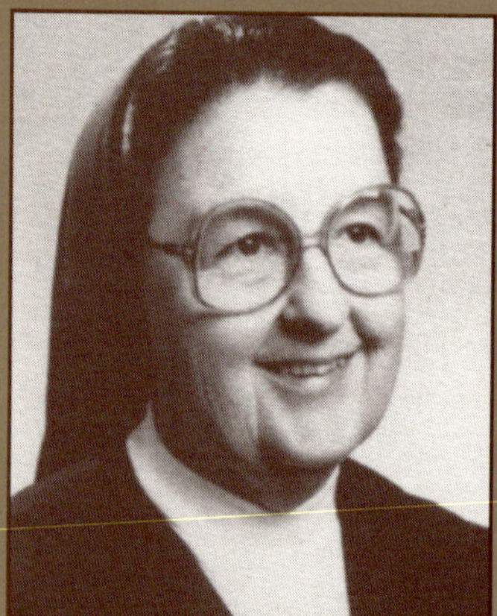

Sister Mary Frances

Sister Mary Frances Loftin had been a regional CEO of the Daughters of Charity National Health System (DCNHS) before serving as the administrator of St. Vincent's from 1987 to 1992. Sister Mary Frances left the hospital to become president of the DCNHS. She is now the chancellor of the Diocese of Birmingham.

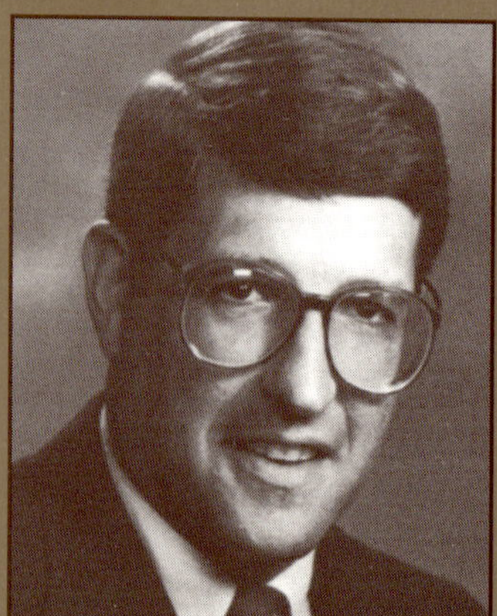

Vincent C. Caponi

Vincent C. Caponi became the first lay administrator of St. Vincent's in 1992. A member of the Council of Regents of the American College of Healthcare Executives, Caponi is president of the board of the Seton Corporation of North Alabama, chairman of the Birmingham Regional Hospital Council and on the board of directors of Regions Bank.

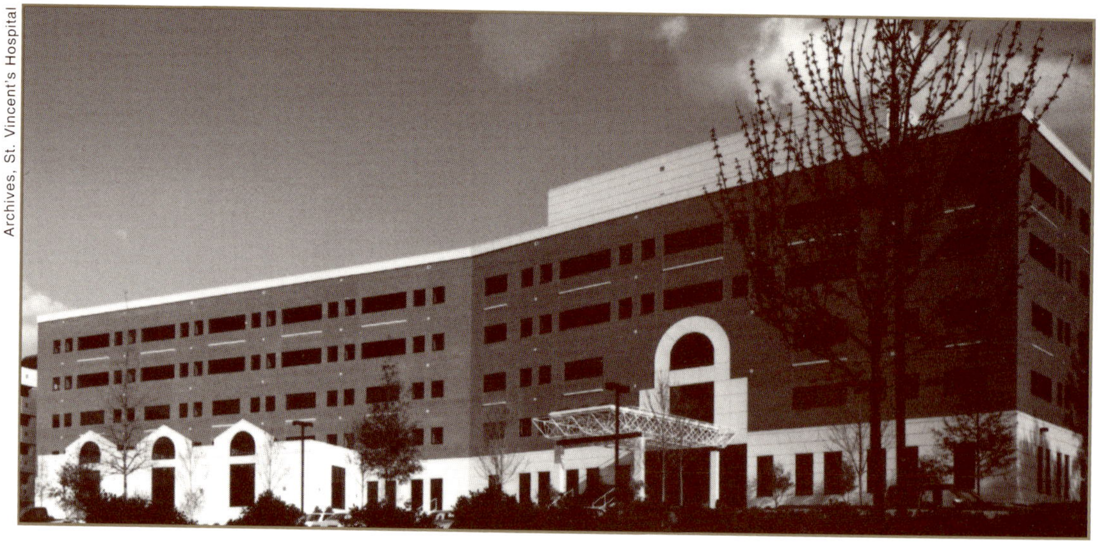

Archives, St. Vincent's Hospital

Professional Building Three

The hospital's second professional building opened in February of 1988, a five-story, 70,000-square-foot structure containing 21 office suites, the practices of about 35 physicians and a Diagnostic Center. A two-level crosswalk linked the building to the first professional building.

That summer, the hospital's renovated third floor became the Maternal and Child Center, with its all-LDR area – the first in Birmingham – a mother/infant unit and specialized nursery facilities.

The Occupational Health Clinic also opened in 1988, and in only six weeks its treatment services for job-related injuries had been retained by companies representing 10,000 local employees.

Ground was broken on January 4, 1988, on the Joseph S. and Theresa R. Bruno Cancer Center. The dedication ceremony on April 5, 1989 was broadcast live worldwide on the Eternal Word Television Network. Governor Guy Hunt gave a keynote address.

The momentum of construction and program expansion continued. The need for both an additional professional building and a larger rehabilitation facility became apparent. In September of 1989 St. Vincent's broke ground on a third professional building and a new 800-car parking deck. Again, a member of the generous Bruno family made a new facility possible.

Lee J. and Nancy Bruno's gift of $4.3 million was not only the largest donation ever made to St. Vincent's, but also it was the largest ever given to a private hospital in Alabama. "St. Vincent's is very important to my family," Lee Bruno said.

Professional Building Three, featuring the Bruno Rehabilitation Center, opened in 1992.

Sadly, Lee Bruno would not live to see the fruit that gift would bear. He, his brother

Angelo, and other members of the Bruno Corporation were killed in a plane crash in 1991. Sister Mary Frances expressed the grief of the hospital family: "There are not words to describe the loss we at St. Vincent's feel."

The Bruno Memorial Heart Care Center was dedicated in 1992 to their memory, as well as to the memories of the many Bruno family members who have been dedicated members of the St. Vincent's family.

St. Vincent's had been approved to perform open-heart surgery in 1991, and the new Heart Care Center made it possible for the varied diagnoses and treatment procedures to all share the same location. Today there are more than 300 open-heart procedures performed at St. Vincent's each year.

The First of His Kind

Sister Mary Frances was known as a fine business person. "She could have been CEO of IBM or General Motors," one St. Vincent's physician said of her.

During her tenure at St. Vincent's, Sister Mary Frances was named "Executive of the Year" by the National Association of Female Executives and one of the "Top 10 Business Women" by the *Birmingham Business Journal*.

So it was not a surprise when, in the Spring of 1992, Sister Mary Frances left St. Vincent's to become the first president of the Daughters of Charity National Health System.

And something unprecedented for St. Vincent's resulted, as Executive Vice President Vincent C. Caponi became the hospital's first lay administrator.

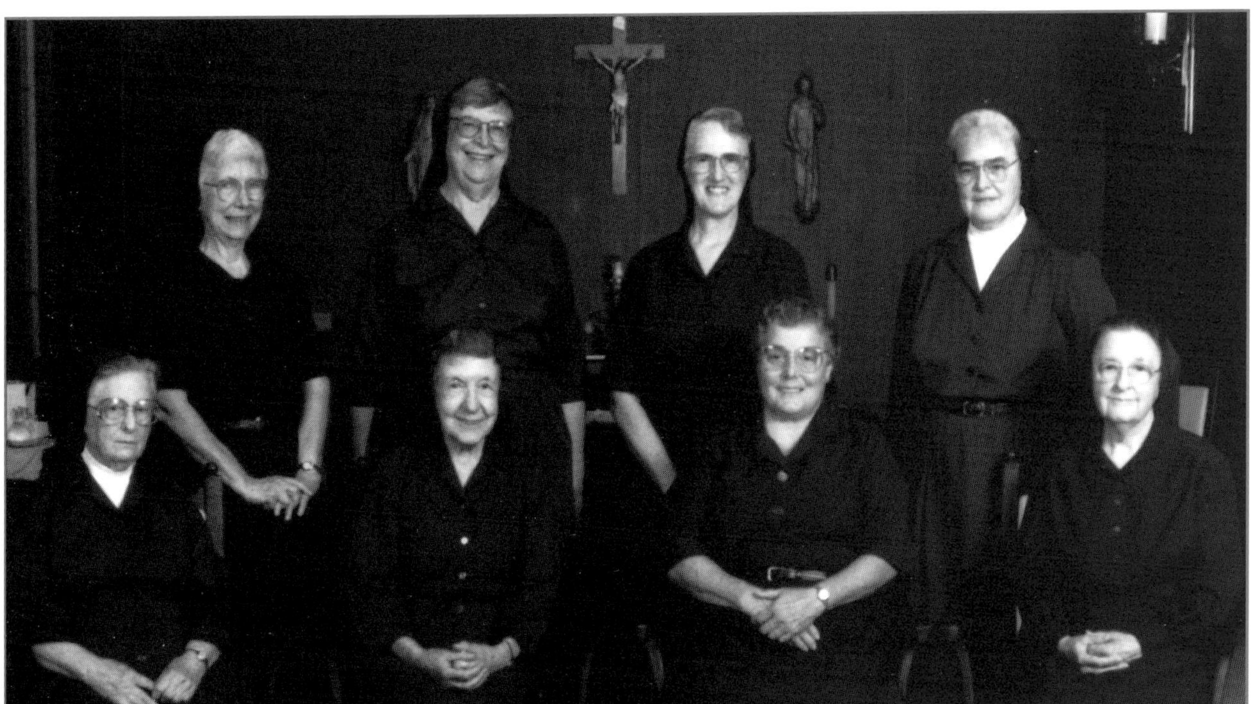

The Sisters of St. Vincent's today (left to right): (standing) Sisters Mary Ann O'Brien, Virginia Delaney, Mary Cecilia Schlebecker and Regina Priller; (seated) Sisters Gerald Mulvanny, Veronica Berg, Almeda Golson and Mary Frances Loftin.

The youthful Caponi, who had been with St. Vincent's for nine months, had already served as CEO or administrator at two other hospitals. Still, "I have some big shoes to fill," Caponi said.

And Caponi began to fill them with strong leadership and vision. By November of 1995 cranes and hard hats were back at the hospital as construction began on another major expansion effort.

The first phase of the new construction was the renovation of the Child Care Center, which had opened in 1989 to serve the families of both hospital associates and the community.

The focal points of the expansion are the Women's and Children's Center and the Bruno Conference Center, scheduled to open in time for St. Vincent's 100th anniversary.

A Century of Caring

As it completes its first century of caring for the people of Birmingham, St. Vincent's continues to broaden its efforts as it remembers its mission.

The "outdoor" clinic Sister Chrysostom started in 1905 has been strengthened through the dedication of Dr. Keehn Berry, whose efforts to keep the clinic running have most often been without compensation.

The watchful eye of the Sisters remains. Sister Almeda returned to St. Vincent's in 1995 to chair the St. Vincent's Board of Directors, Sister Mary Frances is nearby as chancellor of the Diocese of Birmingham. Six other Daughters of Charity hold important positions at the hospital, and equally as vital, continue the tradition of spiritual and emotional support for patients at St. Vincent's.

Never to be moved again, Father O'Reilly rests at Elmwood Cemetery. His monument has a new home at the hospital to preserve his memory into the next millenium.

St. Vincent's Hospital:

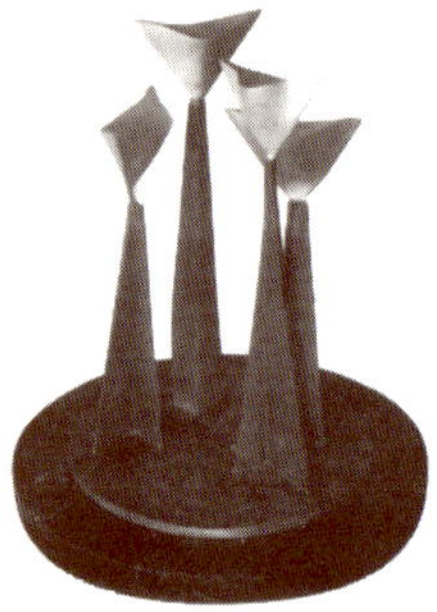

Model of the Centennial Sculpture

Today St. Vincent's is an impressive community medical complex, well prepared to enter its second century of service as it joyfully celebrates its first.

Recent construction necessitated a new hospital entrance, a handsome brick gateway facing University Boulevard, which was the gift of the Vincent J. Bruno family through the Lee J. Bruno Foundation.

Overlooking the new drive is the 16-foot Centennial sculpture, whose imagery was conceived by Dr. Edwin G. Waldrop. The work, by noted local sculptor Brad Morton, is a gift of Dr. and Mrs. Joseph A. Cunningham and symbolizes the original four Sisters who began St. Vincent's.

The joys and trials, heartache and triumph that lie ahead for St. Vincent's and the city it serves are yet to be revealed. But the sculpture will keep vigil during the next 100 years, as Dr. Waldrop said, a "constant reminder that Birmingham is being watched over."

For these past 100 years, this dedication has been the story of St. Vincent's, as it will be throughout the hospital's next century of service.

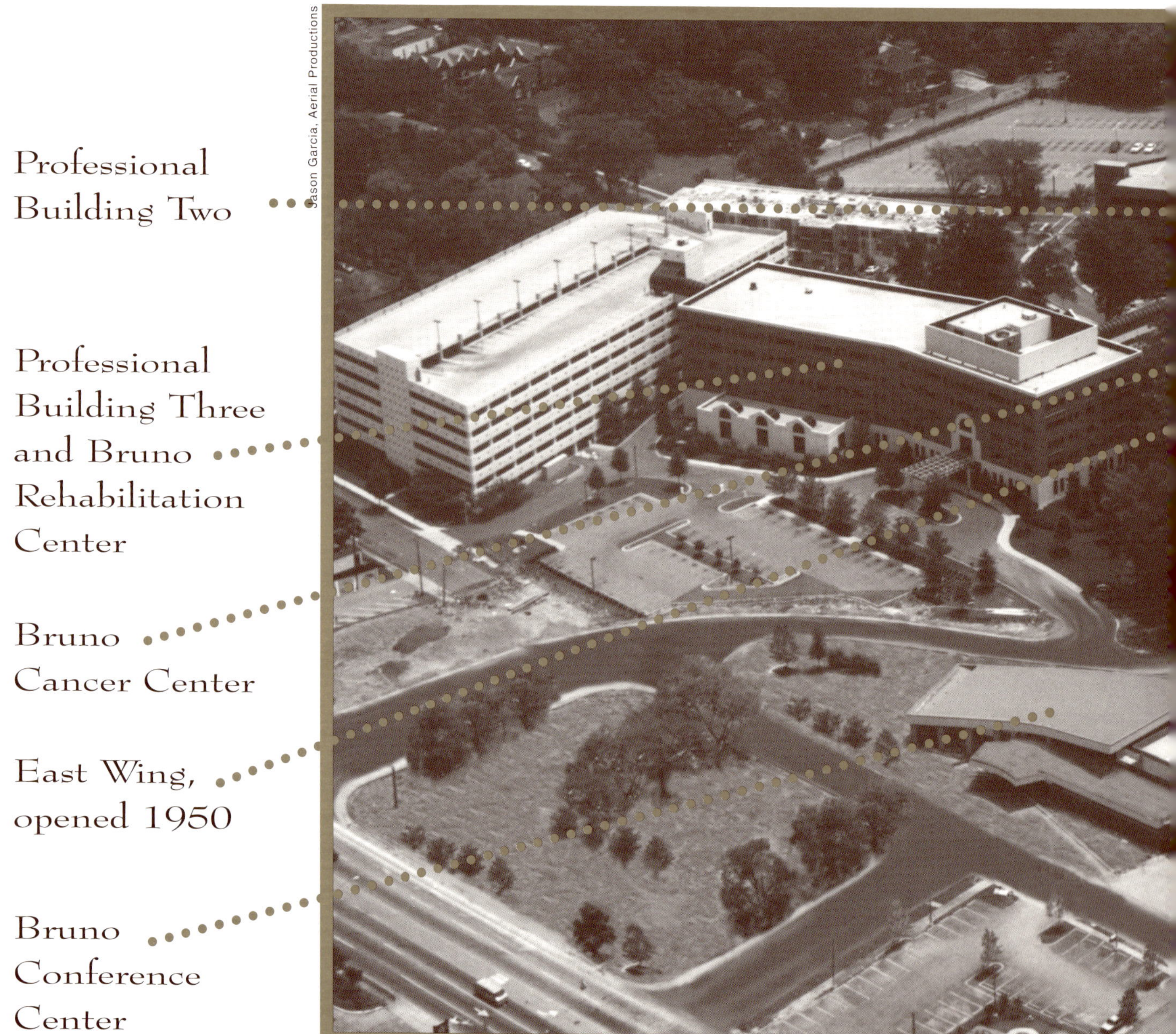

Jason Garcia, Aerial Productions

the first 100 years

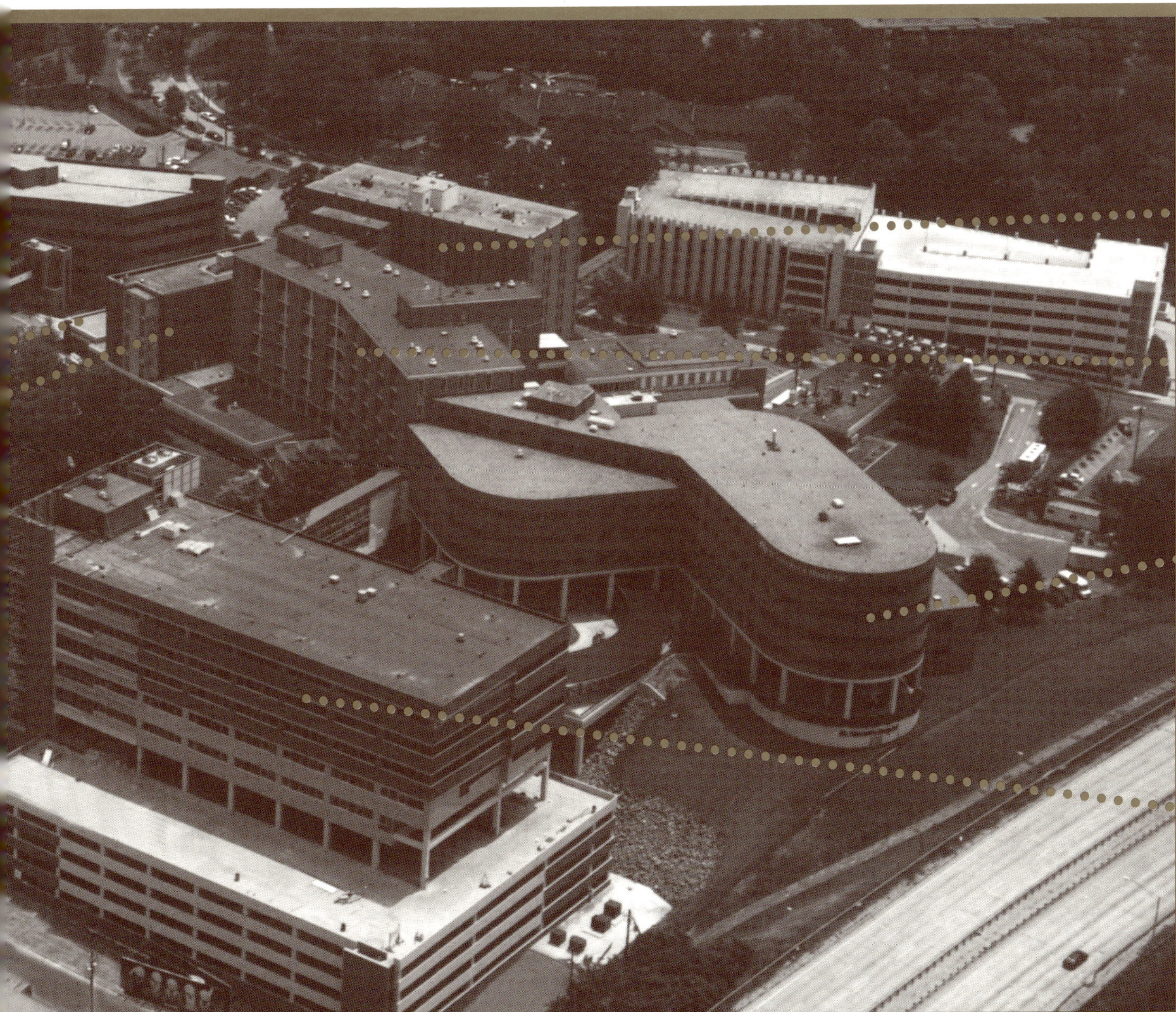

Professional Building One

1972 Hospital Structure

West Wing (Barbara Ingalls Shook Pavilion)

Women's and Children's Center

Remembering the Past...Looking Toward the Future

Medical Staff Presidents

Year	President
1920	Dr. Lewis Morris
1921	Dr. J. M. Mason
1922	Dr. J. M. Mason
1923	Dr. W. F Scott
1924	Dr. E. P. Solomon
1925	Dr. F. A. Lupton
1926	Dr. G. S. Graham
1927	Dr. G. S. Graham
1928	Dr. T. J. Magruder
1929	Dr. Edward O'Connell
1930	Dr. J. A. Meadows
1931	Dr. M. A. Watkins
1932	Dr. W. J. Beddow
1933	Dr. B. S. Lester
1934	Dr. A. C. Cameron
1935	Dr. Cabot Lull
1936	Dr. A. B. Harris
1937	Dr. S. L. Ledbetter
1938	Dr. J. D. Sherrill
1939	Dr. John W. Simpson
1940	Dr. U. J. W. Peters
1941	Dr. F. C. Wilson
1942	Dr. Sid W. Collier
1943	Dr. K. F. Kesmodel
1944	Dr. H. E. Conwell
1945	Dr. S. S. Underwood
1946	Dr. J. L. Carmichael
1947	Dr. J. L. Carmichael
1948	Dr. R. G. Lovelady
1949	Dr. J. A. Cunningham
1950	Dr. E. G. Givhan
1951	Dr. J. M. Mason III
1952	Dr. Bruno Barelare
1953	Dr. Buford S. Word
1954	Dr. John F. Jenkins Jr.
1955	Dr. J. G. Galbraith
1956	Dr. J. E. Linn
1957	Dr. S. E. Upchurch
1958	Dr. T. V. Magruder
1959	Dr. C. H. Wilson
1960	Dr. E. B. Glenn
1961	Dr. B. H. Wiesel
1962	Dr. A. I. Chenoweth
1963	Dr. Wood S. Herren
1964	Dr. William L. Hawley
1965	Dr. Francis A. Marzoni
1966	Dr. Rhodes Johnston
1967	Dr. Alwyn A. Shugerman
1968	Dr. Frank C. Wilson Jr.
1969	Dr. Alfred Habeeb
1970	Dr. James A. Davis Jr.
1971	Dr. Karl F. Kesmodel Jr.
1972	Dr. Samuel K. Cohn
1973	Dr. Henley J. Smith
1974	Dr. Keehn W. Berry Jr.
1975	Dr. Merrill N. Bradley
1976	Dr. Edwin G. Waldrop
1977	Dr. William E. Lawrence
1978	Dr. Walter C. McCoy
1979	Dr. Edward R. Meadows
1980	Dr. Gray C. Buck Jr.
1981	Dr. Harry I. Blaylock Jr.
1982	Dr. Samuel P. Gillis
1983	Dr. Ronald E. Henderson
1984	Dr. Walter N. Pearce Jr.
1985	Dr. William A. Leitner
1986	Dr. Jack W. Trigg Jr.
1987	Dr. Finley McRae
1988	Dr. J. Terrell Spencer
1989	Dr. Ralph Yarbrough
1990	Dr. Michael Grelier
1991	Dr. Philip Walton
1992	Dr. John Mussleman
1993	Dr. Robert Lewis
1994-95	Dr. Robert Lewis
1995-96	Dr. R. Rex Harris
1996-97	Dr. Stephen Coleman
1997-98	Dr. Frank Page

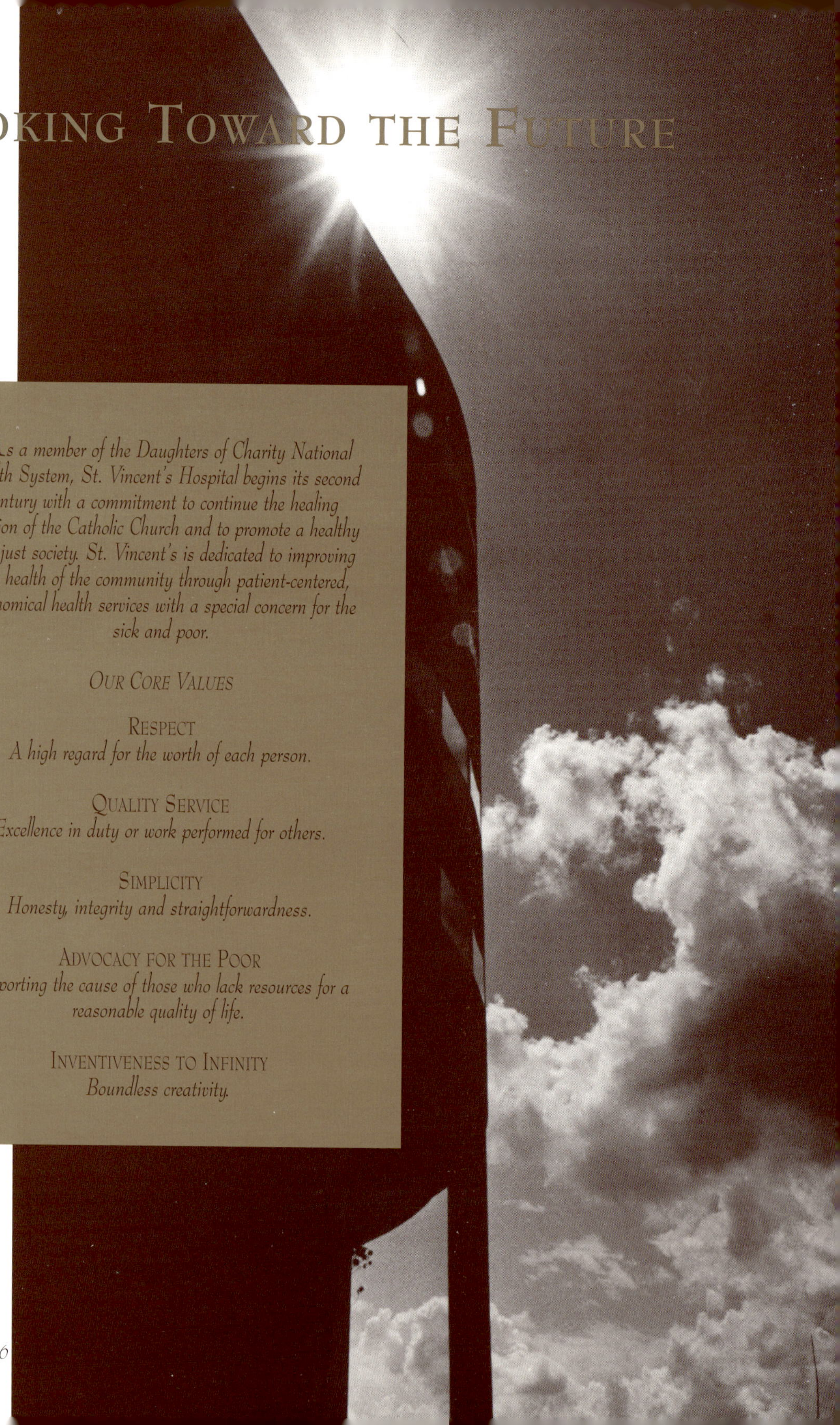

As a member of the Daughters of Charity National Health System, St. Vincent's Hospital begins its second century with a commitment to continue the healing mission of the Catholic Church and to promote a healthy and just society. St. Vincent's is dedicated to improving the health of the community through patient-centered, economical health services with a special concern for the sick and poor.

Our Core Values

Respect
A high regard for the worth of each person.

Quality Service
Excellence in duty or work performed for others.

Simplicity
Honesty, integrity and straightforwardness.

Advocacy for the Poor
Supporting the cause of those who lack resources for a reasonable quality of life.

Inventiveness to Infinity
Boundless creativity.

Bibliography

Leah Rawls Atkins, *The Valley and the Hills: an Illustrated History of Birmingham and Jefferson County*, 1981.

Donald A. Brown, editor, *Birmingham* magazine, Centennial Issue, 1971.

Ann McCorquodale Burkhardt, *Town Within a City: The Five Points South Neighborhood, 1982.*

George M. Cruikshank, *Birmingham and Its Environs*, 1921.

André Dodin, C. M., *Vincent de Paul and Charity: A Contemporary Portrait of His Life and Apostolic Spirit, 1993.*

Frank Joseph Fede, *Italians in the Deep South: Their Impact on Birmingham and the American Heritage, 1994.*

John C. Henley Jr., *This is Birmingham: the Founding and Growth of an American City*, 1960, 1969.

Dr. Mortimer H. Jordan, "Report on Cholera in Birmingham to the United States House of Representatives," 1873.

Jere C. King, *Formation of Greater Birmingham,* Masters Thesis, University of Alabama, 1935.

Martha Carolyn Mitchell, *Birmingham: Biography of a City of the New South,* Dissertation, University of Chicago, 1946, 1972.

Robert S. Newbill, *A Study of the Growth of the City of Birmingham's Corporate Boundaries from 1871 to the Present, 1980.*

Dr. William H. Robertson, a historical manuscript on St. Vincent's Hospital and the practice of medicine.

Many thanks to the following for their assistance in the research of this project:

Aerial Productions
Sister Xavier Ballance
Birmingham Public Library Archives
Birmingham Regional Hospital Council
Sister Veronica Berg
Sister Mary Bourke
Mrs. Zuma Elgin Brentnall
C. J. Bryant
Sybil A. Burton
Dr. Tom O. Caldwell
Mrs. Elizabeth O'Roark Carroll
Dr. Samuel K. Cohn
Dr. Joseph A. Cunningham
Daughters of Charity of St. Vincent de Paul
Sister Virginia Delaney
Linda Dunwoody
Betty Eaford, R.N.
Dr. Hiram R. Elliott
Jean Ellis
Edward Ferrell
Sister Margaret Flynn
Mrs. Claude H. Ford
Mrs. E. B. Glenn
Sister Almeda Golson
Dr. Alfred Habeeb
Lee Isaacs
Larry Johnson
Dr. Karl F. Kesmodel Jr.
Miss Eleanor Kidd
Mary Catherine King
Bill Lang
Sister Mary Frances Loftin
Dr. Thomas V. Magruder Jr.
Sister Catherine Mangan
Lois Martin
Mrs. James M. Mason III
Dr. Walter C. McCoy
Dr. Edward R. Meadows
James J. Monaghan
William Moran
Sister Gerald Mulvanny
Sister Mary Ann O'Brien
Dr. Lamar S. Osment
Linda Ellen Price
Sister Regina Priller
William E. Ricker
Dr. William H. Robertson
St. Vincent's Hospital Archives
Sister Mary Cecilia Schlebecker
Barbara Ingalls Shook
J. Larry Sims
Sister Mary Ellen Sullivan
Ted Tucker
University of Alabama at Birmingham Archives
Dr. Edwin G. Waldrop
J. D. Weeks
Dr. William V. Weldon
Donna Whisenant
Frances D. Wideman
Betty Williams

and the thousands of others who helped create the story of St. Vincent's Hospital.

The author offers special thanks to Barbara Traylor for her guidance and support.

Index

Sponsorship

This history introduces the Centennial celebration of St. Vincent's Hospital in Birmingham. Contributions from Dr. and Mrs. Joesph A. Cunningham, the Joseph S. Bruno Charitable Foundation, the Linn-Henley Charitable Trust and Dr. and Mrs. Edwin G. Waldrop have provided the impetus for the year-long celebration.

The St. Vincent's Story...A Century of Caring

With deepest gratitude, St. Vincent's Foundation acknowledges the contributions of these supporters who have made publication of this book possible.

Gold Sponsors

Nelson and Charleen Kemp Foundation

The Mead Corporation

Silver Sponsors

Bruno's Memorial Classic Foundation, Inc.

Mr. and Mrs. Curtis James

Mr. and Mrs. Ralph Neal

Bronze Sponsors

Mr. Charles W. Ashby
Mrs. Jemile W. Azar
Mr. and Mrs. Stephen H. Berck
Mrs. Evelyn L. Bischoff
Ms. Sybil A. Burton
Mr. and Mrs. Tommy J. Cacioppo
Mr. and Mrs. Vincent C. Caponi
Mr. and Mrs. Clayton C. Carlton
Dr. and Mrs. Samuel K. Cohn
Mr. and Mrs. Richard Crocker
Mr. Sam A. Culotta Sr.
Dr. and Mrs. James A. Davis Jr.
Dr. and Mrs. Hiram R. Elliott
Dr. and Mrs. John D. Elmore
Mrs. Mary F. Fife
Dr. and Mrs. Arthur M. Freeman
Dr. Samuel P. Gillis
Dr. and Mrs. Alfred Habeeb
Dr. and Mrs. James J. Hicks
Mr. and Mrs. Russell Hood
Dr. Eugene H. Howe
Johnson & Johnson
Johnston Properties, Inc.
Dr. and Mrs. Wayne W. Killion
Mrs. Mary Catherine King
Dr. and Mrs. Robert H. Lewis
Mr. Henry S. Lynn Jr.
Mr. and Mrs. Larry W. Masters
Dr. and Mrs. Walter C. McCoy
Dr. and Mrs. Edward R. Meadows
Ms. Nina Miglionico
Mr. and Mrs. William M. Moran
Dr. and Mrs. Frank O. Page
Mr. and Mrs. Steven S. Phillips
Dr. and Mrs. Robert M. Pritchett
Mr. and Mrs. Keith Purdy
Mr. and Mrs. Thomas E. Rast
Dr. and Mrs. Alvin L. Rich
Mr. and Mrs. Wayne M. Rogers
Royal Cup Coffee, Inc.
Mr. and Mrs. Glenn A. Sheffield
Mrs. Herbert E. Smith Jr.
Southern Progress Corporation
Southview Medical Group, P.C.
Mr. William M. Spencer III
Mr. and Mrs. J. W. Traylor
Mr. and Mrs. Stanley Virciglio
Dr. and Mrs. Richard W. Waguespack
Dr. and Mrs. Gilder L. Wideman
Dr. and Mrs. Frank C. Wilson Jr.
Dr. Susan B. Winchester
Dr. and Mrs. Joseph A. Zarzaur

Other Contributors

Mr. and Mrs. Thomas T. Allison Jr. • Dr. and Mrs. J. Maxwell Austin Jr. • Mr. and Mrs. Carl F. Bailey • Mr. and Mrs. A. D. Barnard • Dr. and Mrs. John B. Blalock Jr. • Dr. and Mrs. Marc E. Bloomston • Ms. Martha Clements Brasfield • Mrs. Zuma E. Brentnall • Ms. Elizabeth A. Bridewell • Dr. and Mrs. Arthur I. Chenoweth • Dr. and Mrs. Orville W. Clayton • Mrs. A. Key Foster • Dr. and Mrs. William E. Gathings • Mr. William J. Grayson Jr. • Dr. David B. Hall • Mr. and Mrs. W. Price Hightower • Mr. and Mrs. Thomas A. Hyland • Mrs. Gilbert E. Johnston • Drs. Prakash C. and Santosh S. Kansal • Pediatric Asthma & Allergy • Mrs. Dorothy D. Pigford • Mrs. Sara H. Robinson • Dr. Alwyn A. Shugerman • Mrs. Peter G. Smith • Mr. and Mrs. Robert M. Smith • Mr. and Mrs. Stuart E. Teach • Mr. and Mrs. Leonard J. Weil • Dr. William V. Weldon • Dr. Bert H. Wiesel

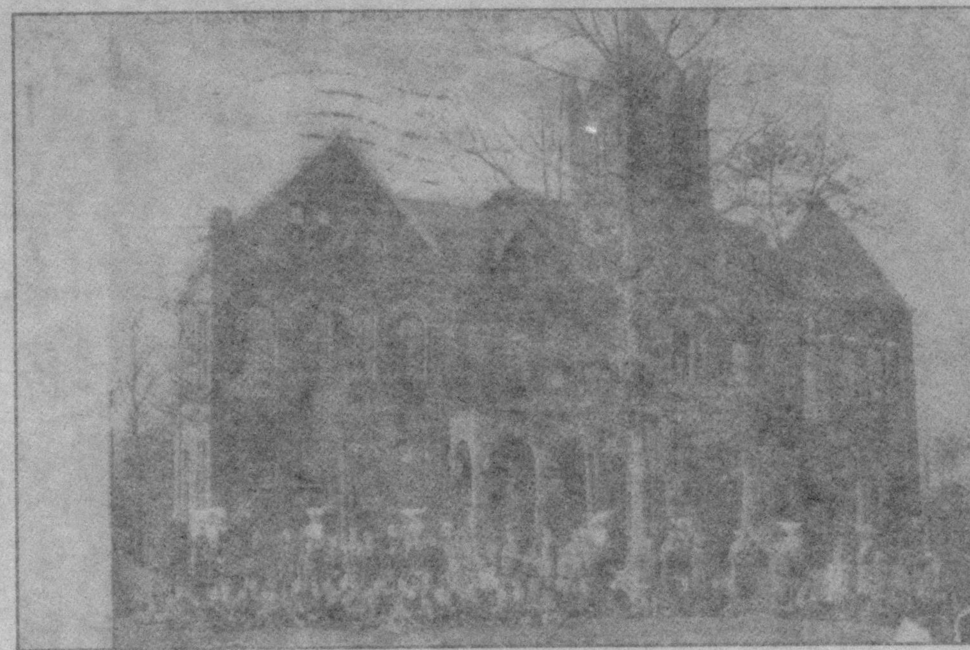

Anthenaeum Orphans Home, Circa 1910

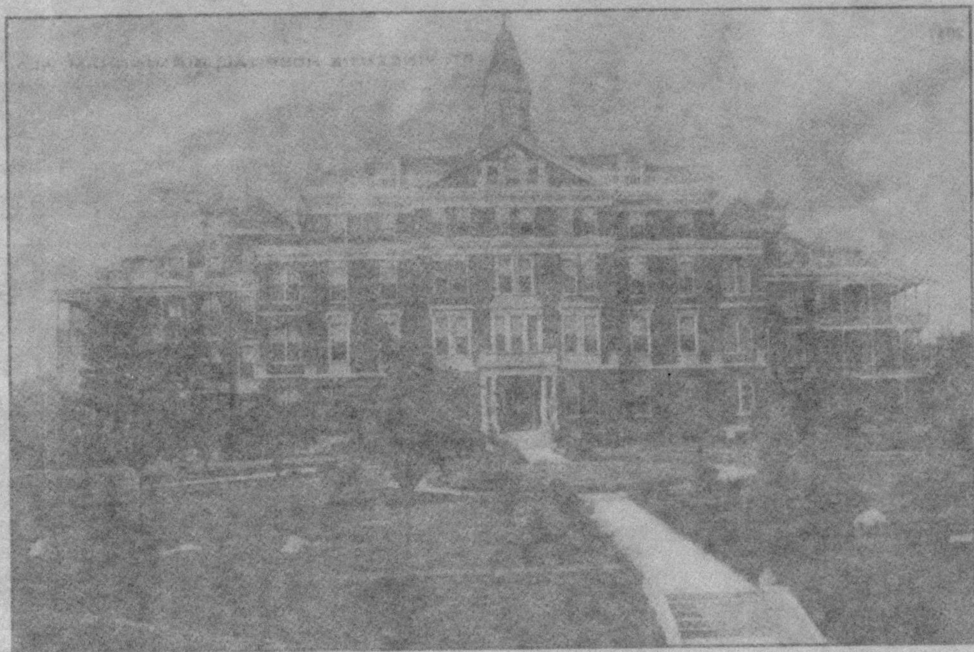

Circa 1915

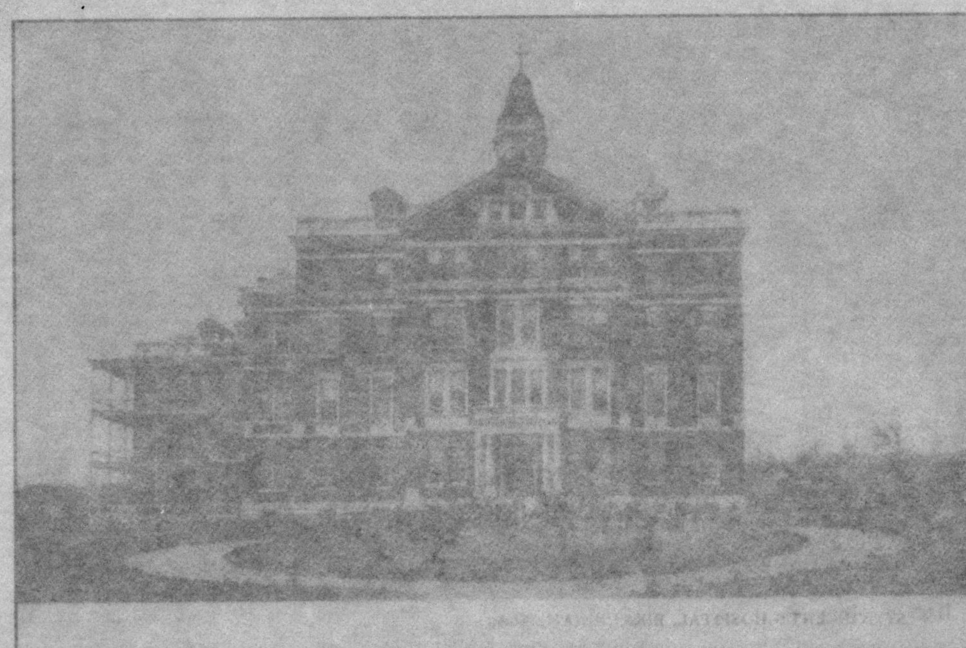

Circa 1908

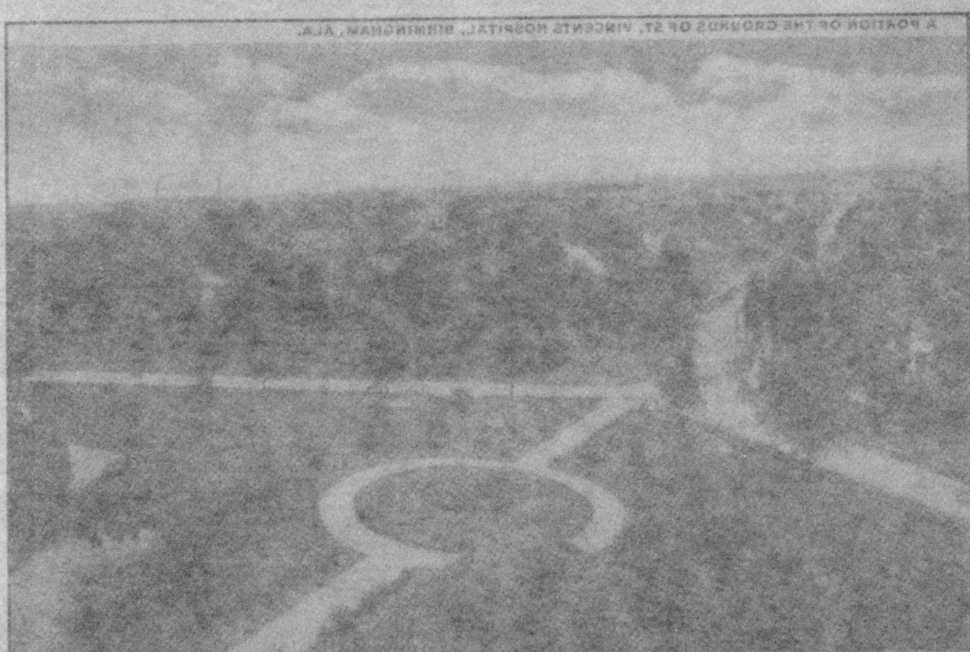

Hospital Grounds, Circa 1910

Historic Postcards: Courtesy of J. D. Weeks and Archives, St. Vincent's

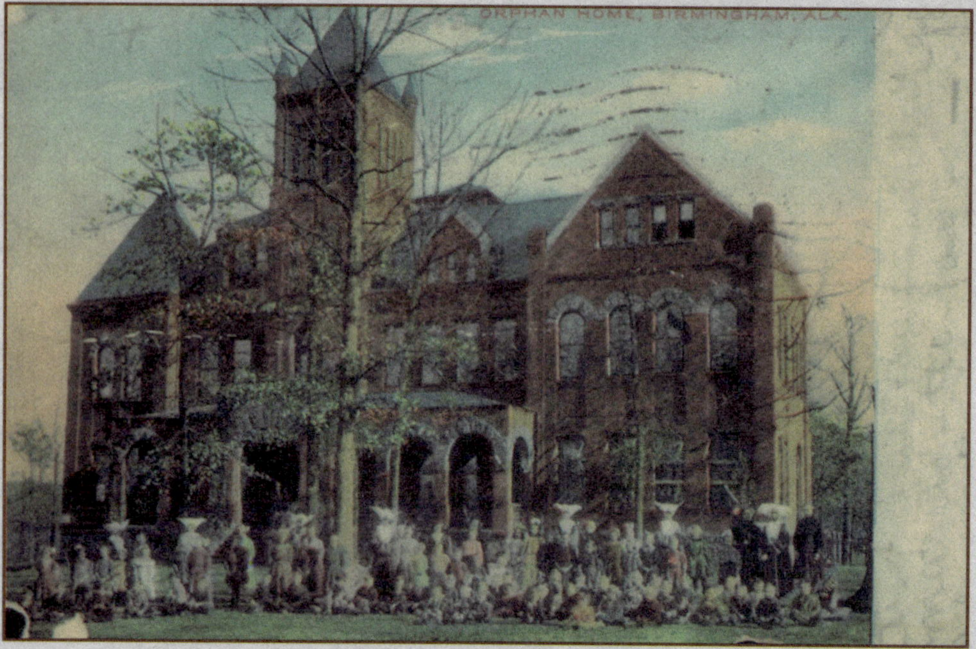

Antheneum Orphans Home, Circa 1910

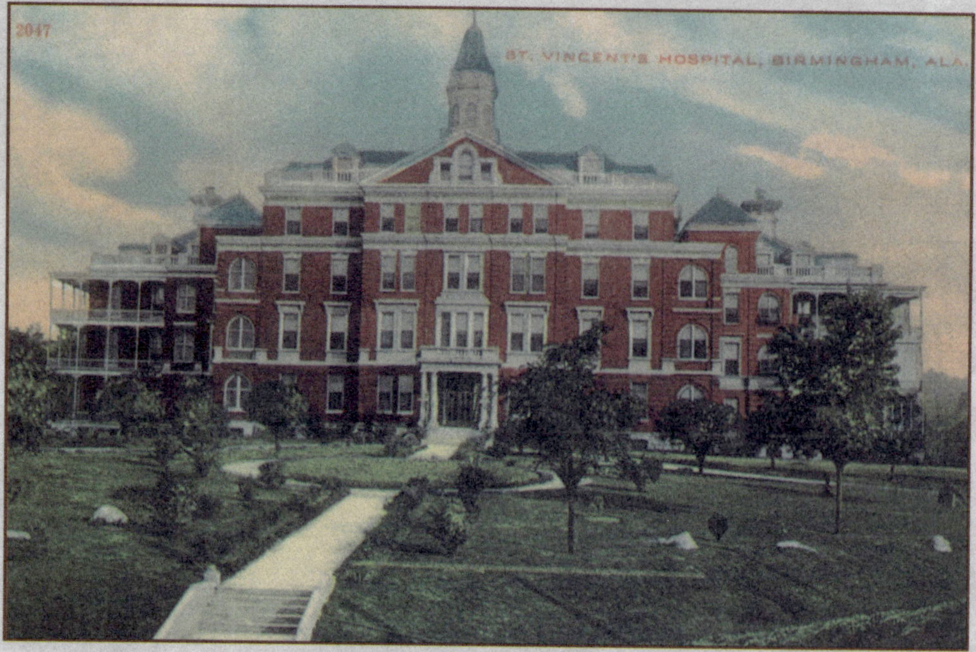

Circa 1915

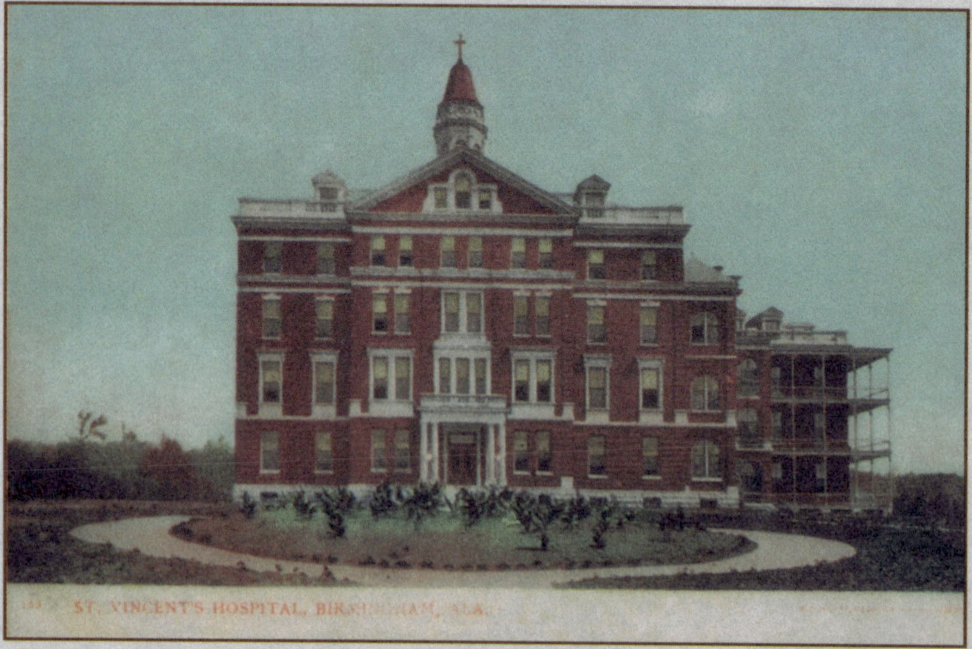

Circa 1908

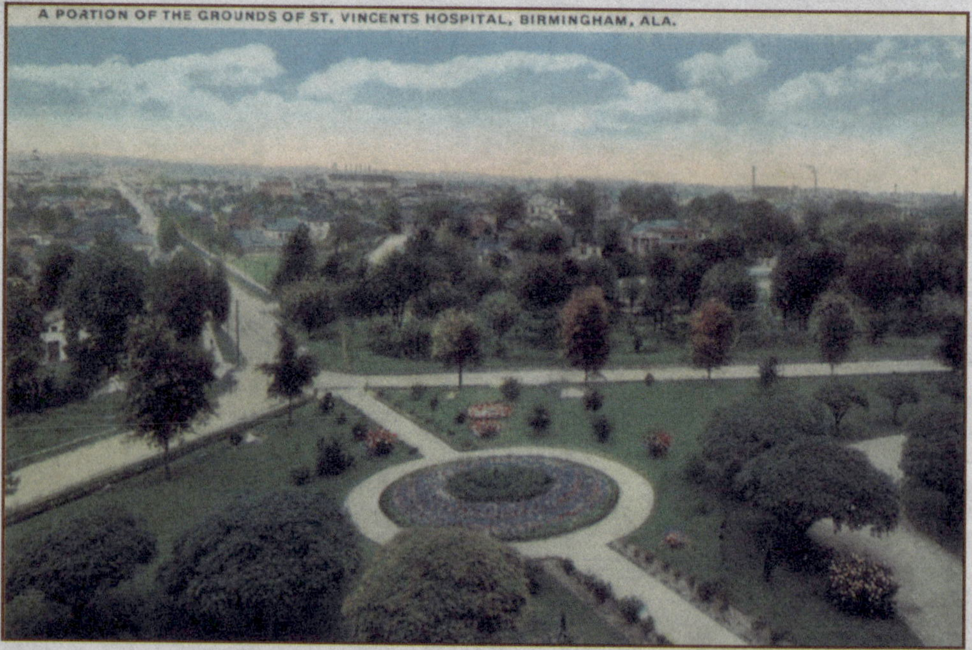

Hospital Grounds, Circa 1910

Historic Postcards: Courtesy of J. D. Weeks and Archives, St. Vincent's